The Legal and Professional Status of Nursing

For Churchill Livingstone:

Senior Commissioning Editor: Sarena Wolfaard
Project Development Manager: Katrina Mather
Project Manager: Jane Dingwall
Design Direction: Judith Wright

The Legal and Professional Status of Nursing

Mary Chiarella RN LL.B(Hons) PhD(UNSW)
Professor of Nursing in Corrections Health,
Faculty of Nursing, Midwifery and Health,
University of Technology, Sydney and
Corrections Health Service,
New South Wales, Australia

Foreword by

Alison Kitson RN DPhil FRCN
Professor and Director, RCN Institute, London, UK

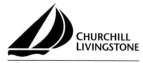

CHURCHILL
LIVINGSTONE

EDINBURGH LONDON NEW YORK PHILADELPHIA ST LOUIS SYDNEY TORONTO 2002

CHURCHILL LIVINGSTONE
An imprint of Harcourt Publishers Limited

© Harcourt Publishers Limited 2002

 is a registered trademark of Harcourt Publishers Limited

First published 2002

ISBN 0 443 07191 8

British Library Cataloguing in Publication Data
A catalogue record for this book is available from the British Library

Library of Congress Cataloging in Publication Data
A catalog record for this book is available from the Library of Congress

Note
Medical knowledge is constantly changing. As new information
becomes available, changes in treatment, procedures, equipment and
the use of drugs become necessary. The author and the publishers have
taken care to ensure that the information given in this text is accurate
and up to date. However, readers are strongly advised to confirm that
the information, especially with regard to drug usage, complies with
the latest legislation and standards of practice.

The
publisher's
policy is to use
paper manufactured
from sustainable forests

Printed in China by RDC Group Limited

Contents

Foreword

This book is one of the most significant contributions to the debate on the development of nursing. From a rich tapestry of life events, Mary Chiarella recounts the tragic stories of patients and professionals, thrown together by chance and yet affecting each other's lives.

The drama of life runs through this book, countless cases immortalised by the accounts from courts of law. And while the examples are mostly from one country – Australia – reflecting one country's legal system, they could have come from any continent in the world.

Chiarella's great skill has been to combine her deep insight and understanding of nursing with an erudition and disciplined approach to case law analysis. As she says in this book, very little attention had been given previously to analysing the many legal accounts that involved nurses, and she has demonstrated how much we can learn from them.

The issues are not unfamiliar to us: nurses as ambiguous commodities, sometimes revered and respected and at others rendered invisible; nurses' work viewed as menial and low level or else substituting for that of medical colleagues; nursing as distinct and complementary to medicine and yet at the same time subordinated. It is not surprising that with this conceptual confusion, come legal and professional confusion.

And while we cannot help but smile when we read the five images of the nurse – the ministering angel, and domestic worker particularly familiar to our western myths and stereotypes – we as nurses, take deeper breaths when we think through the challenge of the autonomous professional role.

Mary Chiarella is challenging every nurse and every legal system in this book. She has laid out the incongruities and with that exposure no legal case involving nurses can, or will, be the same again. Whatever happens, we will be challenged to ask ourselves what sort of professionals we are. But as well as the challenges come the pointers for regeneration and strength. The route towards greater legal and professional clarity is laid out in front of us, waiting for us to respond.

And this is the real test for us all in the profession.

Alison Kitson

Acknowledgements

I wish to record my gratitude to the following organisations for generously providing grants to enable me to undertake a period of full-time study in 1994: The Edith Cavell Trust, the New South Wales Nurses Registration Board and the Joyce Wickham Memorial Scholarship Fund. I would also like to record my appreciation of the New South Wales College of Nursing and the New South Wales Nurses' Association librarians, Graham Spooner and Matthew Platt, and their staff for their tireless enthusiasm and support for my often obscure searches. Thanks go also to the Registration Boards and Coroners in New South Wales, South Australia and Western Australia who provided me with cases and materials. To my colleagues and friends at the New South Wales College of Nursing and the New South Wales Nurses' Association who offered suggestions for and copies of unpublished cases and materials, I am truly grateful.

So many friends and colleagues in the nursing profession have provided support and encouragement that to mention any by name is to risk omitting some of equal importance. However, my sincere thanks must be recorded to Judith Cornell AM, and Patricia Staunton AM. Thanks are also due to my beloved friend, Amanda Adrian, herself a nurse and lawyer; to Kim Walker for his insight into feminist theory when I first began to travel that path; and to Maurice Bessman for his insight into issues of race. My thanks also to the countless nurses in Australia, England and New Zealand who over the years have told me the stories which led me to research this topic. I dedicate this work to those nurses and their patients.

My sincere thanks must also go to both my supervisors. Professor Philip Bates has provided outstanding support in addition to the benefit of his encyclopaedic knowledge of health law. He has been my supervisor, counsellor and advocate and, for undertaking all those roles, I offer him my humble thanks. To Professor Michael Chesterman, my thanks for his constructive criticism, his wonderful sense of humour, his meticulous attention to detail and his preparedness to travel with me on this journey. To Professor Jill Hunter, my thanks for her help in the short time that we spent together, and for her unfailing faith in the worth of my project. To Professor Regina Graycar, my thanks for alerting me to the possibilities of outsider scholarship. To all my friends and colleagues in health law, who have kept reassuring me that the project was needed and welcome, my sincere thanks also.

Finally, my greatest thanks of all go to my wonderful husband, Laurie, who has never stopped believing in me. Without his support, love and faith, I could never have finished. To my children, Ben and Hugo, I offer my sincere thanks for their ability to make me laugh when everything has seemed so difficult, and for their tolerance of a mother who was always working on the computer. My persistence is in part due to Robert Browning, whose Epilogue from *Asolando* inspired me whenever I felt tired or defeated.

One who never turned his back but marched breast forward,

Never doubted clouds would break,

Never dreamed, though right were worsted, wrong would triumph,

Held we fall to rise, are baffled to fight better,

Sleep to wake.

Abbreviations

ACHS	Australian Council on Healthcare Standards
ACHS	Australian Council on Hospital Standards
ACORN	Australian Confederation of Operating Room Nurses
AHMAC	Australian Health Ministers' Advisory Conference
AHTAC	Australian Health Technology Advisory Committee
AIDS	Acquired Immune Deficiency Syndrome
AIN	Assistant in Nursing
AMA	Australian Medical Association
AMO	Admitting Medical Officer
ANCI	Australian Nursing Council Inc.
ANF	Australian Nursing Federation
ANRAC	Australasian Nurse Registering Authorities Conference
ANS	Army Nursing Service
ATNA	Australasian Trained Nurses Association
BHA	British Hospitals Association
BNA	British Nurses' Association
CACCN	Confederation of Australian Critical Care Nurses
CLS	Critical Legal Studies
CMB	Central Midwives Board
CNC	Clinical Nurse Consultant
CNS	Clinical Nurse Specialist
CRT	Critical Race Theory
DHSS	Department of Health and Social Services (UK)
DNS	Director of Nursing Services
DRG	Diagnosis Related Group
DST	Deep Sleep Therapy
ECG	Electrocardiograph
ECT	Electroconvulsive Therapy
EN	Enrolled Nurse
ENT	Ear, Nose and Throat
GP	General Practitioner
HAC	Health Administration Corporation
ICN	International Council of Nurses
NHMRC	National Health and Medical Research Council
NSW	New South Wales
NSWCN	New South Wales College of Nursing
NSWNA	New South Wales Nurses' Association
NSWNRB	New South Wales Nurses Registration Board
NUM	Nurse Unit Manager
PAR	Post Anaesthetic Recovery (room)
PCC	Professional Conduct Committee
PHARM	Pharmaceutical Health and Rational Use of Medicines Committee
PID	Pelvic Inflammatory Disease
RACGP	Royal Australian College of General Practitioners
RANF	Royal Australian Nursing Federation

RCN	Royal College of Nurses (UK)
RCNA	Royal College of Nursing, Australia
RFDS	Royal Flying Doctor Service
RN	Registered Nurse
RVTNA	Royal Victorian Trained Nurses' Association
TAFE	Technical and Further Education
TURP	Transurethral resection of the prostate gland
UKCC	United Kingdom Central Council for Nursing, Midwifery and Health Visiting
VAD	Voluntary Aid Detachment
VMO	Visiting Medical Officer

Table of Cases

Table of Statutes

Midwives Act 1918 (UK)
Nurses, Midwives and Health Visitors Act 1979 (UK)
Nurses Registration Act 1919 (UK)

Victoria
Nurses Act 1993 (Vic)

Western Australia
Nurses Act 1968 (WA)

PART 1

Searching for the 'true' status of the nurse

PART CONTENTS

1

One nurse, four hearings, five images

Sophia (Sophie) Heathcote was an English registered nurse (RN) who trained at the Radcliffe Infirmary, Oxford. She returned to Australia, after a working holiday there, to work as a remote area nurse and obtained employment at Wilcannia Hospital. She had no experience of drug and alcohol management, nor of Aboriginal health. Wilcannia is a remote and isolated town in the Far West District of New South Wales; its Emergency Department provides the only permanent service for 200 km. The hospital has some beds, but the nursing staff have integrated roles with community health and other services (NSW Health Department 1996b p.62). There is no resident doctor; the Royal Flying Doctor Service (RFDS) runs three clinics a week, can be contacted by radio at any time, and is able to attend in cases of emergency, although this obviously takes some time.

The events which occurred in the early hours of 24 June 1987 (eight months after Sophie's arrival in Wilcannia) became the focus of: a Coronial inquiry, the Royal Commission into Aboriginal Deaths in Custody, a disciplinary hearing, and a District Court appeal against the disciplinary decision. The inquest was held at Wilcannia in December 1987 and January 1988 (Inquest touching the death of MAQ 1987/88), and the facts determined at the inquest were not disputed at any later date. The inquest itself attracted intense television and newspaper coverage.

THE FACTS

During the night MAQ, an Aboriginal man aged 22 years, was brought to Wilcannia Hospital hallucinating and shaking, believed to be suffering from alcohol withdrawal. Sister (Sr) Heathcote and a wardsmaid were the only two staff on duty. Sr Heathcote was informed by his relatives that MAQ was 'in the horrors' or 'in the dings', expressions used locally to describe alcohol withdrawal. They asked to leave him with her at the hospital.

She noted that he was somewhat disorientated and went to make him a cup of coffee, during which time he left the hospital. She rang the Wilcannia Police Station and told the police that she was concerned for his safety because the river was close by the hospital. Before the police arrived, MAQ returned, still obviously confused. He was not violent, but Sr Heathcote was worried about the safety of her staff, herself and her patients. She telephoned the police to let them know he had returned, but by this time they were already on their way.

MAQ again left the hospital and at this stage Sr Heathcote telephoned the matron, who was sleeping, to seek advice on handling the situation. Shortly after this two police officers arrived and Sr Heathcote identified MAQ to them. They spoke to him and placed him in the back of the police van. One police officer suggested that he was hallucinating. They spoke with Sr Heathcote who asked if he could stay at the police station, to which the police stated in evidence that they agreed 'if there was no alternative' (Inquest touching the death of MAQ 1987/88 p.000738).

Sr Heathcote telephoned the RFDS and spoke to the doctor there, and consequently checked MAQ's blood glucose levels. As these were satisfactory he was taken to the cells. Later Sr Heathcote made arrangements to attend the police station in the morning as she wanted to check his blood pressure. The police officers left the police station and went home at about 3.15 a.m. When the morning constable came on duty, he found MAQ hanged in his cell. On Sr Heathcote's arrival, she was shown his body and noted that there were no signs of life.

STORIES ABOUT SOPHIE: WOULD THE REAL NURSE PLEASE STAND UP?

Sophie Heathcote (and others) told this story and explained her clinical decision making on four separate occasions in four different legal settings. Many who were not present read the facts and interpreted her behaviour according to their opinions of appropriate nursing behaviour. The atmosphere in the courtroom for the inquest was charged. Sr Heathcote was subject to lengthy cross-examination.

No fewer than nine highly paid barristers crowded into the little non-air-conditioned Wilcannia courthouse, sweltering in conditions well over 40 degrees. Tempers flared—on occasions, learned counsel engaged in 'what can only be described as a shouting match', said the coroner, Mr Graham Johnson.

Barristers referred to the 'atmosphere of rage' at the hearing, to submissions being 'scandalous' and to a witness being 'vilified, scapegoated, witch-hunted … it's an outrage.' (Hills 1990 p.26)

The case illustrates the argument of this book. In the events of one night, recounted in four hearings and some media coverage, one nurse is endowed with or manifests all the images which this book will explore. The expectations of the professions, the response of the media, the representations of the advocates for the parties to the hearings, and the inconsistencies between the courts and tribunals, all lead to the inescapable conclusion that the 'jury is out' on the status of the nurse at law. Indeed, this book will argue that the 'jury' has never really considered the question. Sophie Heathcote was one moment depicted as an esteemed adviser to her medical colleagues, the next a ministering angel, the next a mere handmaiden to the doctor. The resultant quandary for nurses as to what constitutes appropriate nursing behaviour will remain unresolved while such ambiguity continues.

Domestic duties or nursing care?

Although not mentioned within the judgments, for the purposes of this book it is significant that the first thing that Sr Heathcote did after she had spoken to MAQ was to make him a cup of coffee. It would have been an instinctive response in this situation. But not according to the judge Lord Greene MR even some forty years previously.

A nurse, I should have thought, is employed by a hospital to nurse the patients, not merely to carry up the tea; and a patient would expect that the hospital employed a nurse to nurse him. The other duties which the nurse has to perform are incidental to her primary task of nursing, and could as well be performed by anyone else. (Gold v Essex County Council 1942 p.303)

Although courts have dismissed such activities as domestic, this was the first thing Sr Heathcote did, even before she took his observations.

THE FINDINGS OF THE CORONIAL INQUIRY: Sr HEATHCOTE AS AN AUTONOMOUS PROFESSIONAL

In the coronial hearing the first image to emerge was that of the nurse as an autonomous professional. The Coroner considered that Sr Heathcote was the primary professional in this situation (the captain of the ship?) and Dr Ryan from RFDS was her adviser, but dependent on her information and clinical skills. The Coroner's expectations of her clinical skills and judgment were very high, and he clearly perceived her as the key figure in the management of the patient. He spent some considerable time in his decision discussing her actions and the implications of the telephone call to Dr Ryan. The Coroner was critical of the way in which she managed both the telephone call and the patient.

The recorded conversation between the doctor and the nurse was reproduced in full in the decision, and considerable emphasis was placed on the quality of Sr Heathcote's information. She gave the following pieces of information which directly related to the patient:

a) that 'he hadn't been in for three years';
b) that he was 'in the dings';
c) that 'he was seeing things and hearing things and really acting strange'; and
d) that he had escaped on them twice. (Inquest touching the death of MAQ 1987/88 p.000740)

The Coroner felt that as she had the man's medical records before her when she was speaking to the doctor, she should have given the doctor more information about MAQ's past history of alcoholism (Inquest touching the death of MAQ 1987/88 p.000741).

The Coroner was critical of the fact that neither the doctor nor the nurse made the diagnosis of alcohol withdrawal. This is indicative of the expectations of the skilled clinical role which nurses assume in remote areas (Rice 1985 pp.23–4). The doctor also testified that he relied upon nurses to exercise such advanced skills. This defence of reliance upon the clinical skills of nurses is frequently used by doctors and will be discussed later in this book. The Coroner was unequivocal in his expectations of Sr Heathcote.

Sister Heathcote went to great lengths during her evidence to state that nurses do not make diagnoses but only take observations. I find this position difficult to accept. Whilst no one could expect a registered nurse to make a diagnosis with the same competence as a doctor, nonetheless her training and experience would enable her to make a working or provisional diagnosis in many cases. [The doctor] agreed in evidence that nurses in general, and sister Heathcote in particular do make diagnoses and convey clinical impressions. In my view sister Heathcote did in fact diagnose [MAQ's] condition as alcohol withdrawal. (Inquest touching the death of MAQ 1987/88 p.000742)

She was also criticised because it was held that it was she who suggested that he should spend the night in the cells. In her defence she pointed out that she had asked permission for this to happen from both the doctor and the matron. However, the matron had no recollection of this part of the conversation, and it was held that she had put the suggestion as a fait accompli to the doctor. Again the inference is that Sister Heathcote was in charge of the patient, and that she had considerable influence over the doctor.

The quality of Sr Heathcote's observations was also scrutinised. The doctor testified that, had he received better information from Sr Heathcote, he would have managed MAQ quite differently. The Coroner was critical of the paucity of the information which passed between the doctor and Sr Heathcote. He stressed the importance of a nurse conveying all the relevant clinical information to the doctor and was sympathetic to the doctor's decision in the light of the poor information he had received.

He said that if he had known the clinical details, if sister Heathcote had said [MAQ] was 'in the horrors' rather than 'in the dings' (which expression he didn't know) and that [MAQ] hadn't had a drink for a few days, the conversation with sister Heathcote would have taken a different direction and he would have told her to begin a hemineurin regime and to keep the patient in the hospital. (Inquest touching the death of MAQ 1987/88 p.000781)

Sr Heathcote also testified that she was not aware that the police station was unattended during the night, and that she would never have sanctioned MAQ going into a dark room on his own for such a length of time.

However, this statement only attracted further criticism. She was moreover criticised for failing to call the family for assistance. The Coroner, whilst acknowledging that she was working under difficult conditions, referred her papers to the Nurses Registration Board (NRB) as he considered it to be in the public interest to have the Board consider the issue.

THE FINDINGS OF THE DISCIPLINARY TRIBUNAL: Sr HEATHCOTE AS AN AUTONOMOUS PROFESSIONAL

As a result of the Coroner's referral and findings, an inquiry was conducted under s19 of the Nurses Registration Act 1953 (NSW) to investigate the following complaints:

That the said Sophia Mary Ann Heathcote whilst on duty at the Wilcannia and District Hospital on 24 June 1987 did fail to properly perform her duties in relation to a patient [MAQ] (now deceased).

(a) Did fail to adhere to the Nursing Manual which states 'It is important that you obtain all relevant facts about a patient before calling the doctor'.

(b) Did fail to perform basic observations or procedures including temperature, pulse, respiration, blood pressure, neurological observations, and general physical examination and failed to record such observations as may have been made.

(c) Did fail to consult or read the patient's previous clinical notes and/or did fail to inform Doctor Ryan, the consultant medical practitioner of this medical history.

(d) Did fail to obtain a proper medical history from friends or family who brought the patient to the hospital.

(e) Did fail to convey to the consultant medical practitioner, Dr Ryan her diagnosis of the patient's condition as alcohol withdrawal or the results of any observations made.

(f) Did request the police to detain the patient in a police station and did fail to consider alternative options to manage the patient's problem or condition.

(g) Having done (f) did fail to ascertain the suitability of the police station and police supervision for the patient's care and failed to advise the police of necessary precautions and observations they should make in relation to his proper care.

(h) Failed to ask police to stay at the hospital so that she could carry out (a), (b), and (c). (Inquiry conducted under s 19 of Nurses Registration Act 1953 re Sophia Heathcote 1989 p.3)

The findings of the Inquiry were as follows:

The complaint of misconduct in a professional respect in accordance with Section 19 (1) (b) of the Act is found to be proven with particulars (a), (b), (c), (d), (e), (f), and (h) having been established, and only part of (g), namely not informing police of precautions to be taken. (Inquiry conducted under s 19 of Nurses Registration Act 1953 re Sophia Heathcote 1989 p.2)

The Board formed a Committee to hear the complaint and the hearing took place in February 1989. At least two members of the Committee were registered nurses. Two senior nurses who neither worked, nor had worked, in a remote area gave evidence. Both stated during the appeal hearing that they were keen to see the professional advancement of nurses and both testified that nurses ought to undertake the activities listed in the complaint, including diagnosis (Heathcote v NRB and Walton 1991).

The Committee suspended Ms Heathcote's registration for a period of twelve months. However, the New South Wales Nurses Association (NSWNA) lodged an appeal on her behalf to the District Court.

THE FINDINGS OF THE ROYAL COMMISSION INTO ABORIGINAL DEATHS IN CUSTODY: Sr HEATHCOTE AS AN AUTONOMOUS PROFESSIONAL

Before this appeal was heard, the Hon JH Wootten AC, QC, Commissioner of the Royal Commission into Aboriginal Deaths in Custody, submitted reports into 18 deaths in the States of New South Wales, Victoria and Tasmania from May 1988 until December 1990. The Report of that Royal Commission (hereafter the Report) was published in 1991, and was condemnatory of the way in which Aborigines were managed when in custody. One of the deaths examined by the Commission was that of MAQ. The Commissioner was trenchant in his censure of the prevailing attitude towards Aboriginals in the health services in Wilcannia. 'As the events following [MAQ's] death show, even such health services as exist are white dominated and close their ranks rapidly on a racial basis' (Royal Commission into Aboriginal Deaths in Custody 1991 p.379).

The Commissioner considered it extraordinary, and related to his social status, that MAQ was put in jail because he was hallucinating. '[MAQ's] custody was totally unlawful and unreasonable' (Royal Commission into Aboriginal Deaths in Custody 1991 p.76). He was censorious of MAQ's management and suggested that persons of greater standing in the community would not have received such treatment.

He was critical of the actions of both Sr Heathcote and the doctor, not only on professional grounds, but also on grounds of racism. He made it clear that professional people, who by virtue of their standing in the community exercised considerable control over the lives of others, had particular obligations which were not met in this situation. With regard to his criticism of their professional standards, he was explicit.

[MAQ] should never have been taken from hospital to a police cell, and when taken to a police cell, should not have been locked up unattended. In his case there were breaches of duty by a hospital sister and a doctor as well as by two police officers. (Royal Commission into Aboriginal Deaths in Custody 1991 p.64)

Regarding the question of racism, he was equally direct. 'In the case of [MAQ], I find it impossible to believe that the treatment which led to his death would have been given to a white citizen of Wilcannia' (Royal Commission into Aboriginal Deaths in Custody 1991 p.18). Perhaps the Commissioner's outrage was more pronounced because those who sent him to the cells were supposed to care for him and keep him safe. Possibly he considered such behaviour to be doubly reprehensible when perpetrated by those in whom the community places its trust.

THE 'SACRIFICE' OF SISTER SOPHIA:
A MINISTERING ANGEL

However, despite the criticisms of the Coroner, the NRB, and the Commissioner, some people believed that Sr Heathcote had become the scapegoat for the entire incident. An article published in the Sydney Morning Herald entitled *The Sacrifice of Sister Sophia* evoked a completely different image, that of a nurse who was merciful and compassionate, and who had done her best to look after MAQ and the other patients in her care. The article suggested that this good and caring nurse had been sacrificed to save the reputations of the doctor, the hospital matron, and the police. 'She was worried he might fall into the river and drown, worried he might disturb the two seriously ill children [in the hospital] in his wanderings' (1990 p.25). She was described as 'the young English sister,' and it was stated that:

Of them all, she was the one who was ultimately to carry the heaviest burden of blame. It was, submitted one of the barristers, a trial where those responsible transferred the blame down the line—'Truth has suffered in this macabre game of pass the parcel.' (Hills 1991 p.27).

The article revealed that neither of the policemen had been reported to the Commissioner, both were still in the police force and one had been pro- moted to sergeant. It further revealed that the doctor was still free to prac- tise medicine in Minyip, the little town near Ballarat (Victoria) where he had moved following the inquest and subsequent Royal Commission hear- ing. Whilst this information shed no light on his registration status in New South Wales, it indicated that any penalty, if such had been imposed, was not reported on to the Victorian registration authorities, or if it had been, it had not affected his registration. It is interesting to compare their fates with that of Sr Heathcote. Perhaps when an 'angel' is thought to have fallen from grace, society's condemnation is harsher.

But Sr Heathcote was still considered by her peers to be a good nurse. Hills' articles revealed that a letter had been sent from the staff of Wilcannia Hospital, describing her as 'one of the finest, most compassionate and skil- ful nurses (we) have ever had the pleasure of working with'. Sr Heathcote's registration was reinstated pending her appeal, and there was a ground swell of popular support. The NSWNA lodged the appeal on her behalf, and publicly and financially supported her throughout the appeal process (Staunton 1991 p.17). Patricia Staunton, then General Secretary of the NSWNA, was unequivocal in her support.

Reading this article, one has to ask why anyone would choose to work in circumstances such as those in which Sophia found herself on that lonely night. Certainly those who do possess dedication of a unique order. It is not surprising that the Association has received countless messages of support and concern for Sophia Heathcote from nurses throughout the profession. As a member, the Association has and will continue to support Sophia, financially and professionally, in her long and unwavering fight for justice. (Staunton 1990 p.24)

Sr HEATHCOTE: DOCTOR'S HANDMAIDEN OR SUBORDINATE PROFESSIONAL?

Sr Heathcote's appeal against the decision of the NRB was heard by way of rehearing in February 1991 in the District Court in Sydney before Ward DCJ. Several of the expert witnesses from the misconduct hearing were recalled by the NRB, and new expert witnesses were called by Sr Heathcote (Heathcote v NRB and Walton 1991). One of the main planks of the appeal was that Sr Heathcote was not guilty of professional misconduct because, regardless of whether her conduct was less than adequate, it did not amount to conduct which would incur strong censure from her peers (Qidwai v Brown 1984 p.105).

The expert witnesses who had testified in the disciplinary hearing were cross-examined on their experience in remote area nursing and found by the court to be unconvincing. In contrast, Sr Heathcote's expert witnesses had extensive experience of the remote environment and did not criticise her acts strongly. The judge allowed the appeal, dismissing all of the allegations of failure made by the Board on the basis of the evidence before him. She was reinstated.

In the light of my disagreeing with the decision of the Board, I record that it acted upon expert evidence which was largely cut down and based upon inadequate material or without appreciation of the relevance of other material facts. (Heathcote v NRB and Walton 1991 p.17)

Her communications with the doctor, which the Coroner had criticised, were defended by an expert in drug and alcohol (D&A) medicine, as being 'a pretty good summary of the case' (Heathcote v NRB and Walton 1991 p.11). Ward DCJ held that she had sought advice appropriately from her superiors and thus her responsibility for MAQ's removal to the cells was also challenged. Here Sr Heathcote is portrayed not as one in charge, but as one in a position of subordination, who has to seek advice or permission in order to take such an unusual course of action.

The nurse was faced with a situation which 'was something she hadn't come across before' and she did not know what to do at the time. In the difficult management situation, in which I find she genuinely and rightly foresaw the likelihood of safety problems, she sought advice from the Director of Nursing by telephone and then from the Doctor on call. No evidence was given which asserted that the action taken by the appellant was such a failure in conduct in the circumstances that reputable members of the profession would regard it with strong disapprobation. (Heathcote v NRB and Walton 1991 p.12)

Inherent in this appeal judgment is the assertion that, contrary to the doctor's evidence at the inquest, the nurse was unable to take any initiative without the approval of the doctor. There was a very clear portrayal of the nurse's role as limited by her requirement to seek directions from the doctor. The Policy and Procedure Manual was produced in court which stated that the nurse ought 'not to commence any treatment on her own initiative' as she is 'not the doctor'.

The appellant adopted the wisest and proper course of getting in touch with the doctor when the management and necessary treatment could be discussed. She was not allowed in nursing procedure, even at that stage of difficulty in management, to prescribe or administer even sedative medication to settle the patient. (Heathcote v NRB and Walton 1991 p.13)

Sr Heathcote was depicted both by the judge and her own lawyers as unable to act unless so instructed by a doctor. This defence has been used successfully by nurses in other cases and will be discussed later in this book in more detail. The right of the nurse to rely on the instructions of a doctor and to be exonerated if she carries out those instructions, even if they are wrong, was clearly acknowledged. In this situation, she was portrayed as the doctor's handmaiden, unquestioningly performing the doctor's orders.

It was conceded that the appellant, as a nurse, had to follow the doctor's directions and that she had been given directions and that no criticism of the appellant could be levelled after that time. (Heathcote v NRB and Walton 1991 p.17)

However, in other parts of the judgment, her clinical skills were acknowledged, and she seems to have been accorded a more professional role, but one which was still subordinate to the doctor. The D&A expert was quoted as saying that a nurse ought to have some professional responsibility if the orders of the doctor were wrong. He suggested that the nurse ought to have been far more emphatic, 'more assertive' about her expectations of the doctor, which seemed to place some of the responsibility back with the nurse.

The judge considered that a nurse should be able to make a proper assessment of a patient, but did not necessarily view her as a diagnostician. This was further clarified by the D&A expert, who explained the process of 'assessment' and stated that it was a skill taught to both nurses and doctors. However, he too did not comment on whether nurses should be 'diagnosticians'. He grouped both nurses and doctors together in the information which they would receive when taught to make an assessment, and in the manner in which assessment was undertaken.

Thus, in the examination of the same set of facts, Sophia Heathcote, Sister Sophia, Sister Sophie, Sr Heathcote, has been portrayed as a domestic worker, an autonomous professional, a ministering angel, a subordinate professional and a doctor's handmaiden. It has been held at different stages and by different courts and tribunals that she makes diagnoses, and that she does not make diagnoses; that she is exonerated if she obeys the doctor, and that she ought to be more assertive and insist that the doctor obeys her; that she can act independently, and that she cannot act independently. She has been denounced as racist and lauded as compassionate. She has been shown to do everything from making the coffee to making an assessment, and all in the name of nursing care. Would there ever be such ambiguity about the scope of medical or legal practice? How is a nurse to know what entails good nursing practice?

This book will argue that such ambiguity exists because nurses are 'outsiders' to the health law system, and thus have not been contemplated consistently in their own right. They have generally been viewed as 'Other' and their status addressed only consequent to a specific event or issue. In such situations nurses would be scrutinised in relation to doctors, patients, or hospitals, and their status or image would be adjusted accordingly. This single incident viewed through a number of courts and tribunals briefly raises several of the major issues addressed in this book. At the end of the book we shall return to this case.

2

Pulling the images apart

INTRODUCTION

This book was developed from a doctoral thesis and the purpose of this chapter is to explain briefly the question that led to the investigation, the ways in which the research materials were obtained, and the framework which was adopted to make sense of the research findings.

THE RESEARCH QUESTION, THE ARGUMENT AND THE PROCESS OF INQUIRY

This research was undertaken because of a desire to assist nurses with the difficulties and uncertainties which they experience in their political, professional and clinical lives. It was underpinned by the simple idea that if it were possible to determine the status of the accredited nurse (a term which refers to both registered and enrolled nurses under s.3 (1) Nurses Act 1991 NSW) some of these difficulties and uncertainties might be addressed and resolved. Thus my original question was: what is the status of the accredited nurse? Status is defined for the purpose of this book as an amalgam of legal and non-legal factors. These are:

- the nature of the nursing role as it is defined by law and as it evolves in practice;
- whether nursing is regarded as a profession, both at law and in society;
- the legal and actual ability of nurses to exercise power in their professional and clinical lives; and
- the legal and actual responsibilities and duties which nurses are expected to shoulder.

It quickly became clear that there was no single or simple answer to my question. This book will argue that the difficulties which nurses experience in their political, professional and clinical lives are exacerbated by the inconsistency of the law relating to nurses, and the failure of the law to address the reality of nursing practice when there are multidisciplinary influences on such practice. This failure means that nurses are uncertain of their duties and obligations to the patient.

It will be argued that both at law and in health care generally nurses are rarely regarded as central to the delivery of health care. Rather, they are regarded as peripheral, or even invisible, and not regarded at all. There is no consistent view about their status, because they are usually viewed in juxtaposition to other more dominant entities, such as doctors or health care institutions, whose status is fixed more clearly. Furthermore, the responsibilities that they shoulder and the authority that they exercise arise in a climate of medical permission or abrogation, rather than in one of nursing entitlement. Moreover, much of the information which is readily available in health law textbooks discusses civil liability, which rarely affects nurses directly. In New South Wales for example, the majority of nurses are employees and therefore under the Employee's Liability Act 1991 (NSW) s.3 (1) their employers will be vicariously liable for their actions. Nursing has also been considered to be part of a hospital's non-delegable duty of care (Albrighton v Royal Prince Alfred Hospital & Ors 1980). In clinical situations, nurses report that, when disagreements arise over clinical decision making, the fact that doctors are more frequently held to be personally liable for their own tortious acts is often used as a justification for medical dominance and control. Whilst nurses are rarely held to be personally liable for their own tortious acts, there are other forms of sanction, such as professional disciplinary actions, which are potentially more damaging than tortious liability, given that one can insure against civil liability.

Both nurses and doctors can and do carry professional responsibility for their actions, either through employment sanctions (such as dismissal), professional sanctions (such as those stemming from the decisions of disciplinary tribunals), or through coronial criticism. This book will demonstrate that the professional sanctions on nurses are often excessively severe, and that employment sanctions on nurses were extremely oppressive for many years, and rarely challenged. In addition, the considerable clinical responsibility with which nurses are vested in practice is not commensurate with the amount of power or control they are able to exercise over their environment or the events for which they are responsible.

Defining the role of the nurse

Mullighan J observed in Versteegh v Nurses Board of South Australia (1992 p.142) that '[t]he court has no familiarity with many of the aspects of the work of the nursing profession'. However, authorities such as the International Council of Nurses (ICN) (1969 amended 1975) and the National Health and Medical Research Council (NHMRC) (1991) have attempted to define the role of the nurse, and these definitions are available to inform courts and tribunals. Yet in a case where a definition of nursing was required, the judge, Mahoney J, turned to a dictionary, rather than to any of the available professional definitions (Thomas v Ferguson Transformers P/L 1979 p.221).

There are also few descriptive statutory definitions of a nurse. The Nurses Registration Act 1953 (NSW) and other statutes such as the Human Tissue Act 1983 (NSW) provide no definition of the terms 'nurse' or 'nursing'. The Nurses Act 1991 (NSW) s.3 (1) defines an accredited nurse as 'a registered nurse or an enrolled nurse' and then defines registered and enrolled nurses as persons who are respectively registered or enrolled under the Act.

However, despite the fact that there are more recent definitions, still the most popular and frequently reproduced definition of the nursing role seems to be that developed by Virginia Henderson for the ICN in 1969. It is of particular value to this book as it explicitly defines the unique function of the nurse both in relation to the patient and to other members of the health care team. It is as follows:

The unique function of the nurse is to assist the individual, sick or well, in the performance of those activities contributing to health or its recovery (or to a peaceful death) that he (sic) would perform unaided if he had the necessary strength, will or knowledge. And to do this in such a way as to help him gain independence as rapidly as possible. This aspect of her (sic) work, this part of her function, she initiates and controls; of this she is master. In addition she helps the patient carry out the therapeutic plan as initiated by the physician. She also, as a member of a medical team, helps other members, as they in turn help her, to plan and carry out the total program whether it be for the improvement of health, or the recovery from illness or support in death. (Henderson 1969 p.4)

THE STUDY OF NURSING AND THE LAW
Nursing as a subset of medicine or health

There are quite a number of books written about nursing and the law, which provide a comprehensive statement of the existing medico-legal situation, drawing mainly on the major medical negligence cases, with specific nursing information being provided in areas such as registration and poisons legislation, and documentation policy. These texts are extremely useful as a means of informing nurses about general health law matters, such as the age of consent, or the requirements for tissue donation. However, most of them contain little case law specifically about nursing.[1] Furthermore, very few of them attempt to critique the law from a nursing perspective.[2] This is not surprising, as specific legal material relating to nursing is often

---

[1] Patricia Staunton and Ross Whyburn are an exception to this, in what is probably the most popular NSW 'law for nurses' text *Nursing and the Law* (4th ed, 1997). They provide some specific nursing examples, particularly in relation to documentation, and use a number of unreported cases from the New South Wales Nurses' Association archives.

[2] One of the most thorough critiques has been undertaken by a nurse ethicist, Megan-Jane Johnstone. In her book *Nursing and the Injustices of the Law* (1994), she employs feminist jurisprudential inquiry to provide an insightful critique of a large collection of (substantially) American cases and a smaller number of English, Canadian and Australian cases.

difficult to obtain. Many of the existing statutes relating to health care pay little or no attention to the role played by nurses, according decision making power to medical practitioners.

In addition, there has been a tendency to focus on medical practice and issues when organisations and courses have undertaken to address health law issues. These organisations and courses often originally called themselves departments of, or courses in, law and medicine, although some are now adopting the term health law. This is not to suggest that medical law per se is not a valid or important field of study. It is simply to indicate that, if one wishes to address legal problems which nurses encounter, clinical life is not the same for nurses as it is for doctors. Thus, although the medical law cases and materials are informative, they rarely address specifically nurses' concerns and/or potential contributions, because nurses are not usually evident in them.

Collecting a body of case law

The book initially set out to explore the scope of the nurses' legal duties and responsibilities through an analysis of case law, in the hope that by 'gather[ing] large numbers of opinions together, the law [would] emerge from the crowd' (Papke 1991 p.206). Collecting a body of nursing law over the 20th century has presented its own difficulties. To collect a body of case law which addressed the scope of nursing responsibility it was necessary to search a number of doctrinal areas, including civil negligence cases involving hospitals, coronial hearings, industrial award decisions, and appeals against decisions of professional tribunals. A significant number of these cases were unreported. In order to develop a body of nursing law, it was necessary to identify the issues which affected nurses and to work backwards from there. Graycar and Morgan (1990 pp.5–6) have described similar strategies (and difficulties) in developing a book of law 'whose focus is the concrete realities of women's lives'.

Sources of case law and supplementary materials

Although originally my focus was the nurse in New South Wales, I have included cases from English and Canadian jurisdictions where they address issues similar to those found in the Australian situation. The collection of case law spans 1904–1998.

For the first half of the century the negligence and disciplinary case law is gathered from the civil jurisdictions of Australia, Canada and England. These three jurisdictions were drawn upon particularly because there was much cross citation from one judgment to another. A small number of Scottish and New Zealand cases are also included in the first half of the century because they were referred to frequently in the major cases.

Australian, Canadian and English civil negligence cases and appeals against decisions of disciplinary tribunals from the second half of the last century are also used. Whilst Canadian and English cases are now, at best, persuasive precedent in Australia, those selected are illustrative of the practice situations in which Australian nurses might find themselves. The other judgments include industrial decisions, almost exclusively from New South Wales, and Australian coronial decisions. The fact that a significant number of the judgments are either unreported or not in official reports is characteristic of the invisibility of the nurse in law. A wide range of supplementary legal materials has been used.

The book also draws on texts and materials from a broad selection of other disciplinary sources. Nursing and health care literature is examined from the time of Florence Nightingale to the present day. The use of English nursing history as well as Australian sources is appropriate, as Australian nursing is founded on the Nightingale model.

The recurrent images and their chronology

What became evident from this investigation was that there were a number of recurrent images of nurses in the case law. Some of the images were directly contradictory to others. Some of the images emerged more frequently than others, and some were more dominant than others at different periods of history. But all are recognisable to some extent in the realities of the lives of nurses today.

There must always be a caveat when using relatively simple images to describe extremely complex situations (Morgan 1997 p.4). However, by employing a number of conflicting images and by identifying the elements within each image (see Appendix for a full presentation of the images and their elements), hopefully the complexity of the situation will still be evident.

In the first half of the 20th century, when nurses rarely gave evidence, the dominant images of the nurse which emerged from the case law were feminine images: the domestic worker, the ministering angel, the doctor's handmaiden. All of these images were subordinate constructs, defined in relation to and often by the (usually) male doctor. But one must remember that nurses had actively promoted the ministering angel image at the turn of the century to evince an appearance of respectability for the nursing workforce. In this way, it was an image which nurses themselves fostered and controlled in order to achieve their goals at that time.

The images of domestic worker and doctor's handmaiden often emerged through the case law by default, because the issue of the status of nurses was not the central consideration of the court. The question of civil liability was often pivotal in these early cases, and the notional status of the nurse was a side issue. Yet these images and the subordinate status which they implied emerged because they lay dormant in the minds of the lawyers involved in the cases—they were constructs which were 'always already' present (Lather 1991 p.170).

In the second half of the century, there has been greater societal recognition of nursing as a profession, brought about mainly by the efforts of professional and industrial nursing organisations. However, the extent of this acceptance and recognition has varied. Nurses have pressed for professional autonomy, but this has often been actively opposed by the medical profession. From a legal perspective in more recent times, where nurses have been the sole focus of the 'judicial gaze' and nurses have given evidence, the extensive scope of nursing responsibility has been acknowledged. However, in courts or tribunals where the focus of the judicial gaze does not rest exclusively on the nurse, and a doctor is also present, the nurse is invariably viewed as a subordinate professional, and the dilemmas which such a position might present for nurses are very seldom addressed. In health care practice, power over clinical decision making continues to be the domain of the medical profession, and financial power is now exercised predominantly by administrators. In health policy and legislation, it is often as though the nurse does not exist.

THE THEORETICAL FRAMEWORK

The remainder of this chapter is concerned with the theoretical approach used in this book. It describes briefly the theoretical approaches that have been used to analyse the case law and emergent images in this book: feminist jurisprudence, critical race theory, and the use of narrative scholarship.

The value and relevance of feminist jurisprudence

Finding a theoretical framework within which to analyse the images that emerged from the case law also required an acknowledgement of the paradoxes relating to the status of nurses. For example, the images of domestic worker, doctor's handmaiden and ministering angel invite a feminist jurisprudential analysis, and feminist jurisprudence has been most valuable in shaping this book. Nursing is predominantly a female profession,[3] and is still dominated by the medical profession, which until recently was predominantly male.[4] In addition, nursing work is still viewed by many as 'women's work' because of its caring nature, and has been similarly devalued as a result (Chesterman 1983 pp.43–64, Graycar 1985 p.22).

---

[3] The 1996 NSW Nurses Registration Board Annual Survey showed that 93% of the nursing workforce was female.
[4] Although 54% of entrants to Australian medical schools are now female (ABS 1996), the majority of medical specialists are still male, with female medical practitioners working in part-time or general practice positions. Since the majority of nurses still work in hospital settings, the senior medical officers would still be predominantly male.

Feminist lawyers who critique the law from a feminist perspective adopt a position as 'outsiders' to the legal system. They examine the law as lawyers (who become the 'insiders' for the purpose of such a critique), but from the perspective of their outsider experience as women, who they believe have been discriminated against by mainstream (or 'malestream' (Graycar & Morgan 1990 p.6)) legal thought and analysis. This may be argued to be a form of academic schizophrenia, but the law is such a complex discipline that it would be difficult to provide an adequate critique without a grounding in the discipline. Women lawyers have described their experiences of feeling a sense of 'otherness' within the legal profession and thus are well placed to expound the problems which women face both within and from the legal profession (Thornton 1996). Feminist lawyers state that 'sexism is all pervasive in legal life' (Sachs & Hoff Wilson 1978). They point out that the law has been formulated from the dominant paradigm of the white middle class male, but it has traditionally presented itself as both rational and gender neutral. Catharine MacKinnon describes this invisibility of sexism in the law. She states that it is 'perhaps the most pervasive and tenacious system of power in history ... it is metaphysically nearly perfect. Its point of view is the standard for point of viewlessness, its particularity the meaning of universality' (1983 p.35).

The need for a further dimension

However, a purely feminist analysis would fail to address adequately the complexity of nurses as professionals. Throughout the 20th century, nurses viewed themselves as professionals who traditionally had a great deal of professional pride (Russell 1990, Schultz 1991). They were one of the earliest recognised 'female' professions (as in a profession which originally was only for women and which still has an overwhelming predominance of women), the first 'female' profession to have professional registration (Abel-Smith 1960), and the first to be organised industrially (Dickenson 1993). Although in the early part of the century nurses clearly deferred to their (mostly male) medical counterparts (Gladwin 1930 p.21), they also had a considerable amount of influence for women of that time. For example, the ICN, which was established by Mrs Bedford Fenwick in 1899 (ICN 1973 p.12), provided links for nurses to travel and exchange ideas throughout the world. In terms of financial control, the Matrons of the hospitals at that time controlled substantial nursing and housekeeping budgets (Schultz 1991 p.178) at a time when women were still disadvantaged in society in innumerable ways (Scutt 1994). They also had a considerable amount of freedom and license in their interactions with men. Their access to men and their knowledge of men's bodies were probably matched only by married women and prostitutes, and nursing offered a career ladder and an escape from their own homes which was one of few alternatives to marriage or holy orders. They were viewed as adventurous and brave, particularly in relation to their war-time efforts (Adam-Smith 1996 pp.8–35). Nurses also derive considerable pleasure and satisfaction from the core work that they undertake and from their interactions with patients (Wicks 1999 pp.75–90).

The feminist movement, in its early stages in the 20th century,[5] did not address these benefits of nursing, but rather characterised it as one of a limited number of archetypal female careers. Thus nursing, along with housework, to some extent became an allegory for female oppression (Salvage 1985, Gardner 1989, Daniel 1990). Because nurses had viewed themselves as professional and had valued their caring role, this was a difficult experience for some, who experienced feelings of shame and embarrassment about their profession. Nursing recruitment fell as more career choices opened up for women, and the queues of young women waiting to become nurses no longer exist (NSW Health Department 1996a). However, nursing still provides significant job satisfaction and has a proactive and dynamic professional core (Knepfer & Johns 1989, Dickenson 1993, Taylor 1994). This ambivalence toward nursing can still be evidenced by the Letters pages in *The Lamp* (the official journal of the New South Wales Nurses' Association) which are full of questions such as 'Why do we say we are "only" nurses?' As Franz Fanon (1963) has identified, oppressed groups tend to internalise their oppression and turn it into a form of self-hatred. Matsuda (1990 p.1772) describes this as 'false consciousness'.

Thus, to examine nursing solely from a feminist perspective would not address fully the contemporary phenomenon of nurses as professionals. Feminism has been a most illuminating and empowering movement for nurses, in that it has highlighted many of the difficulties which nurses-as-women encounter, and has provided us with a framework from which to understand and deal with our oppression (Delacour 1991, Parker 1991, Speedy 1991). But it has also disadvantaged nursing both from a recruitment perspective and as a profession, insofar as it has devalued nursing work.

The value and relevance of critical race theory

A useful complementary theoretical framework in which to analyse these diverse nursing images is critical race theory. Critical race theory has similar origins to feminist jurisprudence, in that it deals with the way the law affects oppressed and minority (outsider) groups. Both belong to a school of

---

[5] There is beginning to be a change in this attitude now. See for example Jocelynne Scutt 'Women and the power to change' in *The Sexual Gerrymander* (1994 p.243).

legal scholarship sometimes referred to as 'outsider scholarship' (Matsuda 1987 p.323).[6]

The particular relevance of critical race theory is that it provides some extra dimensions to the nature of oppression which help to analyse the paradoxes inherent in the study of case law involving nursing. An example that provides a useful analogy for nurses is the way in which critical race theorists use the notion of 'double consciousness' (Du Bois 1903 cited in Delgardo 1995). This mechanism explains how people of colour view themselves in two ways: in the view of their oppressors, in which they are an underclass, and in their own view, where they see themselves as normal. Similarly nurses know that they do not have the same professional status as the medical profession, and have (in the past) accepted the inequalities of power and decision making which this status differential has caused. Yet they also view themselves as a profession, deserving all the rewards and privileges accorded to other 'normal' professions.

Through feminism nurses have learnt that their oppression is partly due to the nature of their work, which has been devalued because it is women's work; and also due to the fact that doctors, the dominant group in the health care hierarchy, were until recently predominantly male, whereas nursing is predominantly female. However, the feminist movement also had negative effects for the consciousness of nurses, in that nursing was one of the only professions to which women had access in the pre-feminist days. Thus the profession suffered what nurses felt to be a devaluation in status when women (understandably) wanted to enter other (previously male) domains such as business, law and medicine in greater numbers (Lumby 1991). Pringle has observed that 'there is a recognisable class discourse that now connects doing medicine with being bright and doing nursing with being dumb' (1998 p.194).

As a result nurses have developed what Matsuda has described as 'multiple consciousness' (1989 p.7) a term she has used to depict the difficulties of women from minority groups, such as lesbian women and women of colour. This term is used to illustrate the feeling of belonging to a group that shares the same basic values and concerns but, for some reason, of also being inferior and/or different to that main group. For example, if women of colour join a predominantly white, middle class, feminist movement, they may share many of the concerns of the group. Yet they may still feel like outsiders, because their particular 'other' concerns either may not be addressed or may make them feel in some way unacceptable to the group

---

[6] It is interesting to note that these scholars tend not to refer to the work of Michel Foucault in any depth, although his writings on knowledge *The Archaelogy of Knowledge* (1972) and power *Power/Knowledge: Selected Interviews and Other Writings* (1980) seem to underpin, or at least mirror, much of the writing of critical race theorists. However, it is beyond the scope of this book to address the issue further.

(Delgado 1995). However, critical race theory does not assert that women such as these ought to be subsumed into the white, middle class, group: rather, it focuses on their difference, and 'the richness of their ethnic and political diversity' (Minda 1995 p.178). Writers such as Hallam (2000) have demonstrated how oppressed outsider groups such as nurses can also discriminate against nurses of colour.

The use of outsider scholarship

A technique used by both feminists and critical race legal scholars is that of narrative scholarship (Scheppele 1989), also called voice scholarship (Sarmas 1994), outsider scholarship (Matsuda 1987), or storytelling (Delgado 1989). It is a useful technique for oppressed and/or minority groups.[7] It propounds a counter approach to the positivist school of thought that the findings of authoritative institutions, such as courts, constitute the authentic truth, which accordingly suggests that all other parties' accounts become devalued in formal decision making processes.

The development of this technique in law is mirrored in academia in general. Post-modernist thought and deconstructionism have led the academy to challenge the way in which knowledge is accepted and received (Davies 1993). Legal scholars who embrace the movement express a degree of dissatisfaction with the positivist or scientific method of legal analysis (McKenzie 1992), legal scholarship (Matasar 1992, Austin 1993), and legal education (Meyer 1992). Matasar argues that:

Legal scholarship that relies on this pseudo-objective and falsely scientific rhetoric doubly distorts: it abstracts legal problems from the real people who have those problems and it pretends that law provides answers to problems without reference to the particular social context in which any given legal problem arises. The language of neutral principles, rationales, and holdings may be perceived as a cover for actual reasoning, the influence of culture, and the hold of ideology. Thus, today, many legal scholars are searching for a new rhetoric that more candidly reveals the way that law is a reflection of very personal matters. (1992 p.355)

The central tenets of outsider scholarship

To understand the way in which outsider scholarship analyses case law it is necessary to become familiar with some basic concepts, including outsiders or outgroups, stock stories, outsider stories and the aims of outsider scholarship. Although these concepts, if studied in depth, require a knowledge of legal process, they are also instantly recognisable to anyone who, for whatever reason, has felt like an outsider.

---

[7] It seems odd to describe women as minority scholars, and nurses as the minority in health care.

Outsiders

The criticism which feminist and 'minority' legal scholars make of trad-itional legal scholarship is that it treats judicial decisions as though they are fact (Matasar 1992 p.353). Despite being 'inside' the law in that they are members of the legal profession, they adopt 'outsider' positions for the pur-poses of legal and social critique. This notion of 'outsiders' can become quite complicated. Outsiders are variously described, but a useful broad definition which will be adopted for the purpose of this book, is provided by Sarmas who describes them as 'those who are not part of the dominant culture' (1994 p.703). Scheppele is more specific and applies the definition to case law stating that outsiders are 'those whose perspective has been excluded in the law's construction of an official story for the particular case' (1989 p.2074). Matsuda points out that defining those who are oppressed or outsiders can be problematic. She states that the oppressed/oppressor dichotomy can cause problems of identification, because 'subordination is a dynamic, not a static' (1990 p.1772). Hallam makes this very point in relation to black nurses (Hallam 2000).

'False consciousness', also described as 'recycled hate', is the way that oppressed groups tend to despise themselves because they know them-selves to be despised by others. However, Matsuda argues that just because it may be difficult to identify a group as perpetually oppressed, we should not deny what we do know about a group's subordination. She points out that 'the dynamic quality of intragroup and intergroup relations does not necessarily destroy the intellectual power of group categorisation' (1990 p.1774). People may belong to several groups or may be a subset of a larger group, as in the women of colour example used earlier. This notion of belonging to more than one group contingent on the issue to be addressed is described by Kimberle Crenshaw (1989 p.167) as 'intersectionality', the point where two critical issues intersect for a given group. She refuses to allow the similarities which an outgroup might share to be discredited by its differences. Matsuda acknowledges the fact that categorising outsiders into groups often meets with a great deal of opposition, and seems to be very threatening for those who become 'insiders' by virtue of the categor-isation. However, she points out that the argument that no two people are alike (and therefore cannot belong to a group) is a fiction. 'Complexity is not the same as chaos. No two snowflakes are alike, but when it is snowing it is cold outside.' (1990 p.1776)

Stock stories

Feminist and 'minority' scholars who embrace outsider scholarship chal-lenge the belief that legal method is supposedly a process which finds rules for new cases inductively by applying cases and statutes by analogy, and applies existing written rules deductively to factual situations (Matasar 1992 p.353). They argue that this 'pseudo-objective approach' disguises the true nature of the law, since 'all law is political, and no amount of theorising on its objective and neutral quality can alter its fundamental character' (O'Byrne 1991 p.491). O'Byrne explains this by stating that 'legal questions, no matter how technical, are really about giving benefits to some people or taking them away from others.' (1991 p.355)

Trials are not about 'things' and 'people'. They are about communication about people and things. In trials, decisions cannot be made about individuals, but only about information about individuals. This information is only available to a trial's decision maker via the persuasive messages presented to them.

Trial outcomes, then, depend upon communication about the world, not upon the actualities of the world. Thus, communication practices of the trial participants will directly affect trial outcomes. This is not to suggest that reality has no effect on trial outcomes, but only that it has less to do with trial outcomes than most people would believe. (Dowling 1993 196–97)

Espinoza explains that all legal problems begin with a story, but the story becomes distorted by the legal process. She explains that the legal system 'freezes the story' so that it becomes the 'official story', but that in the freezing the broader sociopolitical narrative of oppression is lost because 'language as a product of a hierarchical society often renders mute the experience of oppression' (Espinoza 1997 pp.913–14).

The narrative aspects of judicial decision making are too often overlooked (Hayman & Levitt 1996 p.401). Justice Margaret Beazley, in her opening address to the Australasian Association for Quality in Health Care (1998) stated that '[t]here can be no doubt, in my view, that the outcome of cases can be due, not to the hard analysis of medical and other evidence, but to the life experiences and philosophies of the judges who decide the case'.

Delgado defines a stock story as 'the one the institution collectively forms and tells about itself. The story picks and chooses from among the available facts to present a picture of what happened: an account that justifies the world as it is' (1989 p.2421). Sarmas describes stock stories as 'those that are part of, and reinforce, the dominant discourse' (1994 p.703) and Scheppele says that a stock story is 'one that makes sense, is true to what the listeners know about the world, and hangs together' (1989 p.2080). Delgado points out that the stock stories which ingroups tell reinforce the perceived superior position of ingroups to outgroups in subtle ways. He points out that most oppression does not seem like oppression to oppressors (1989 p.2438).

He argues further that because of the way in which society is structured, these mindsets which form the dominant world view are like contact lenses. Judges and lawyers look through them without seeing them or realising that they are affecting their vision (Delgardo 1989 p.2413). Justice Heerey, an Australian judge, acknowledged that the law is about storytelling and accepted the forensic constraints of evidence and the way in which trials are conducted. However, he expressed his belief that the judge's task, which he described as the 'judging craft' is to '"find" ... the true facts or, more accurately, the facts more likely than not to be true' (1996 p.20). Scheppele explains that this is problematic for outsiders because these stock stories, when they become judgments of the court, then become accepted and viewed as truth.

There are few things more disempowering in law than having one's own believed story rejected, when rules of law (however fair in the abstract) are applied to facts that are not one's own, when legal judgments proceed from a description of one's own world that one does not recognise. (Scheppele 1989 pp.2089–90)

Matsuda points out that the difficulty for outsiders is that this acceptance of the stock story as truth becomes a way of establishing and reinforcing further their subordination. 'Power at its peak becomes so quiet and obvious in its place of seized truth that it becomes, simply, truth rather than power.' (1990 p.1765)

Outsider stories

Delgado (1989 p.2413) offers outsiders the technique of story telling or counter storytelling, as he calls it, as the cure for these perspectives 'the bundle of presuppositions, received wisdoms, and shared understandings against a background of which legal and political discourse takes place'. When these stories are told publicly they become outsider or counter stories, stories which are told 'to attack and subvert the very "institutional logic" of the system' (1989 p.2429). Furthermore, storytelling by outsiders can have both destructive and creative effects. It can break down a prevailing ideology by demonstrating that it is biased, stupid, selfish or cruel (Delgado 1989 p.2415). It can expose what Scheppele (1989 p.2082) calls 'the perceptual fault lines', an uncomfortable awareness that our society is actually built on somewhat unstable foundations, that some groups are not enjoying the privileges and freedoms which we believed our legal system made accessible to everyone. In this way, outsider stories can be seen as troublesome, upsetting or interfering, and the natural tendency is to ignore them, because the established order already works very well for those in power.

What emerges is a jurisprudence of nostalgia based on the story of a cohesive past. In the face of change, there arises a yearning for an imagined past, a beckoning back to a history constructed largely without the benefit of counter stories, to a simple, more stable, time when cultural discourse was not confounded by the sound of dissonant voices. (Hayman & Levitt 1996 p.413)

Outsider stories can also be creative. They can be a valuable and noncoercive way to identify an alternative viewpoint. Delgado (1989 p.2435) explains that storytelling is also a way to pull the readers into the story, making them 'vacillate between their own world and that of the storyteller'. They can be illuminating and educative. They can quicken and engage our consciences because 'narrative ... corresponds more closely to the manner in which the human mind makes sense of experience than does the conventional, abstracted rhetoric of law' (Winter 1989 p.2227). Narratives provide a way for us to order our thoughts, to cope with difficult issues which we might otherwise prefer to ignore (Scheppele 1989 p.2075). Stories can convey truths without confrontation, and enable the reader to view the world through other eyes (Matsuda 1990 pp.1781–82). Thus the value of outsider storytelling is that it provides for the decision makers an alternative to the stories of the dominant groups from the perspective of groups whose voices might otherwise not be heard.

Matsuda also points out that by advocating outsider stories she is not suggesting an 'either/or' perspective. She states that part of the challenge for outsider theorists is not to choose sides when faced with the question: 'Is law and liberty an oxymoron?' (1990 p.1771). There is an inherent danger in a binary approach, which is that it assumes that all arguments have only two sides. Of course, the world is much more complex than that, and arguments that adopt the binary approach are usually, at best, unsophisticated and, at worst, dangerous and misleading.

Aims of outsider scholarship

There are a number of schools of thought on the aims of outsider scholarship. Delgado (1989 p.2436) points out that stories can have both therapeutic and activist purposes. First, they can be a means of psychic self-preservation and secondly, they can be a means of lessening the outsiders' subordination. McCrystal Culp (1996 pp.70–71) explains that outsider scholarship provides a 'means to alter the contours of public debate'. He identifies three objects of narrative—to educate, to prevent discussion, or to force public discussion on a particular set of stories. Sarmas states that 'legal storytelling poses a radical challenge to established ways of thinking and writing about the law.' (1994 p.701)

However, other legal scholars point out that narrative is not solely the domain of those who wish to challenge established ways of thinking in the law; authors can use narrative scholarship as a means 'to highlight and celebrate diversity' (Scheppele 1989 p.2074). Matasar maintains that outsider scholarship has exactly the same aims as traditional legal scholarship.

Legal scholars advocate positions. They rely on law as an instrument for social reorganisation. And that they do so has nothing to do with science or objectivity. The legal scholar is a social actor using all available rhetorical tools to achieve a desired result. (Matasar 1992 p.357)

Techniques of outsider scholarship

Because outsider scholarship is a comparatively young area of legal scholarship there are a number of techniques which seem to be prevalent. However, if it is accepted that the aim of outsider scholarship is to present an outsider story, one that is viewed from the perspective of a person or group whose story is different from the dominant group, then a number of techniques can be used. The techniques are modified according to the type of narrative chosen and the topic to be addressed.

The narrative voice can be used in several ways. It can be used to bring outsider analysis to a particular case, or as a metastory which is designed to address a particular issue rather than a particular case and provides a different form of critique. For example, in *The Alchemy of Race and Rights: Diary of a Law Professor*, Williams (1991) contemplates the quality of her great-grandmother's life as a slave who was sold for breeding purposes at the age of 11 and was pregnant to her master by the age of 13. Matsuda (1990 p.67) tells the story of Darlene Leach, a poor African-American woman.

Although various writing styles can be used and the topics which can be addressed by this critique draw on literature from multiple sources, the purpose is always to challenge the accepted wisdom of the 'stock story' and the dominant world view. This literature is then juxtaposed against the 'truth' of a judgment or the purported effects of a piece of legislation to provide the excluded view (Graycar & Morgan 1990, Scutt 1994). Yet another technique is to take a single judgment, apply the implications of the 'stock story' revealed in that judgment to society in general, and then, by the use of a third voice, offer a counter story (e.g. Hayman & Levitt 1996).

Not all outsider stories are told 'out of court'. Sometimes, although the outsider story gets told in court, the matter before the court means that the injustice which is evident in the outsider's story is not the focus of the case, but is seen as 'incidental' to the issue (Sarat & Felstiner 1986 p.107). Sometimes an outsider story gets told in court and might even achieve a 'win'. However, here the role of the metastory in such a situation might be to point out how the 'win' in the courts was eroded either by government policy or institutionalised discrimination or both, and thus in reality the stock story prevailed (Delgado 1995 p.152).

The application of outsider scholarship in the context of this book

When finding cases in which nurses were mentioned or implicated, it became obvious that they did not often figure as central to the concerns of the court. Where nurses' actions or omissions were part of the facts of a case, the task of the court might have been to determine the liability of a hospital or a doctor, or to determine the nature and cause of death of a patient. But unless the cases were industrial or professional in nature, they rarely addressed the lives and/or concerns of nurses specifically. Thus the depictions of nurses in the case law have predominantly been those which were 'always already' present in the minds of counsel and the judges, or which were told and accepted by the dominant power groups, such as doctors or administrators. Where nurses have been implicated, depictions used on occasions by counsel for nurses to exonerate them from blame were often unflattering and (ultimately) damaging to nurses. This is because the images used condoned a power differential which in practice can cause nurses considerable angst.

Although an individual nurse might be pleased to be exonerated, outcomes based on unfavourable representations of nurses do little to address the day to day inconsistencies and injustices in nurses' political, professional and clinical lives. The purpose of outsider scholarship is to raise inconsistencies and injustices which are of importance to outgroups. These inconsistencies may not occur to, or may have little import for, the dominant group. Delgado (1989 p.2421) stresses the fact that when ingroups are challenged about their mindsets, their received wisdoms, they often respond by addressing procedural, rather than substantive issues. This is not to deny the constraints which (for example) the rules of evidence place on the stories which can be told in court. However, it is to argue that these constraints contest the claim of positivists to a search for 'an absolute truth' through the legal process (Dowling 1993 p.218).

Another response to raising the inconsistencies and injustices which are the concerns of outsider scholars has been to insist that judgments are not (usually) about groups, but about individuals, and thus to make broad claims for particular groups is to miss the point of the law. Heerey proposes that 'much of the criticism [of outsider scholars] involves replacing one alleged stereotype with another and using litigation as a weapon for the correction of perceived injustice to classes within a society rather than justice according to law between the parties in a particular case' (1996 p.2). There is a feminist expression which states that 'the personal is political' and a central tenet of feminist jurisprudence is that it takes women's lives as a starting point for any legal analysis. As Graycar and Morgan illustrate, the private/public dichotomy has always created problems for women because society still perpetuates the dominant male paradigm by a seemingly neutral stance (1990 p.30).

The position of the author

In order to use outsider scholarship, the author must adopt the perspective of an outgroup. For the purpose of this book, the nursing profession is designated as an outgroup, and the perspective adopted by the medical profession and hospital administrators is designated as the dominant 'world' view, particularly within the 'world' of the health care system, where many of the stories in this book are told. Nurses, despite their majority in the health care workforce, are significantly less powerful and less influential in all aspects of health care decision making (political, professional and clinical) than are other key professional groups.

I have had twenty years of clinical experience as a nurse, and in my role as a teacher of law to nurses have regularly heard their concerns and difficulties. Often when I have tried to answer these concerns by reference to existing law or policy, there was no obvious solution, because the relevant law or policy was silent on the nurses' role or responsibilities. This is very frustrating because nurses do not know where they 'stand', and they often receive conflicting messages about others' expectations of them, as demonstrated in Chapter 1. Hence my desire to present a nursing voice for the purpose of the legal analysis of these cases and materials.

The book does not attempt to be 'objective' in the sense of being uninvolved and dispassionate about the experiences of nurses. Rather, from the beginning it is important to acknowledge my situatedness both as lawyer and insider to the law, and as nurse and outsider to the health system and the law which governs it. That this book will be political in that respect is unquestionable. Indeed, Davies argues that 'it is one of the political tasks of feminism not only to ensure that women get access to the position of subject, but also that the non-situated, non-subjective paradigm of knowledge is challenged' (1993 p.176).

It is also recognised that, for some who may read this book, the arguments it advances will be seen as an 'impertinence' (Thornton 1996 p.vii).[8] I hope that the arguments will challenge traditional beliefs about the objectivity of medical knowledge and the exclusivity of medical control over health care. However, Davies further states that such challenges are important for the very reason that 'the ideal of objective knowledge has ... worked to silence or stigmatise as "subjective" views which do not reflect the orthodox epistemological order' (1993 p.176).

THE STOCK AND OUTSIDER STORIES IN THE FIVE IMAGES OF THE NURSE

Five themes or images of the nurse have emerged from the case law, and these themes are further categorised into two groups: themes that are stock stories, and those that are outsider stories. The stock stories tend to emerge from the case law, and the chapter structures which address them are a

---

[8] In the Foreword, Mary Jane Mossman quotes the words of Elizabeth Elstob, a self taught Saxon scholar who commenced her translation work by apologising for her 'impertinence' and 'neglect of household affairs'.

reflection of this. The stock story chapters tend to focus on an analysis of the case law which generates the stock story. These stock stories tend to be at odds with the outsider stories of nurses, the stories 'from the bottom'. By contrast, the outsider stories are usually generated from the nursing literature or from accounts provided by nurses in employment or other research studies. The outsider story chapters commence with a description of the outsider story and then explore the extent to which this story might have been accepted by the courts and tribunals.

What is significant for narrative scholarship is that in the groups of cases where the stock stories emerge, the evidence about nurses and nursing work is not usually provided by nurses but by doctors or administrators. Thus, in the cases which are examined in this group, sometimes the nursing voice has not even been heard. Where nurses and doctors give evidence together, the stock stories commonly prevail.

The stock stories: nurses 'under control'

The images which form the stock stories, stories which accept without comment 'the way the world is' are those of domestic worker, doctor's handmaiden and subordinate professional. These are all images where the nurse is considered to be 'under control': either the control of the doctor or of the hospital. The critical factor about these images of the nurse is that their application is inconsistent and unpredictable, and they emerge as a consequence of trying to fit the nurse into a pre-existing dominant relationship.

The domestic worker image has been particularly damaging for nurses. It emerged from a series of cases which examined the liability of hospitals, and for which purpose the work of nurses came under scrutiny. Depending upon the facts of the particular case, the nursing role was fragmented arbitrarily and delineated as either domestic or professional (or both), with no regard to contemporaneous nursing evidence about the status of such work for patient well-being.

In the doctor's handmaiden and subordinate professional images, the status of the doctor or hospital is a given, a constant, so the status of the nurse needs to be manipulated to 'fit' the prevailing orthodoxy. Thus the fate/liability of the nurses tends not to depend on their own behaviour, but rather on the behaviour of the 'key' players. If the doctor has behaved heinously and the nurse did not challenge that behaviour, it seems usually to be sufficient to 'get' the doctor. Thus, the nurse is exonerated because she (and nurses are usually females) was only the doctor's handmaiden (e.g. Report of The Royal Commission into Deep Sleep Therapy 1990). If the doctor's misdemeanor was marginal and they can argue that they relied on the nurse, then the nurse is likely to be criticised because, although the doctor was in charge, she ought to have had sufficient skill to provide at least a warning (Inquest touching the death of TJB 1989), if not an assertive prompt

(Heathcote v NRB & Walton 1991). It will be demonstrated, however, that it is most unusual for such judgments to exonerate the doctor without safeguarding his position of control.

The outsider stories: nurses 'in control'

The images which form the outsider stories, stories which nurses have actively promoted through their own writings and endeavours, are those of ministering angel and autonomous professional. These stories have been promulgated by nurses at differing times in history with the purpose of nurses trying to set the agenda on the public perception of nurses. They are dealt with in their respective chapters first by addressing the development of these images by nurses and then examining the extent to which they are reflected in the case law.

At first glance the ministering angel image is another archetypal female image, and its place as an outsider story might be questioned. But this image was marketed quite flagrantly by nurses before and at the turn of the last century to counteract the stock image of 'Sarey Gamp', Dickens' archetypal drunken, dissolute woman of no education and little hygiene, who was more of a danger to the patient than a benefit. Although its status as an outsider story was clearer in those days than it is now, as the years have progressed this image has been somewhat more of a hindrance than a help to nurses. It has tied them into problematic stereotypical roles and has meant that they have been expected to exhibit a degree of forebearance and self-sacrifice, particularly in relation to their pay and conditions, which has not been expected of other health care professionals. Yet this book will demonstrate that the image is alive today, and is still employed by nurses on occasions. However, its current status as an outsider story is debatable, as will be discussed further in the text. Significantly, in 1999 in the UK, delegates of Unison, a large health workers' trade union which represents some nurses, have voted 'to ditch Florence Nightingale as the founding mother of modern nursing' (Brindle 1999). Paradoxically, this is indicative of the fact that nurses have seen this image as one which was within their control (and, in this case, disposal).

Promotion of the other outsider image, that of the autonomous professional, has been a deliberate endeavour by nurses to be seen as a profession equal in status and authority to medicine, a movement which has gained momentum over the last century. This has manifested in several ways, including bids for self-regulation, better education, control over the nursing workforce and recognition of their clinical equality and validity in the work place. This movement has found varying degrees of acceptance in the courts and tribunals, depending on the proximity of nurses to other more dominant groups within the scrutiny, such as medicine, whose images are far more fixed and constant.

Usually (although not exclusively) these outsider images are nurse initiated and driven, as opposed to the stock stories, which are usually (although not exclusively) initiated and driven by other dominant groups, such as doctors and hospital administrators. Where these outsider images are accepted by the courts and tribunals, the evidence given about nurses and nursing work is generally provided by nurses. However, this evidence is frequently provided in courts and tribunals where nurses are addressing nursing matters, for example, industrial courts and professional tribunals, and where the issue of medical dominance is not in question.

Accordingly the images can be grouped as follows:

Stock stories (nurses under control)	Outsider stories (nurses in control)
The nurse as a domestic worker The nurse as the doctor's handmaiden The nurse as a subordinate professional	The nurse as a ministering angel The nurse as an autonomous professional

The application of both feminist and critical race scholarship

As a result of the feminist movement, nurses have realised that one of the main reasons for their oppression and segregation is that nursing is predominantly a female profession. It will be demonstrated that, in both judicial decisions and literature, some of those images which present nurses as archetypal women have contributed to the exclusion of their voices from critical health care discourse. Accordingly, as already indicated, much of the legal analysis in this book has its origins in feminist philosophy and legal thought.

However, as previously discussed, although feminism has helped nurses to analyse and understand the reality of their exclusion, it has also diminished the value of nursing as a career, as many more careers open up to women, and nursing is viewed as a stereotypical female career. For this reason critical race theory, with its added dimension of intersectionality, is also used extensively to analyse the case law.

These two domains of scholarship have been used throughout the book to explain and explore the different issues which arise. Graycar and Morgan's (1990) insights into the male-oriented structure of legal studies have been fundamental to the validation of this nursing perspective on what has hitherto been predominantly the field of medical law. Feminist studies of language analysis have been most informative, and surface intermittently throughout the book. Throughout the book there is also a recognition that nurses have not always been kind to or supportive of each other, and the work of Franz Fanon (1963) and his successors on racial lateral violence has been illuminating.

In those chapters which identify the outsider stories of ministering angel and autonomous professional, critical feminist and race theorists inform the analysis of the way in which outgroups are seen as deviant or problematic if they complain or adopt a 'different' stance. The concept of 'false consciousness', which has been a dominant theme in critical race theory, is instructive in the understanding of the effect of the domestic worker image on the fragmentation of the nursing role. The use of a narrative approach is instrumental in the analysis of Hillyer v Governors of St Bartholomew's Hospital (1909) and the feminist jurisprudential literature informed the approach to women's work. In the discussions on doctor's handmaiden, the strategy of senior nurses to accept and on occasions actively seek medical domination to further their own professional ends is elucidated by the research of Margaret Thornton on women working in the law (1996). The descriptive and (for nurses) instantly recognisable notion of 'microaggressions' (Grillo 1997 p.749), a concept developed by critical race theorists, provides rich ground for the discussion on professional subordination. The ongoing racial affirmative action debate in America also surfaces in this chapter and provides a useful backdrop to the discussion on the determination of merit in health care decision making (Delgado 1995 p.78). Pringle's (1998) recent research on women doctors and their relationships with nurses provides further insights into the concept of 'intersectionality' and the way in which nurses are seen to be subordinate professionals even by other women. The theories of equality on which feminist action might be based provide valuable insights into the way in which nurses have striven for professional equality with medicine (Sheehey 1987).

Factors defining the status of the nurse

1. The role of the nurse

The focus of the nursing role and the consequent nature of nursing work emerge in several of the images. The 'ministering angel' image addresses the intimate nature of nursing work and the resultant need for clinical invisibility. The 'domestic worker' image raises the tension between a holistic and a fragmented role. If nurses need to do work which might be thought of by society and the courts and tribunals as domestic, ought all nurses to do it, and if not, then which nurses ought to do it? The 'subordinate professional' image identifies the overlap of tasks between nurses and other health care professionals, and the subsequent confusion about whether a role either is no more than a collection of protected tasks, or is constructed as a particular focus whose tasks might constantly be changing and evolving. The 'autonomous professional' image addresses nursing's own ongoing debate as to whether nursing is an art or a science, what research methods most appropriately explore the nursing role, and whether the emotional aspects or the technical aspects of nursing should be privileged.

2. The question of whether nursing is a profession

The ministering angel and, to a lesser extent, the doctor's handmaiden images raise the tension between nursing as a vocation and as a profession. The question whether basic nursing care—frequently described as traditional women's work—could be classed and remunerated as professional work is explored in the sections which examine the image of the domestic worker. Abraham Flexner's (1910) early criteria for a profession are examined briefly in the discussion on the subordinate professional image and nursing meets some, but not all, of those criteria. Two types of professionalism are identified. Where professional status was ascribed to nursing because of its association with medicine, this vicarious professional status is described as 'extrinsic' professionalism. When nurses are recognised as professionals because of the specific nature of nursing care, this is described as 'intrinsic' professionalism. The contemporary quest for nursing to achieve professional status as a result of higher educational status, better pay and conditions, new theoretical frameworks and new care delivery models is scrutinised in the autonomous professional image.

3. The duties and responsibilities of the nurse

This vexed issue appears in almost every image, but is particularly prominent in the doctor's handmaiden, subordinate professional, and autonomous professional images. Questions arise such as the extent and nature of the nurses' legal and moral duties and responsibilities to each other, the medical profession and their patients. Another pressing question is whether the nurses' duty to the patients flows directly from their own association with the patient or indirectly through a duty to carry out the doctor's orders. In addition to the confusing and often contradictory legal expectations which emerge from the case law, the questions of moral duties and obligations which nurses confront are addressed. Issues are explored such as the ambiguity surrounding the nurses' right to intervene or to exercise moral autonomy, as is its effect on the nurses' ability to intercede on behalf of a patient when the power differential between the nurse and the doctor is so uneven.

Sources of stock and outsider stories about nurses

Analysis of different aspects of contemporary nursing, legal and health care literature, health policy and legislation occur at different points of the book and provide the opportunity to compare the experiences of nurses with the experiences and observations of feminist and critical race theorists. In the stock story chapters, the stories which are told and accepted in the courts and tribunals are described, and other sources which provide support for these stories such as Hansard, legislation, policy documents and literature are also examined.

The outsider stories appear in the nursing literature, and are initiated and told by nurses. These stories provide opportunities to hear the voices of nurses describing their own problems and difficulties and enable the reader to relate to those problems and difficulties first-hand. In the outsider story chapters, after the stories have been described, relevant case law is examined to ascertain the extent to which the courts and tribunals accept these stories. Thus the chapters addressing the stock stories of domestic worker, doctor's handmaiden and subordinate professional consist predominantly of legal materials, whereas the chapters addressing the outsider stories of ministering angel and autonomous professional contain predominantly contextual materials from the professional nursing literature.

The stock and outsider stories are not always clear cut. The most obvious analysis of stock and counter stories is that they can be seen to be political strategies employed by either insider or outsider groups. But, as previously stated, they have also been employed as tactical devices by those groups who would normally be expected to oppose them. Some stock stories, such as the domestic worker, have been so powerful that they have been adopted and actively pursued by nurses (for better or worse) in certain situations. On other occasions, stock stories such as the doctors handmaiden and subordinate professional stories have been used as tactical devices by lawyers to maximise the (nurse) clients' chances of success within the forensic constraints of the courtroom. Some outsider stories, such as the ministering angel, have been so successfully 'marketed' that they have captured the public imagination and almost become stock stories. Other outsider stories, such as the nurse as autonomous professional, have also been used strategically by lawyers for dominant groups such as employers and doctors. Some issues, such as the nurse practitioner debate, straddle both the subordinate (stock) and autonomous (outsider) professional stories, according to the perspective from which the story is told. An outsider story can be told in the courts and be successful, and this has been so to some extent in the industrial courts and tribunals, where the specialist knowledge and clinical skills of nurses have received considerable acclaim. However, just as with major civil rights cases such as Brown v Board of Education (1954) the reality can often amount to a Pyrrhic victory (Delgado 1995). This has been the case with nurses. Professional domination and segregation in health care still means that nurses, the majority group, are substantially disenfranchised, despite recognition of their responsibility and competence in the industrial courts and tribunals.

CONCLUSION

This chapter has set out to identify the purpose and process of this inquiry, and to define the term 'status' for this purpose. The chapter has identified the theoretical framework which is used to analyse the case law and supporting materials. A synopsis of the developing school of legal theory known as outsider scholarship has been provided, which has identified the central tenets of outsider scholarship and given an overview of its application to the book. Finally, the chapter has outlined a structure for the book, including the framework in which the five images are examined, and the elements of the images which are identified and explained.

PART 2

Images of women in the workforce

PART CONTENTS

3

The nurse as a ministering angel

Elements of the image

- Nursing is a quasi-religious calling, and nurses are most like women in holy orders, therefore:

  - Nurses are unlike witches, and unlike Sarey Gamp;

  - Nurses are expected to demonstrate high moral standards and to be abstemious and sober; they embody all that is good and proper and their lives must be strictly controlled;

  - Because nursing is a practical skill which comes from the heart, it is better learnt 'at the bedside';

  - Nurses must be asexual beings, because the work they do involves them in extremely intimate physical activities;

  - Because nurses are so good, their acts or omissions could not be malicious.

- It is a privilege to serve as a nurse, and therefore nurses should not complain about poor living and working conditions and huge workloads.

INTRODUCTION

This chapter argues that the image of nurses as ministering angels is an 'outsider story'. It was actively fostered by Florence Nightingale and her cohorts earlier last century to counter the predominant worldview of the mid-nineteenth century that nurses were disreputable, drunken and debauched. It was also promoted by the media during the Crimean War. Today it is almost a stock story, as each year in Australia nurses top the opinion polls as the most honest and ethical professionals (Anon 1998a). However, it is only 'almost' a stock story: when the words *nurse* and *professional* were entered into the Newslink computer program, 75 references appeared; when the words *nurse* and *sex* were entered, there were 866 references (Moait 1998 p.5). Hallam (2000) also identifies the sexual image of the nurse as predominant in the media, which might suggest that the goal of promoting the ministering angel image has not been completely successful. However, despite the populist sexual image of the nurse, it is not one which appeared at all in the case law researched for this book. Indeed, the only case which touched on a nurse's sexual relations portrayed her as the innocent victim of a predatory medical superintendent, unable to rebuff his amorous advances (Hoile v Medical Board of South Australia 1960).

The image of the nurse as a ministering angel has become central to nurses' self-image, and has often dictated both their industrial and political demeanour. It has created advantages and disadvantages for nurses in their treatment by the courts and tribunals. Because the image has been promulgated by nurses, this chapter traces its genesis through the nursing literature and then examines its application in law. The elements of the story which emerge through an exploration of the literature and the case law are listed at the opening to this chapter.

THE CHRONOLOGICAL EMERGENCE OF THE ELEMENTS OF THE IMAGE

Not all of these elements of the image arose simultaneously. The need for nurses to be devout arose as a backlash to the image of the women who worked as nurses in England in the nineteenth century, and also as a result of the piety of Florence Nightingale and her Victorian counterparts. Most of the elements were present at that time to some degree, but some developed further as the century progressed. The image is not as dominant now in the nursing literature as it was even up until the 1960s, but vestiges still remain (Kalisch & Kalisch 1982, Kalisch et al 1982, Bonawit 1989, Hallam 2000, Walker 2000).

Although nurses have written much about the need to change this image (Clark 1989, Lumby & Zetler 1990, NSW Health Department 1995, 1996a), and government campaigns have been undertaken to give nursing a more modern persona (Hallam 2000), there is still a tendency for nurses to be viewed as 'good women'. Perhaps this is because a conspicuous alternative seems to have been the 'naughty nurse' image discussed previously, which nurses have actively discouraged and denounced whenever it has arisen.

Another possible reason for the persistence of this angelic image may be found in the type of work that nurses do. It will be argued in Chapter 4 that the development of nursing as a career was the professionalisation of traditional women's work, and that nurses deal with many aspects of life that are traditionally within the domestic domain. Thus it is perhaps easier to trivialise nursing and dismiss it as kindness or goodness, rather than to recognise it as expertise or professionalism. Graycar and Morgan (1990) and others (e.g. Finley 1989, Cox 1996) have argued that much of women's work, experience and business is trivialised in this way and relegated to the private, rather than the public, domain.

This chapter explores the extent to which the courts and tribunals accept the elements of this image. It demonstrates that judges who invoke this image usually adopt a relatively benign approach to the nurses under scrutiny. However, when nurses are found to have behaved unconscionably or maliciously, there is little leniency shown, as such behaviour runs counter to community expectations (Schroeder & Ors & Health Services Union of Australia v Mildura Base Hospital 1997).

NURSING IS A QUASI-RELIGIOUS CALLING, AND NURSES ARE MOST LIKE WOMEN IN HOLY ORDERS

Florence Nightingale: the 'angel' is born

Wherever there is a hospital, big or little; wherever in a long ward in a quiet room a nurse fights for the life and well-being of her patient; wherever there is a woman in a nurse's uniform, in the slums of a great city, in far-away Alaska, or on the sparsely populated mountainside, in the school, the factory, or the clinic, there floats the banner of Florence Nightingale. (Gladwin 1930 p.266)

The concept of 'The Lady with the Lamp', the ever available, ever watchful presence of the nurse, was popularised by the media during the Crimean War (Seymer 1949 p.84). Florence Nightingale, in the genre of women of her class, was a devout and chaste woman. Her letters reveal her soul-searching, her constant prayers for guidance and the deeply held conviction that God wished her to become a nurse (Vicinus & Nergaard 1989). However, her need for devotion and chasteness in her nursing staff was as much the product of her shrewd political acumen as her religious beliefs. During the Crimean War, Florence Nightingale's old friend, Sydney Herbert, who was Secretary at War, wrote of the idea to send women as nurses to Crimea.

If this succeeds, an enormous amount of good will be done now, and to persons deserving everything at our hands; and a prejudice will have been broken through and a precedent established, which will multiply the good to all time. (Vicinus & Nergaard 1989 p.82)

The idea to have women nurses with the British Army was not only controversial at the time, it was 'immodest, unthinkable, revolutionary!' (Abel-Smith 1960). The stakes were very high, and Nightingale strategised to make these women acceptable.

Nurses are unlike witches and unlike Sarey Gamp

The need for a new image—no more witches or 'Sarey Gamps'

In pre-Nightingale times, nursing care was delivered by a motley assortment of people. Long before there were accredited nurses many people were involved in nurturing, and in making the experiences of sick and suffering human beings as bearable and acceptable as possible. These people undertook their tasks for a range of reasons: for maternal or familial reasons; for altruistic or religious reasons; for reasons of duty or demand; for pragmatic or financial reasons; or for pure interest or a search for meaning. Thus those who nursed may or may not have been socially acceptable.

Some had very high social status. In ancient Irish civilisation, there were physicians, and also midwives, known as wise-women, whose role it was to assist intra- and post-natally (Dolan 1963 pp.65–66). The deaconesses of the early Christian church were also highly esteemed, and visited the sick similarly to district or community nurses (Griffin & Griffin 1969).

Under the feudal system in the early European Middle Ages, the ladies of the manor were responsible for caring for those sick and wounded under the protection of their feudal lord. After the Crusades, and with the establishment of the Knights Hospitallers of St John, more men went into nursing due to the formation of military nursing orders (Griffin & Griffin 1969). They acknowledged the importance of sanitation and hygiene and sought to introduce drainage systems, garbage collection and rapid burial of the dead. The Crusades were the first of many wars in which nursing proliferated, the Crimean being the most famous. There was also significant recruitment to nursing in the American War of Independence, the American Civil War, and World Wars I and II.

However, not all those involved in nursing work were accorded such high social status, particularly if they were not of the ruling classes themselves, and notwithstanding the fact that they may have been providing a valuable service. There is a feminist argument that women have always been healers; because they were denied access to universities and political power bases, they were never recognised as such, and their traditional knowledge base was actively taken over during the Middle Ages.

The witch hunts

In their history of women healers, Ehrenreich and English (1973) state that in the Middle Ages it was women who were experimenting with new herbs and adopting humane and empirical approaches to healing, while men clung to ritualistic and outdated procedures, such as leeching, mercury and purgation. They suggest that the witch craze, which lasted from the 14th to the 17th century, was basically a ruling class campaign of terror against the female peasant population. In the seminal text on witch hunting, the *Malleus Maleficarum* (the *Hammer on Witches*) and the ensuing trials in which it was used, witches were identified and accused of three possible sets of crimes. Ehrenreich and English argued that two of the charges related closely to nursing. These were: possessing magical powers to affect health positively and negatively; and possessing medical and obstetric skills.

From a primitive perspective, one can see that the argument would be quite compelling, even attractive, in its simplicity. Since illness was sent from God, and suffering was a means of expiation for sin, anyone who made that easier, must be anti-God, and therefore for the Devil. The numbers of witches executed is estimated to have been in the millions (Ehrenrich & English 1973 p.8). Thus it is not surprising that nursing fell into disrepute by the 18th century, and the only women who were accorded any status for being involved in nursing were again those in holy orders.

Nursing's 'dark ages'

During this time midwifery, which had previously been the domain of women who were licensed by the bishops, was taken over by licensed physicians, who realised that including midwifery into their practice had economic advantages (Luxford 1996 p.73). Nursing care was delivered by characters who were epitomised by Charles Dickens' 'Sarey Gamp'— drunken, dirty, unscrupulous characters who expressed a predilection for payment in gin. Nightingale, being an astute politician, knew that she would never enable nursing to receive any social esteem in Victorian England unless she advanced the image of the nurse as docile, obedient and, of course, chaste. Nurses had to be so far removed from witches as to give no sniff of a stake, and from temptresses as to give no cause for moral concern.

> *Nurses are expected to demonstrate high moral standards and to be abstemious and sober; They embody all that is good and proper and their lives must be strictly controlled*

The need for sobriety

This new image fostered by Nightingale had some dramatic industrial effects for nurses, although these were invariably dealt with outside of any formal framework. A single episode of drunkenness could result in a nurse being summarily dismissed and, if overseas, returned to England, regardless of her worth. Nightingale wrote to Elizabeth Herbert of such an incident:

I am so sorry to be obliged to tell you that Thompson & Anderson, two of the Presbyterian nurses from Edinburgh, went out drinking with an Orderly on Saturday night. Anderson was brought back dead drunk ... This was such a catastrophe that there was nothing to be done but to pack them off to England directly—& accordingly they sail this morning by the Gottenburg. It is a great disappointment, as they were hard working good-natured women ... Only one week's wages was due to them, which I have not given them, of course, as by rights they ought not to have a free passage home. (Vicinus & Nergaard 1989 p.113)

The need for chastity

Concern for protecting the morality of nurses was also paramount, and a nurse who became emotionally involved with a patient would likewise be dealt with most severely. Lucy Osburn wrote to Florence Nightingale in 1868 of her management of Sister Bessie Chant, a nurse at the first Sydney hospital. She had intercepted and read Sister Chant's letter from an ex-patient wishing to marry her, which was expressed in terms such that 'it made the perspiration come out all over my head as if I had been in a shower bath'. Miss Osburn wrote to the man herself and threatened to inform the Colonial Secretary if he persisted with his suit. After four weeks of correspondence between the two of them Miss Osburn informed Sister Chant that she had been in contact with the man. Osburn advised Florence Nightingale that Sister Chant 'was penitent quite saw it must be given up and said she would write and tell him so, this she did today'.

The fact that Sister Chant expressed neither outrage nor anger that both her marriage prospects and her privacy had been violated is indicative of the control which matrons exercised over their nursing staff. There is no doubt that Nightingale modelled her nurses on the Sisters of Kaiserwerth, where she undertook her own initiation into nursing. It was also where she first met the idea that nursing could be undertaken by women of any class, provided that they possessed the vocation to undertake nursing (Vicinus & Nergaard 1989 p.53). She was to observe later that, 'Never have I met with a higher tone, a purer devotion than there. There was no neglect. It was the more remarkable because many of the Deaconesses had been only peasants—none were gentlewomen (when I was there)'. The working regime at Kaiserwerth was intense, and the days were long, followed by Bible readings in the evenings. It was perhaps for such reasons that Nightingale herself was opposed to the notion of nursing as a profession, preferring to call it a vocation or calling (Vicinus & Nergaard 1989 p.425).

The influence of the church and the army

Certainly the regimes which Nightingale instituted for her nurses were strictly disciplinarian, and nurses' uniforms bore a strong resemblance to those of women in holy orders until very recently. The dresses were very plain and tailored, with the only form of adornment being the nurse's cap. This need to ensure that the nurses' uniform was very chaste and asexual was no doubt due in part to the intimate nature of the work which nurses have always performed. In Nightingale's time, the only other group of (unmarried) women who would have had such unlimited access to men's bodies would have been prostitutes. Hence the need to differentiate and desexualise the intimate work of nurses that was paramount in the minds of those early matrons. They enforced strict controls on any social relations with the opposite sex (Barber & Shadbolt 1996) and there was total intolerance of any expressions of interest in appearance (Vicinus & Nergaard 1989 p.83). Thornton acknowledges this need to manage women's bodies in a non-sexual way for woman lawyers today (1996 p.223).

In New South Wales, legislative provisions relating to the wearing of nurses' caps were still in force until the 1991 Nurses Act. These caps were actually known as 'veils' and their use has only been discontinued in New South Wales within the last twenty years. They were worn by qualified nurses, significantly at their graduation ceremony when the tradition was that the newly qualified nurses recited the Nightingale 'Pledge'. The language of this pledge had deeply religious and sacrificial overtones. It commits the nurse to 'pass her life in purity', to practise 'faithfully', to assist the physician 'with loyalty', and to 'devote' herself to her patients.[1]

It has been said that nursing was 'born in the church and bred in the army' (Gillespie 1990), a reference to the equally important influence of the military. When Nightingale first went to the Crimea, she was instructed by Sidney Herbert to observe 'strict attention to … the preservation of that subordination which is indispensable in every Military Establishment' (Smith 1982). Cordery, writing of Nightingale's militaristic organisation of nursing, captures the strict regulation of morality which was so predominant:

Nightingale was influential in the development of a system of nurse training in which discipline and punishment were institutionalised—discipline was ceaselessly monitored and indiscretions punished … To Nightingale, discipline was 'the essence of training' which embraced order and method, but in her sanitised vision, discipline was rewritten as 'womanly self-regulation'. (Cordery 1996 p.195)

Because nursing is a practical skill which comes from the heart, it is better learnt 'at the bedside'

This image of nurses initiated by Nightingale was actively fostered over the next fifty years or more by the nursing profession itself (Gladwin 1930). If a Legislative Assembly can be taken to represent the views of the general public, the image was certainly accepted at the time of the passing of the Nurses Registration Act 1953 (NSW) (NSW Hansard, 9 September 1953). Following World War II there was a campaign to safeguard the status of nursing through legislation, as the early Registration Acts were permissive, rather than exclusive (Bendall & Raybould 1969). The end of the war brought many unemployed Voluntary Aid Detachments (VADs), untrained women who had been used to swell the nursing ranks (Abel-Smith 1960 p.100). The nursing profession was concerned that these people might call themselves nurses

---

[1] Published in the front of the *Australasian Nurses Journal* from 1904 to 1954. It is unclear as to the source of this pledge, as it seems unlikely that Nightingale herself wrote it, being opposed as she was to the idea of describing nursing as a profession.

and set themselves up in business. Tighter controls were demanded in nursing education and registration, and concerns were expressed about the calibre of women who might call themselves nurses (Abel-Smith 1960 p.98).

The esteem in which nurses were held in 1953 was evidenced by the second reading speech of Dr Parr, the Honourable Member for Burwood—a speech that he described as eulogistic.

[F]or over thirty five years [I have] been closely associated with the great nursing profession, whose lips have been touched with the live coals from the altar of unselfish humanity. In war and peace, the members of this noble calling have never wilted in their duty, and in a period when leisure, pleasure and selfishness are vying with one another for the allegiance of the youth of our land, their example shines out as a bright light of service for all to see. (NSW Hansard 1953 p.487)

The profession whose skills must be learnt 'at the bedside'

The laudable skills of these selfless women were nevertheless resolved by the Honourable Member to be quintessentially practical, with no academic input necessary for their development. In discussing the reduction of the nurses' working week to forty hours, Dr Parr expressed concern.

There must not be any lowering of standards. Of course, when hours of work were reduced to forty a week the practical training of nurses was reduced by four hours a week. Therefore, since 1947, there may have been some difference in the training that nurses receive because nursing is a very practical profession and the loss of four hours per week cannot be dismissed as a mere nothing. Nursing is learned not out of textbooks, but at the bedside. (NSW Hansard 1953 p.447)

Nurses must be asexual beings, because the work they do involves them in extremely intimate physical activities

'Body work'

Nursing is an intensely private and personal activity, as nurses deal with people's bodies as part of their daily work. Lawler, in the preface to her seminal text *Behind the Screens*, explains that she found this body work to be central to her understanding of nursing, the way people responded to nursing work and the taboo which was generic to the lives and work of nurses (Lawler 1991 p.v).

The type of work which nurses have to do—caring for people's bodies in their most intimate and messy detail—means that nurses are privileged in the access which they have (to a far greater extent than probably any other group) to men's and women's bodies (Chiarella 1990). Although other groups of professionals also deal with people's bodies for the purpose of treatment, they usually focus on one part of the body, rather than the body as a whole. But for nurses so much of the care is a form of nurturing, and is sensual by the very nature of the nursing role. Activities such as bathing, massaging, holding and cleansing patients are integral to the sense of well-being which nurses seek to instil in the sick and dying. Lawler (1991 pp.179–86) describes the 'recovery trajectory' indicating that, as patients recover, there is a tendency for sensuality to develop into sexuality. At this point the physical distance between the nurse and the patient increases, and the nurse hands back control of the patient's body to the patient.

In order to undertake the intimate work they do without embarrassing the patient, nurses need to be asexual, so that patients do not feel embarrassed and so that they can obtain access to the patient's body without fear of compromise on either part. At their most intrusive, really skilful clinical management renders nurses almost invisible and eminently forgettable. Lawler describes the different strategies which nurses use to achieve this 'invisibility of nursing care', which she describes as 'creating environments of permission' (1991 pp.166–69).

The invisibility of nursing care (and nursing)

It is perhaps for reasons such as these that the public feels most comfortable thinking of nurses as ministering angels. (After all, who would want anyone less than such a character giving them a bedpan, washing their genitalia, or holding them while they cry?) But invisibility brings its own problems in other spheres. Finley writes of the problems of black women in the law, and describes them as 'twice removed from the norm'. The difficulty for them of 'slipping into invisibility' in a legal sense is that they are perceived as a minority group, different from the mainstream, regardless of their numbers, and are often forgotten when law or policy is being made, unless a special effort is made to include them. This means that as a group they are seen as 'problematic' or 'deviant' (Finley 1989 pp.886–87). Bell explores the problem of invisibility for blacks in general when he notes that often, if he recommends a black colleague for promotion, the question is asked: 'Who else likes this person?' Bell points out that 'both parties know who 'who else' is' (1992 pp.11–13). Nurses will recognise this phenomenon instantly, but it is important also to recognise that the problem partially has its origins in the invisibility of nursing care.

> *Because nurses are so good, their acts or omissions*
> *could not be malicious*

The 'misguided, innocent woman'

In a number of cases there has been either overt recognition of this image in the judgments, or a degree of sympathy or leniency which has indicated a judicial reluctance to 'think ill' of nurses.

The decision in Mahon v Osborne (1939)[2] provides a good example of this protective attitude. The case is one of the 'failure to remove swabs' cases. The deceased patient was operated upon by the resident surgeon for a perforated duodenal ulcer with the assistance of a Nurse Ashburner, who was chief nurse at the operation. Both were sued by the deceased's family, but it appears that the nurse did not appreciate the extent of her involvement. Scott LJ noted this in the appeal judgment.

[I]t is reported, (she) had no spare money, imagined that her interest would be looked after by the surgeon, never consulted a solicitor, and failed to enter an appearance. Interlocutory judgment was signed against her in November, but no notice of it was sent to her. She attended the trial solely because the defendant's legal advisers wanted her evidence. (Mahon v Osborn 1939)[3]

Scott LJ described the trial judge's observations of her as 'very favourable' and his summing up of the case as 'even more favourable' towards her and noted that the jury 'not unnaturally held that she had not been negligent'.[4]

On appeal all three judges found that part of the responsibility for the error rested with Nurse Ashburner and that a new trial should be held. One can only speculate on why the trial judge should have treated Nurse Ashburner so favourably. It may have been her naive dependence upon the surgeon to look after her and her lack of money, but clearly the trial judge influenced the jury to find that there was no evidence against her, a decision with which all three appeal judges disagreed.

The 'sweet gentlewoman'

In a 1990 unfair dismissal case (re Australian Nursing Federation) there was disagreement between the nurse, Ms Howden, and her employer, Ms Poperechney, as to the tone of the termination interview. Garlick DP was sympathetic to Ms Howden and demonstrated, in his assessment of her as a witness, his impression of the compassionate nature of nursing work. Although this matter did not go to the heart of the unfair dismissal allegation, the description serves to illustrate the influence of the ministering angel story.

Ms Howden's description of it [the termination interview] presented an intimidatory setting. Ms Poperechney's description of it presenting a compassionate setting. As a witness, Ms Howden presented as a quietly spoken person and imbued with a care-giving spirit which was not surprising for her occupation. As a witness, Ms Poperechney presented as articulate but excessively emphatic

---

[2] The most authoritative citation for this case is *Mahon v Osborn* [1939] 2 KB 14.
[3] *Mahon v Osborne* [1939] 1 All ER 535, 538. This piece of information is not included in the KB Reports. Whilst it is acknowledged that the KB Reports are the more authoritative, it seems unlikely that such information has been fabricated, and the information is of relevance to this book.
[4] p.538. This portion of Scott LJ's judgment is also omitted from the KB Reports.

and highly assertive. I do not believe that the interview was compassionate. It probably was not as grim as the impression given by Ms Howden, for whom such a meeting would have been very different from the care-giving environment in which she usually works. (Re Australian Nursing Federation 1990 pp.318–9)

The 'girls' who were led astray

In the Canadian case of Lahey v St Joseph's Hospital (1992) the doctors and nursing staff in the emergency room were found not to have negligently caused the death of a 55-year-old lawyer by failing to manage an asthma attack properly. However, the Chief Executive Officer and the Director of Nursing were held to be negligent for failing to manage the smooth running of the emergency department. In addition, all the staff involved were found to have exposed themselves to the possibility of criminal prosecution for making false documents. The extent of the deception was quite shocking, as the patient had died in the emergency department, but the staff intubated him and transferred him to the Intensive Care Unit, where he was ventilated for nine days. The records were fabricated, as were reports from so-called independent experts. Due to the extraordinary nature of this case, there is little to be gained by reporting on the judgment in detail. However, two matters within the judgment are worthy of comment. The first was the criticism which Cummings J made of the deputy head nurse's use of the term 'the kids' to describe her staff.

In a hospital context the term 'the kids' is not the gender-neutral equivalent of 'the girls', a traditional informal collective noun for a group of nurses that was used by many of the women who testified. In my view Cathy Goodin's use of the term 'the kids' is not appropriate.

The expression 'the kids' implies very low expectations. It reflects negatively on her ability to motivate and lead a team of responsible health care experts. That she would use that expression after having been head nurse of the emergency department for three years also reflects negatively on her superiors. They should have corrected her long ago. (Lahey v St Joseph's Hospital 1992 p.190)

It seems extraordinary that his Honour should have condoned the use of either term, as the expression 'the girls' similarly does little to conjure up an image of 'a team of responsible health care experts'. His Honour considered it important to correct one term, which implies a group of children or young people, but did not condemn the other more sexist term. In order to have graduated as a nurse, all the nurses, male and female, would have been over the age of 21, which would have qualified them as men and women, rather than as boys and girls. There was accordingly a reluctance to condone the use of slang, but an acceptance of the immaturity or even innocence of the nursing staff.

Cummings J also seemed reluctant to implicate the nurses fully in the cover-up of the death, despite the acknowledged fact that they tried to cover up the missing Ventolin. The language in the ensuing passages is telling: the nurses 'followed the bad examples of the doctors'—they were corrupted (a more passive implication), whereas the doctors 'joined ... to help' (a much more active concept).

In my opinion the evidence proves that seven physicians on the medical staff of St Joseph's Hospital were involved in the cover-up of the death of Edward J Lahey in February 1985 ... A number of nurses appeared to have followed the bad examples of those doctors and thus helped cover up the death.

The emergency room nurses also wanted to cover up that they could not find the Ventolin. The respiratory therapist did not report to chart his delay and error in starting the Ventolin aerosol on air instead of oxygen. The doctors appear to have joined the tangled web to help cover up the Ventolin problems, the time of death and the throat injury. (Lahey v St Joseph's Hospital 1992 p.256)

The language used by the judge indicates a more tolerant attitude to the 'girls' who 'followed bad examples' than to the doctors who 'set' them. This is evident in the way in which his Honour made the pejorative finding that the doctors 'were involved in the cover-up of the patients death', whereas he found only that the nurses 'wanted to cover up that they could not find the Ventolin'. Despite the fact that it was the inability to find the Ventolin which actually caused the patient's death, it would appear that the judge was reluctant to blame these 'girls' for their wrongdoings, and preferred to believe that they were led astray. Implicit in this is the forfeiture of independent moral agency on the part of the nurses, which is discussed later in more detail.

Sympathy in the Coroner's Court: the 'halo' effect

Nurses are often called to give evidence in the Coroner's Court. Although they do not always receive sympathetic treatment, there have often been expressions of sympathy for their difficult and demanding working environment. There is almost a 'halo effect' in operation. Because nurses do caring work, they must be caring people. While this may often be the case, and nurses under scrutiny seem to have acquitted themselves very favourably, there is a tendency to move from the general to the particular, and to use similar language to describe all nurses.

In the Inquest touching the death of BRC (1989), a young mentally handicapped person was found drowned after he had wandered away from his nursing home. The then State Coroner, Mr Waller, spoke with compassion about the difficulties for nursing staff and family during a coronial hearing such as this.

I, likewise, I might say, have admiration for people like nurses who care for the sick and the ailing and the dying and the handicapped in our community. I just don't know where we would be without them. I am, I would agree, somewhat defensive of them. I don't like them, seeing them (sic) called before the Court and attacked over their behaviour in a particular case, particularly when the attack is so often based on hindsight. (1989 pp.1–2)

The nurses were criticised by the relatives, but Mr Waller expressed his support for them.

Sister B. (?) (sic) has been singled out for criticism. I really think when one has seen these ladies in the witness box giving evidence, they present as solid, reliable and caring persons. There is just no evidence that they treated this matter with any callousness or indifference. They adopted an attitude, I think, of responsibility. (1989 p.5)

Similarly, in a number of other cases, words such as sincere, dedicated, reliable, caring and competent are used to describe the nurses (Inquest touching the death of JCF 1987, Corley v NW Hertfordshire HA 1997). The reluctance to criticise nursing staff is based to some extent on the nature of the work which nurses do. Thus the work of nurses has a certain 'halo effect' in these cases. The ministering angel image is obvious.

The reluctance to sue an 'angel'

In the early 20th century the law was that hospitals would not be liable for the professional acts of nurses (Hillyer v Governors of St Bartholomew's Hospital 1909, Vuchar v Trustees of Toronto General Hospital 1937). However, in reality nurses were hardly ever held to be personally liable for their professional acts, Strangeways-Lesmere v Clayton and others (1936) being an exception, perhaps because of a reluctance to 'take on' the nurses. To bring an action against a nurse or to find a nurse personally liable would have required a plaintiff (or at least their lawyers) to be seen to attack the popular mythology of the courageous, ministering angel, the 'Lady with the Lamp'. This could have proven particularly troublesome in situations where the services administered by the nurse had been given at a charitable institution, and thus at no cost to the plaintiff.

> *IT IS A PRIVILEGE TO SERVE AS A NURSE, AND*
> *THEREFORE NURSES SHOULD NOT COMPLAIN*
> *ABOUT POOR LIVING AND WORKING*
> *CONDITIONS AND HUGE WORKLOADS*

Nursing work is not 'rendered for profit'

There have also been negative aspects of the 'halo effect' as a consequence of the maxim that goodness should be its own reward. This has been most evident in the industrial arena.

The industry is one of a most unusual character; indeed, one to which the word industry would not in ordinary parlance be applied at all ... the work carried on by these institutions is not industry in the ordinary sense of the word, but consists in providing medical and surgical services for the sick, and providing them with accommodation and expert care and attention during illness, and in some cases also services designed to prevent illness or ward off future suffering.

These services in a large majority of the institutions with which the award deals are not rendered for profit, but as social services provided by means of funds from the State, from charitable donors and from fees in the case of those who can afford to pay them. (In re Hospital Nurses (State) Award 1936b pp.250–251)

These comments, made in an appeal judgment of the first NSW nurses award, are indicative of the perception of hospitals' work as charitable work, services to society. The nurses who undertook the work were described in this judgment as 'devoted' women, 'willing to make sacrifices in the work which they have undertaken' (1936b p.252).

It was determined that these devoted women 'must not be asked to submit to conditions that may impair their health or are more onerous than they should reasonably be asked to bear'. However, what they could 'reasonably be asked to bear' was significantly more onerous than that which the general public might reasonably be asked to bear. Concerning their living conditions, it was held that the trainees 'in most cases' were provided with a good home (1936b p.253). A 'reasonable measure of elasticity' meant that ordinary working hours may be balanced 'over eight weeks' (1936b 249), that the nurses' day ought not to finish until nine o' clock at night because that 'was in the interests of the patients' (Hospital Nurses' (State) & c (State) Conciliation Committee 1936a p.99), and that a 44+ hour working week was 'in the public interest'. The decision to make no provision for sick leave or holiday pay was reasonable because 'there was no suggestion that any nurse had not been sympathetically treated by her employer when ill' (1936b p.102) and that working on Sundays, holidays and weekends was 'indispensable to the industry' (1936b p.92).

The 'guilt factor' in wage fixing principles

There was an acknowledged reluctance to pay nurses too much because it placed an undue financial burden on hospitals. Webb J, the Industrial Commissioner, condoned a refusal to pay overtime for 'the carrying out of duties on Sundays, holidays and at night' by the fact that 'such work ... will be compensated by the granting of adequate annual leave' (1936b p.92). What 'adequate' meant is questionable. The nurse historian Russell reports that in 1927 a nurse in training at Royal Prince Alfred Hospital, Sydney, would be working 'up to 12 hours a day, six days a week, for 49 weeks of the year' (Russell 1990 p.27). However, on appeal, the Full Bench of the Industrial Commission held that even this might impose too great a burden on the hospital, stating that the Commission should 'walk warily' when setting awards for the first time (1936a p.252).

Demanding compliance with regulations reasonable and desirable in themselves might impose on some of these institutions financial burdens greater than they can bear without jeopardy to the health of many of the sick in the community or even causing loss of life that might otherwise have been saved. (1936a p.251)

Nursing is a labour-intensive occupation, and even a 1 per cent increase in nursing salaries can affect the payroll dramatically. The argument that an increase in nurses' salaries might affect the lives of patients would have been a powerful deterrent to any industrial demands which nurses might have wished to make. Moral pressure such as this was repeatedly brought to bear until it became a part of the nursing culture (Hindwood 1991 p.48). In addition, caring was so central to notions of womanhood that to demand significant recompense for it would have risked nurses being perceived as heartless by the general public (Gladwin 1930 p.34). Thornton, discussing the way in which caring has shaped notions of the proper work of women, points out that such ideology 'has been a very effective device for disempowering ... women' (1996 p.25).

The 'taint' of money

Nurses, still paying for the privilege of being trained as late as 1924, and receiving 'no pay, and ... no limitation of hours of work except that conceded by the ward sister', would probably have agreed that it was improper to seek recompense for womanly work (Miller 1985 p.31). Gladwin, writing in 1930, conceded that nurses had the right to live decently, but was anxious to put the receipt of wages into its proper perspective—a necessary evil which could only be counterbalanced by dedication to one's work.

The money making possibilities of nursing have been much advertised and a profession cannot fail to suffer when this happens. The question of earning a living confronts an increasing number of young girls and, having chosen nursing from among other gainful occupations or having been thrust into it with no choice at all, one is expected to give unselfishly of her best efforts and to consecrate herself to her work as did the saints of old ... However, she is headed straight for trouble if the money to be earned is her chief consideration.

She attempted to help the nurses assuage their guilt at making money:

For our comfort, we should remember that some of the world's best work is prompted by the necessity of earning money. It is good work, because, forgetting the economic compulsion, the doer throws her heart and soul into it. (1930 p.34)

The responses of nurses: exodus or industrial action

Although later decisions of the NSW Industrial Commission were somewhat more favourable, nurses' wages have often fallen behind the average living wage. The industrial history of nursing is one of poor conditions and low wages, with nurses enduring such arrangements until they became intolerable, and then leaving in large numbers. As Abel-Smith stated:

Underfed, overworked and underpaid, they struggled on rather than break a 'professional' code of honour. Activism was unprofessional, worse still it would have undermined the cherished spirit of vocation: it smelt of hard bargaining and the pursuit of selfish material interests. It was also unfeminine. (1960 p.245)

There has been a cyclical nature to these exoduses, in that they have resulted in nursing shortages, which in turn have caused the over-stretched remaining nurses ultimately to demand better pay and conditions. At such points successive governments around the world have been forced to intervene and deliver substantial wage reforms (Abel-Smith 1960, Dickenson 1993). Dingwall et al (1991 p.205), writing of the establishment of the Briggs Committee in England, stated that it was 'set up against a background of industrial unrest. In this respect it resembled most of the major policy initiatives in nursing since the Nurses Registration Act 1919 (UK).'

Nurses never contemplated strike action in New South Wales until the 1970s, but even then it was voted out by the general nurses (Dickenson 1993 p.189). A series of bans were introduced, which were strongly criticised by the Sydney Morning Herald (29 May 1976) describing them as 'irresponsible', despite the fact that the same article acknowledged nurses' exploitation. The only nurses to take strike action at this time were the psychiatric nurses, who have a larger percentage of men in their workforce. They organised a series of 24-hour stoppages, with skeleton staff coverage.

In the Inquest touching the death of MO'D (1973) the Coroner found that the patient died from burns sustained in a scalding hot bath. This incident occurred during the nurses' strike at a psychiatric hospital in 1973. The Coroner found no criminal negligence, but he was critical of the actions of the strike committee. In his caveat about his criticisms there is a sense that he also did not consider it appropriate for the nursing staff to be industrially active in this way.

I must say from the outset that I am disturbed by the evidence adduced at this inquest. Having said that, I must guard against comments which would be borne of feelings I have from a humane and social point of view, rather than from views I would be required and obliged to take in my position as Coroner.

Normally it would not be the province of a Coroner to concern himself with the rights or wrongs of a body involving itself in strike action. However, the circumstances surrounding the death of MO'D have made it necessary for me to give every consideration to the strike action by the nursing staff of X hospital.

It is my view that the strike action committee, whatever the grievance, acted irresponsibly in calling the strike, when one considers the fact that normal attention was denied to patients, in the order of 770, of a mental hospital. I am prepared to give credence to the fact that a minimum nursing staff was placed in each ward to carry out certain duties on a voluntary basis but the duties undertaken to my mind, fell far short of the norm. (1973 p.1)

CONCLUSION

This chapter has explored the image of the nurse as a ministering angel, an outsider story initially fostered by nurses in the past and accepted over time by the general public and the courts and tribunals. It is a story whose roots are to be found more in the nursing literature than in case law, but its influences, both positive and negative, can be detected in Parliamentary debate, and judicial and coronial decisions. This image has been valuable for nurses. It served in Nightingale's time to differentiate them from the disreputable poor house nurses. But its greatest benefit has been to enable nurses to undertake the intimate and private work, which is the foundation of their practice, in an atmosphere of compassion with distance.

The difficulties that have arisen from this image relate to the invisibility of nurses undertaking this work, and to the dissonance this image can create for nurses in certain areas of their work. Such an image and its concomitant invisibility have, on some occasions, rendered nurses morally invisible, too. There has been a reluctance on the behalf of some judges to blame nurses for behaviour which was morally reprehensible. Perhaps this was because they were sympathetic to these 'ministering angels' or perhaps because the nurses' involvement was also invisible to their eyes. The other difficulties have occurred in the past because nursing has been associated with notions of self sacrifice and dedication. The sense that 'goodness has its own rewards' seems to have given rise to a degree of complacency when the question of tangible financial and industrial rewards has been before the courts or wage-fixing bodies.

4

Introducing the nurse as a domestic worker

Elements of the image

- Nurses are domestic workers to the extent that they do cleaning and cooking, undertake tasks which provide personal comfort, and get their hands (and clothes) dirty. These domestic tasks are to be viewed as separate from, and intrinsically inferior to, 'true' nursing work—rather than as an integral element of holistic nursing care.

- Such tasks could not possibly be performed by professional, upper or middle class people; they could only be undertaken by domestic workers or people of the lower classes.

- People who do such work would be less likely to give reliable evidence in court than professional medical men, so this should be imputed to nurses generally.

- People such as nurses who do such work do not deserve the same pay or living conditions as professional, middle or upper class people.

INTRODUCTION

This is the first of the 'stock story' chapters, the nurse as a domestic worker. It is a relatively uncomplicated image, based on a preconception of the nature of a particular aspect of nursing work. The elements of this image have all been present since early last century. However, the critical issues surrounding this image are the effects its perception has had on the fragmentation of the nursing role, the way in which nurses have felt about these aspects of their work, and the subsequent ways in which nurses dealt with these perceptions and feelings.

The 'domestic worker' stock story

The next two chapters demonstrate that in the early 20th century the patient-centred view nurses held did not represent the prevailing ideology. In fact, the nursing role was segmented in early judgments for legalistic concerns far removed from patient care. They related to determinations of liability for injuries to patients in hospital. This reductionist approach to nursing work led to a devaluation and erosion of the nursing role over the century, while the voices of nurses have been either silent or disregarded in those discussions of nursing work. The 'domestic' work which nurses have performed has not been treated as an integral part of a wider professional skilled occupation. Instead, it has been compartmentalised and given sufficient prominence (in the stock story) to pull the rest of nursing work 'down' to the level of domestic work, which has made it harder for nurses to obtain recognition as a profession.

The key elements of the domestic worker stock story discussed in the ensuing two chapters are listed at the opening to this chapter. This chapter examines the effect of the domestic worker image on nurses over the twentieth century. It begins with a brief introduction to vicarious liability, as much of the early case law involving nurses relates to the question of a hospital's liability for the tortious acts of its staff. It then addresses some resultant general themes which recur throughout the book. These are chiefly the argument that nursing is the extension of a knowledge base for traditional women's work, and the formal abdication (but informal retention) of this domestic work in the search for professional status. They also include the impact of the proximity of medicine to the status of an industry as a profession or para-profession, with its associated concepts of intrinsic and extrinsic professionalism, and the inclusive nature of nursing as a discipline.

The doctrine of vicarious liability

It is necessary briefly to address the doctrine of vicarious liability because of the effect of the judgment in Hillyer v Governors of St Bartholomew's Hospital (1909) (hereafter Hillyer) on the future treatment of nursing work in negligence cases. Hillyer specifically addressed the question of whether a hospital was vicariously liable for the tortious acts of its nurses. It will be clear from the discussion of the judgment that this was a vexed question for the English Court of Appeal in 1909. Although questions of a hospital's liability for the wrongs of its professional staff are now settled at law, some understanding of the doctrine will inform the case law within this book.

The concerns of the judges in the early liability cases were far removed from the status of nursing work. However, the 'stock stories' about nurses, which the judges accepted (even if subconsciously) influenced their decisions significantly, and indirectly affected the holistic conception of nursing work. The nursing role was dissected in most cases specifically for the purpose of fixing liability, but the incidental repercussions of that dissection were to have a far-reaching influence on the way in which nurses and society perceived their work.

The phrase 'vicarious responsibility' was coined by Pollock in the late nineteenth century (Williams & Hepple 1984 p.132). Luntz and Hambly describe the doctrine as follows:

In certain situations the law of torts allows the victim of one person's wrong-doing to recover damages from another for the loss occasioned thereby. Such liability for the consequences of the conduct of others is described as 'vicarious'. (1995 p.867)

The basis of the doctrine is that, on establishing the existence of the special relationship between employer and employee, the employer will be liable for the wrongful acts of the employee, provided that they were performed in the course of the employee's employment (Luntz & Hambly 1995). It is implicit in the maxim *respondeat superior*, meaning 'let the master answer'. Thus to demonstrate vicarious liability it has been necessary to prove two major facts—whether there was a relationship of employer and employee; and whether the wrong was committed in the course of the employee's employment.

The determination of employee status, also known as a 'contract of service' has been difficult at times; but around 1909, when the discussion of the topic begins for this book, some sort of 'control' test was applied. At that time, professionals were not considered to be employees, as their highly skilled activities were not deemed to be within the control of anyone but themselves (e.g. Evans v Liverpool Corporation 1906, Hall v Lees 1904, Hillyer 1909). So hospitals were not vicariously liable for the wrongs of their professional staff, but were considered to have discharged their duty if they had selected them with due care.

The rationale for vicarious liability: the protection of charity hospitals?

Later judges such as Lord Denning LJ (Cassidy v Ministry of Health 1951 p.361) and Justice Kirby (Ellis v Wallsend District Hospital 1989 p.566) and academic writers such as Picard (1994 pp.313–14) have suggested that the underlying rationale for this early attitude to a hospital's liability for its professional staff was a reluctance to impose liability on the hospital because it was a charitable institution. Payment of compensation for injuries was problematic for hospitals in the early part of the twentieth century, as the majority were charitable institutions. These hospitals provided care free of charge and were hard pressed by the rising cost of medical care, often depending on the state for subsidies (Chesterman 1979).

In the pivotal case of Hillyer v Governors of St Bartholomew's Hospital, Mr Hillyer, who suffered severe burns, sued the hospital for the negligent acts of its nursing staff while they were working with a surgeon in the operating theatre. In the English Court of Appeal the judges did go to considerable lengths to exclude the hospital from liability. Kennedy LJ alluded to the hospital's charitable status as a possible basis for his reluctance when he noted that Dr Hillyer was admitted 'to enjoy in the hospital the gratuitous benefit of its care'. He held that the hospital was not vicariously liable for the nurses while in the operating room because at that time (although emphasising that they were not always professionals) they were professionals and therefore under their own control. Farwell LJ found that the hospital was not vicariously liable for the nurses because they were under the control of the surgeon, not the hospital, while they were in the operating theatre.

However, if a reluctance to fix a charity hospital with liability was the only or indeed, true, underlying policy reason for their decisions, then the simplest course for all the judges was to have accepted the argument of the hospital's lawyers, which was that all the staff were professional. In fact, Farwell LJ seemed prepared as a general principle (although not in this case) to fix hospitals with liability for the wrongs of their staff, despite their 'charitable functions'. In the early cases explored in this book, there is only one direct acknowledgement of the undesirability of burdening hospitals with liability due to their charitable nature (Lavere v Smith's Falls Public Hospital 1915b p.360). However, Partlett (1985) has identified a reluctance by the courts at that time to articulate underlying policy influences.

Resolving the matter: the liability of hospitals for the torts of professional staff

By the late 1940s there was a growing willingness throughout the Commonwealth to find hospitals vicariously liable for all the actions of their nurse employees, thus making redundant the dissection of the nursing role. Following the decision in Gold v Essex County Council (1942), there has been much judicial deliberation and learned writing on the nature of the tests required at law to determine vicarious liability. They are outside the scope of this book, but are well covered by eminent legal academics (e.g. Luntz & Hambly 1995).

In relation to the determination of vicarious liability for hospitals, the Court of Appeal's decision in Gold v Essex County Council (1942) is a landmark case. At trial, a radiographer was found to have negligently caused burns to a child's face as a result of using lint instead of a proper shield over the face during an X-ray. Although the department was supervised by a Dr Allen, there was no suggestion that, at the time of the incident, the radiographer was acting under his instruction. In initial argument for the plaintiff, Mr Denning KC had challenged the 'contractual' method of determining liability, arguing that '[t]his duty does not arise out of contract and Hillyer v Governors of St Bartholomew's Hospital errs in this respect' (1942 p.296).

On appeal, Lord Greene MR found that Farwell LJ's judgment in Hillyer was relevant only to the operating room. His Lordship referred almost exclusively to nurses in his decision, although the case concerned a radiographer. He did not dissect nursing work into professional or ministerial duties, but held that a hospital would be liable for all the acts of a nurse, both professional and domestic.

However, he did make a distinction between professional nursing duties, i.e. a nurse acting in her capacity as a nurse, and delegated medical tasks, where a nurse is carrying out the orders of a doctor. Even in this differentiation, he still sought to protect the hospital from liability. He suggested that if the nurse were acting on the instructions of the surgeon 'she is not guilty of negligence if she carries out the orders of the surgeon or doctor, however negligent those orders may be' (1942 p.300). This contradicts earlier case law which had identified the need for nurses to scrutinise closely the orders of doctors (Lavere v Smith's Falls Public Hospital 1915b, Nyberg v Provost 1927, Henson v Board of Management of Perth Hospital and another 1938), but is a defence which nurses have used to good effect in later cases (e.g. Report of The Royal Commission into Deep Sleep Therapy 1990).

Lord Greene did not suggest that the nurse became the employee of the doctor in these circumstances. He held that '[t]here is no room in his [the radiographer's] case for the theory of a transmutation in the nature of the employment such as, in the view of Farwell LJ, takes place in the case of a nurse once the door of the operating room has closed' (Gold v Essex County Council 1942 p.300). The rejection of the 'theory of a transmutation of employment' was an important and sensible development.

Differing degrees of influence exerted by doctors and nurses

The application of the doctrine of vicarious liability to hospitals has developed in response to a number of underlying policy factors. These are becoming more explicit now in the judgments, but there is still a degree of forensic obfuscation which clouds these policy objectives.

In addition to the problems caused by Hillyer, the absence of nurse witnesses and the evidence of medical practitioners have also influenced decisions concerning hospital liability for nurses. Partlett, writing on the history of the development of professional liability, states that professionals such as doctors have always influenced law making (1985 p.16). By contrast, the development of the doctrine of vicarious liability has paid little attention to, and shown little concern for, the professional status of nurses. This is despite the fact that nurses have been repeatedly (if inconsistently) referred to and used as examples throughout the case law. On occasions, they have even been key players in the story, although rarely have they been parties to the action. However, because of the effect of the evolution of the case law on the fragmentation of the nursing role, the 'relic of Hillyer' has had far-reaching effects on the nursing profession.

This next section addresses a number of recurrent issues which arise from the domestic worker image, but which are central to the quest of nurses for professional recognition and an understanding of nursing work. The themes recur throughout the book.

The professionalisation of traditional women's work

Work such as cleaning, cooking, caring and comforting was always under-taken by women. Florence Nightingale envisaged that her nurses would undertake such work as part of the totality of nursing care. She always maintained that these tasks required skill and knowledge and could not simply be performed by anyone.

[T]hese things are not done by drinking old females, but by respectable women. Yet we are often told that a nurse needs only to be 'devoted and obedient'. This definition would do just as well for a porter. It might even do for a horse. It would not do for a policeman. Consider how many women there are who have nothing to devote—neither intelligence, nor eyes, nor ears, nor hands. They would sit up all night by the patient, it is true; but their attendance is worth nothing to him, nor their observations to the doctor. (1952 pp.140–1)

The development of nursing as a form of paid employment is discussed earlier. But once this had occurred, the extent to which this work should be deemed professional arose for consideration. Mrs Bedford Fenwick was a Nightingale trainee, founder of the British Nurses' Association and the pion-eer of nursing registration legislation in England (Bendall & Raybould 1969). When she began to lobby for the registration of nurses, nurses had ele-vated the status of the full range of the work they did in an endeavour to par-allel that of traditionally male professions. The development of nursing as a career was seen by Mrs Bedford Fenwick and her supporters as the pro-fessionalisation of a number of traditional women's responsibilities, just as traditional male responsibilities such as fighting, witch doctoring, and dispute resolution had been professionalised into soldiering, medicine, and law. The work which nurses undertook, such as the care of the sick and the manage-ment of large domestic establishments, would once have been performed by wives, housekeepers, and the ladies of the manor (Seymer 1949). Nurses have taken these roles, adapted them and brought them up to date with know-ledge originally garnered from experience but also from developments in public health and science (Ottley Forword in Nightingale 1952 pp.6–8).

However, at the turn of the 20th century, one of the difficulties for nurses was that society (and the courts), although prepared to accept the minister-ing angel image to some extent, were not at all prepared to accept that women's work might be on a professional par with men's work.

The acceptance by nurses of the fragmentation of the nurses' role and the emergence of non-nursing duties

The fragmented approach adopted by the courts and tribunals to the role of nursing seems to have originated in Hillyer v Governors of St Bartholomew's Hospital. Gradually, this demarcation of various aspects of nurses' work and its subsequent devaluation of the status of aspects of their role and work were internalised by the nursing profession. Industrial claims in the second half of the last century reflected this division of nursing work into 'nursing' and 'non-nursing' duties.

This provides an example of what Matsuda (1990) describes as 'false consciousness' where the outsider group starts to see itself through the eyes of the dominant group and consequently learns to despise and devalue itself. Nurses became prepared to denounce and disclaim previously important aspects of their work in order to seek recognition for themselves and their work with the dominant group, a strategy which they saw as the way to achieve improved pay and conditions.

Prominent Australian nurses have since deplored the way in which nursing divided its domain in this way (Staunton 1993). They have argued that it is inherently damaging to nurses to deny any aspect of their work, because it will not improve the status of nursing per se, but simply undermine the existing nursing role so that cheaper alternatives may be found to perform nursing work (Staunton 1989).

These concerns are well founded. Today, although the question of the liability of hospitals is resolved, the debate about the status of domestic work and its relation to nurses still continues, particularly in relation to accident and workers compensation claims. In practice, nurses still undertake informally much work that would fall within the classification of 'domestic'. They do so simply because the focus of nursing work, namely patient well-being, still demands that nurses do whatever needs to be done to make the patient comfortable.

Financial considerations have also continued to be the force behind the characterisation of nursing as domestic work in accident and workers compensation claims. If the work required to be undertaken for the claimant can be shown to be domestic, rather than nursing work, it attracts less or, under some statutes, no compensation at all for the injured party. A rearguard action within the nursing profession to reclaim and embrace its lost territory by [re]adopting a more holistic approach to nursing care over the past twenty years has not been reflected in the judgments of the compensation courts and tribunals. This may in part be due to the fact that medical practitioners, rather than nurses, are usually the professionals called to give expert opinions, even in cases where the matter under review is the need for nursing care.

Intrinsic and extrinsic models of ascribing professional status

Much has been written about the identification and recognition of professions by both sociologists and lawyers (Albon & Lindsay 1984, Cotterell 1984, Daniel 1990, Lupton 1995, Field & Taylor 1998, Petersen & Waddell 1998). It has been suggested that the groups organised around a dominant profession are actually para-professions, who gain their professional status from their proximity to the dominant professional group (Gardner & McCoppin 1989 pp.304–306). This notion of ascribed professional status for nursing by virtue of medical proximity has arisen in case law. I have described this phenomenon as extrinsic professionalism because the status is generated medically and delegated to the nurse. In the cases where it is acknowledged that nurses have professional skills which are peculiarly their own, I have labelled such attribution of status as intrinsic professionalism. Throughout the book there are numerous examples of the way in which the courts and tribunals reward nurses (particularly financially) for taking on medically delegated or generated work. In addition, nurse leaders originally used a medical model of professionalism as the yardstick against which they measured themselves as a profession (Short & Sharman 1995 p.239) and thus themselves saw certain medical activities as being symbolic of professional status.

Nursing as an inclusive rather than exclusive discipline

Nursing work has never been carried out exclusively by nurses, but has always also involved teaching others to care for the sick. Many unqualified carers, usually women, care for their sick families, and nurses in hospitals and community settings have supported and educated them. In this way, nursing, unlike many other professions, could be described as an inclusive, rather than an exclusive, discipline. To some extent this has been problematic for nurses, as it is well-nigh impossible (and highly undesirable) to exercise any monopoly over certain aspects of caring activities. Life would be very difficult if lay persons were not involved in caring for the sick. In addition, other health professionals, including some doctors, are keen to demonstrate their commitment to caring and their nursing skills (Little 1995, Baume 1998). Because of this inclusive nature of nursing practice, it has also been difficult to proscribe nursing or caring activities by legislation, as has been the case with aspects of, say, medical or chiropractic practice.

However, the difference is that nurses have become professional carers, employed and expected to deliver skilled care to the sick with a similar degree of devotion and compassion. This confers on nurses special rights of access to the patient given to very few others, access which is given on trust because the person seeking access is designated 'nurse'. This right of access has been described as the 'privilege of intimacy' (Chiarella 1990, Lawler 1991). With this privilege comes special duties, some legal, some moral. They are outlined succinctly in the ANCI Code of Professional Conduct for Nurses in Australia (1995). This proximity as a professional carer means that nurses have always worked in very intimate circumstances with their patients and, as a result, have undertaken a wide range of tasks. These tasks range from the mundane to the highly specialised, and occur because of the proximity and the continual nature of the relationship between the nurse and the patient. Nurses are still the only accredited health professionals to provide a twenty-four hours a day, seven days a week, presence with hospitalised patients.

As a result of this continuity and proximity, work which might in other circumstances have been designated as domestic work has always been considered by nurses to be an integral part of nursing work. Nurses believed that tasks which were recognisable at one level as domestic duties could at another level be elevated to professional work. Gladwin, writing in 1930, acknowledged that 'a servant is able to do many things, which a nurse does for the patient, and to do them quite acceptably'. However, she maintained that 'the difference lies in the trained facilities which enable the nurses to understand reactions, to read symptoms ... and to interpret needs' (1930 p.110).

The comprehensive nature of nursing work

The 'stock story' became that much of nursing work was of a routine or domestic nature, and required no special skill. This stock story, through its influence on the dominant view of what nursing entailed, has to some extent jeopardised claims which nursing might have made to be viewed as a profession, different from, but on an equal footing with, medicine. In this way, the 'fragmentation' of the nursing role into 'domestic' and other tasks evolved into a dominant stock story in which the whole nursing role was characterised as domestic. Stock stories which 'are part of, and reinforce the dominant discourse' (Sarmas 1994 p.703), 'that make sense' and are 'true to what the listeners know about the world' (Scheppele 1989 p.2080), are very persuasive, especially when they emerge from the courts and tribunals.

The outsider story was, however, that nurses viewed their role as being to care for the whole patient, which would mean doing whatever needed to be done for the safety and well-being of the patient. Nurses would not have determined their status on a piecemeal basis according to which task a nurse was performing at a particular point in time. Rather, the early nurses considered many so-called 'domestic' tasks to be central to their professional nursing role. Yet these were the tasks which were differentiated from 'true' professional work in the judgments.

Because of the nature and intimacy of nursing work, the fact that one possesses a particular skill does not preclude one from undertaking unskilled activities. Thus, if the focus of nursing care is to take care of a person who is ill, then part of that care-taking may be to remove their dirty dishes because this may ultimately benefit their well-being. Because the focus of nursing is on people's well-being, rather than on tasks, it makes it difficult to make any demarcation on what constitutes nursing care. Perhaps a better way to define nursing is by examining the intent behind the action, to ask whether the work was performed with a *mens nutricia*, a 'nursing mind'. Thus if the work is done with the intent to optimise patient well-being, and it is performed by a nurse, then it becomes nursing. Certainly, Virginia Henderson defined nursing in terms of intent, rather than in terms of tasks (1969).

Today, while nurses still bemoan the loss of the control over the cleaning of the wards (Gaze 1992), most cleaning work in hospitals is now contracted out (Sadler 1990). In some health services, cleaning duties have now been realigned under nursing management, although no longer predominantly carried out by nurses.

The necessary persistence of 'domestic' work in nursing

A recent workers' compensation case demonstrates the continuing potential breadth of the nursing role and the difficulty in distinguishing nursing work from domestic work in certain situations. St Basil's Nursing Home v Eliza Duff-Tytler (1993) demonstrates that there may still be circumstances where very senior nurses are required to perform domestic duties. The case concerned the Director of Nursing who had fallen from a tree sustaining a head injury while collecting apricots at a friend's house for the Nursing Home's Christmas party. It was held that she suffered a compensable disability arising out of or in the course of her employment on the grounds that she had an extensive discretion and extensive responsibilities. Her lengthy list of identified responsibilities included such obvious requirements as 'proper medical (sic) care of the patients including the keeping of records, the maintaining of appropriate staffing levels ... the proper oversight of treatment and nursing care of the patients ... and the control of medicines and drugs' (1993 p.393).

However, in addition to these requirements, a further job description existed which included 'housekeeping, economy and pastoral care'. In addition, she gave evidence to the effect that she was also responsible for garden maintenance, electrical equipment checks and shopping! Parsons J held that 'in these circumstances where the employer required such overall responsibility and discretion ... it is untenable to suggest that if she decided on a Sunday to collect apricots for the nursing home that such an enterprising activity for the benefit of the patients and thus indirectly for the benefit of her employer was not within the scope of her employment' (1993 p.394). The responsibilities of this 'matron' in 1993 do not differ significantly from those of Lucy Osburn on her arrival in Australia in 1868 (Bowd 1968).

CONCLUSION

This chapter has introduced the image of the nurse as the domestic worker and explored its genesis in the case of Hillyer v Governors of

St Bartholomew's Hospital. It has also examined how the fragmentation of the role occurred for the purposes of fixing liability in negligence cases, and discussed briefly the ramifications of such fragmentation. It also introduced a number of themes that recur throughout the book. Two such themes are the concept of nursing as the professionalisation of traditional women's work, and the formal abdication (but informal retention) of domestic work in the search for professional status. The impact of the proximity of medicine to the status of an industry as a profession or para-profession, with its associated concepts of intrinsic and extrinsic professionalism, and the inclusive nature of nursing as a discipline are also broached.

5

The nurse as a domestic worker

Elements of the image

- Nurses are domestic workers to the extent that they do cleaning and cooking, undertake tasks which provide personal comfort, and get their hands (and clothes) dirty. These domestic tasks are to be viewed as separate from, and intrinsically inferior to, 'true' nursing work—rather than as an integral element of holistic nursing care.

- Such tasks could not possibly be performed by professional, upper or middle class people; they could only be undertaken by domestic workers or people of the lower classes.

- People who do such work would be less likely to give reliable evidence in court than professional medical men, so this should be imputed to nurses generally.

- People such as nurses who do such work do not deserve the same pay or living conditions as professional, middle or upper class people.

INTRODUCTION

This chapter examines further the starting point for the domestic worker image—the incoherent judgments of the English Court of Appeal in the 1909 case of Hillyer v Governors of St Bartholomew's Hospital (1909). Factors, other than the protection of charitable hospitals, which might have led to the decision (such as gender and class) are also explored.

The chapter also examines the consequences of the domestic worker image through a series of cases described as 'the burns sagas' which attempted (somewhat inconsistently) to apply Hillyer and caused further fragmentation of the nursing role. It examines the concept of 'false consciousness' and the persistence of the fragmentation of the nursing role, Finally, the poor pay, living and working conditions which nurses have experienced are discussed, and the extent to which the domestic worker story may be responsible is examined.

The stock story of the nurse as domestic worker, which was probably 'always already' (Lather 1991 p.170) present in the law, did not really become evident until the decision in the English case of Hillyer v Governors of St Bartholomew's Hospital in 1909.

Hillyer: the facts in detail

The plaintiff Hillyer was a doctor who had recently returned from West Africa and was very poor and in ill health. The consultant surgeon agreed to examine him under anaesthetic as a non-paying patient at St Bartholomew's Hospital. Hillyer was injured during the examination and brought an action in negligence against the governors of the hospital. During the course of the examination, it was claimed that as a result of his incorrect positioning, one of his arms was burned and the other was bruised, and that he had also suffered traumatic neuritis and paralysis, which had caused him to be unable to earn a living. Hillyer's lawyers argued that, since all the staff were servants or agents of the hospital, the hospital was liable for the negligent actions of all of them. The argument of the hospital's lawyers was that hospitals are only responsible for the selection of their professional staff, not their actions, and if they had exercised due care in their selection they should not be liable. At the trial it was held that, as the law stood, organisations were not liable for the torts of [professional] people, but were only responsible for selecting them with due care.

The appeal

On appeal, Mr Hillyer's lawyer modified his argument slightly, as lawyers are wont to do if they can see that a particular line of argument is not likely to be successful (Meyer 1992 p.129). He drew a distinction between: the relationship of the governors to the operating surgeon, Mr Lockwood; and their relationship with the remainder of those present at the operation, who were described as 'the staff'. The hospital's lawyer's argument remained the same: namely, that it was not appropriate to distinguish between the operating surgeon, the house surgeons, and the nurses. They were not servants but agents (meaning independent contractors), and accordingly the only responsibility of the hospital was to select these agents with due care.

There were three appeal judges. The first two, Kennedy and Farwell LJJ, differed markedly from each other in the reasons they gave as to why the hospital was not liable for the tortious acts of its nursing staff. Incredibly, the third judge, Cozens-Hardy MR, agreed with the reasons given by both in dismissing the appeal (1909 p.824).

Kennedy LJ held that the only duty of the hospital was to exercise due care in the selection of the staff. They would in turn be able to exercise professional skill as independent professional people. His Lordship, in dismissing the appeal, described surgeons, physicians and nurses as 'experts' able to provide 'the privilege of skilled ... nursing aid' (1909 pp.828–29). His Lordship held that the operating room was an area where nurses were presumed to practise this 'expert aid'.

However, the important factor for this book is that later in his judgment he established that nurses actually did two classifications of work. Effectively, he segmented the nursing role by differentiating between nurses 'conducting themselves in matters of professional skill', for which the hospital was not liable, and the 'due performance of hospital servants', for which the hospital would be liable. This work performed by 'servants' he described as 'ministerial or administrative', but all the duties he listed would have been performed by nursing staff. These duties included 'the attendance of nurses in the ward, the summoning of medical aid in cases of emergency, the supply of proper food, and the like' (1909 p.829).

What is unclear is why the judge should have chosen to make this observation. Neither side's lawyers seem to have made an argument to differentiate between various aspects of nursing work in this way, which suggests that this was a gratuitous observation which the judge felt it necessary to make. But one has to ask—for what reason? It is unimaginable that his Lordship might have compartmentalised the work of a medical practitioner in this way yet he obviously felt unable to let the matter rest without making some differentiation.

The second judge, Farwell LJ, would certainly not have behaved toward a medical practitioner in such a fashion. He began his judgment by stating that it was 'impossible to contend' that 'Mr Lockwood, the surgeon, or the acting assistant surgeon, or the acting house surgeon, or the administrator of anaesthetics, or any of them' were servants because they were 'all professional men' (1909 p.825). His Lordship asked whether 'any of the persons present at the examination [were] servants of the defendant?' However, he distinguished the status of doctors from the other personnel present. He held that the three nurses and the box carriers (porters) were servants of the hospital for general purposes, but then further differentiated between these purposes and the purpose of an operation. In this sense, Farwell LJ's judgment was the narrower of the two, confining the question of liability to a matter of location, rather than to the status of the practitioners.

[A]s soon as the door of the theatre or operating room has closed on them for the purposes of an operation ... they [the nurses and box carriers] cease to be under the orders of the defendants, and are at the disposal and under the sole orders of the operating surgeon until the whole operation has been completely finished; the surgeon is for the time being supreme, and the defendants cannot interfere with or gainsay his orders. (1909 p.826)

This concept is described in a later case as a 'transmutation of employment', and criticised as an incorrect ground upon which a hospital might avert liability (Gold v Essex County Council 1942 p.297). From this second judgment it could be inferred that a surgeon might be vicariously liable for the acts of the assisting staff during an operation. But the research undertaken for this book revealed no case where a surgeon was actually held to be vicariously liable for the acts or omissions of a nurse (although if a doctor were to be the nurse's employer, this would be the case). Farwell LJ explained that, during an operation, the hospital 'only suppl[ied] qualified persons to act as nurses and assistants under the control of the operating surgeons' (1909 p.827) which meant, of course, that the hospital could not be liable for their tortious acts.

The fragmentation of the nursing role in Hillyer's case

In Hillyer's case, three distinct aspects of the nursing role appear:

1. Nurses are considered to perform routine, ministerial work. Kennedy LJ described nursing activities such as 'the attendance on wards, the summoning of medical aid in cases of emergencies and the supply of proper food' as servants' work—routine or ministerial.

2. Nurses perform expert work as assistants to surgeons. Farwell LJ said that nurses were servants for general purposes, but undergo a change in employment or liability status as a result of the activity in which they are involved. So when they are assisting a surgeon with an operation, they cease to be a servant of the hospital, but are transferred to the control of the surgeon. Although he changes their locus of control because of their proximity to the surgeon and the existence of their 'expert assisting' skills, he does not really bother to address the question of their status. However, in later cases (e.g. Vuchar v Trustees of Toronto General Hospital 1937) the proximity to the surgeon has been of significance in determining or contributing to the professional status of a nursing act.

3. Nurses perform professional work in their own right. Kennedy LJ stated that nurses 'exercis[e] professional judgment in matters of professional skill' and that assisting in the operating room was an instance of such an activity.

The common element within the two judgments is that the nursing role is segmented, but the two methods of segmentation are very different and have far-reaching consequences.

Factors which may have influenced the decision in Hillyer

Why should their Lordships have chosen to reason in such a convoluted manner in Hillyer? Their reasons do not reflect the arguments offered by either the patient or the hospital lawyers. Hillyer's lawyers argued that all the professional staff except the surgeon were servants; the hospital lawyers argued that none of the professional staff were servants. But their

Lordships developed a new story, woven from some of the threads of those presented to them (Heerey 1996). They unhesitatingly found that the hospital was not liable for its operating surgeons, because they were professionals, yet they clearly hesitated to accord identical status to the nursing staff.

Three possible underlying policy reasons are suggested. First there is the reluctance to burden charity hospitals as discussed in Chapter 4. The other two related reasons, both of which would have precluded nurses from being classed as professionals, are that nursing was traditional women's work, and many nurses were working class women.

The devaluation of nursing because its substantial 'domestic' element was perceived as women's work

There was obviously reluctance on the part of both their Lordships to accord professional status to certain aspects of nursing work, 'the attendance on wards, the summoning of medical aid in cases of emergencies and the supply of proper food'. Both already held the view that some or all aspects of the nursing role were routine, domestic or administrative, as opposed to professional, and wished to put such a determination on the record. In order to achieve this, they 'pick(ed) and cho(se) from among the available facts to present...an account that justifies the world as it is' (Delgado 1989 p.2421).

This classification of those aspects of nursing work was part of the stock story, the 'dominant discourse' (Sarmas 1994 p.703) of the day, because tasks such as feeding and attending to patients on the wards would not have been considered professional but rather domestic tasks, traditional women's work (Probert 1989). Such work would have been both undervalued (Graycar 1992 p.1995) and, from a theoretical perspective, unexplored. The judges would have equated that kind of work with the work their domestic servants undertook at home, and it would have been preposterous to them to compare such work with the work of an operating surgeon. Being 'in attendance' (Hillyer 1909 p.829), albeit on the wards, was a term used to describe servant work.

It is not surprising that activities such as cleaning floors, serving meals and tea should be regarded as domestic duties in 1909. In wealthy households such tasks were, and still are, carried out by servants. Only poor and working class women would have served their own meals or cleaned their own floors. In addition, nursing's professional status was a politically volatile question at this time. Many, though not all, medical practitioners saw the increasing professionalisation of nursing as posing a threat to their livelihood. It was also a matter of concern for hospital administrators, due to the potential increase in costs (Bendall & Raybould 1969). Finally, in the absence of any input in Hillyer from nursing experts themselves, there was no opportunity for nurses' views to be heard on the importance of their work.

The significance of social class

The factor of class must also be taken into account. Not all women entering nursing would have come from the middle and upper classes, whereas other male professionals, such as doctors and lawyers, usually had privileged backgrounds. Women such as Florence Nightingale and Ethel Bedford Fenwick were from the upper or middle classes, and Nightingale envisaged that these women were to be trained to lead. But nursing is a labour-intensive activity, and many nurses were required. Since not all well-bred young women had a taste for work, there was a need to swell the nursing ranks from the other classes. Nightingale considered that there should be four types of 'probationers', the name then given to entrants into nursing.

Probationers included the 'ordinaries', who received a salary of 10 pounds per annum, the 'Free Specials' who had no salary, the 'Free Specials' who received a small salary, and the 'Specials' who paid 30 pounds for room and board ... Nightingale determined that her 'Specials' become leaders, was assiduous in forwarding their careers—and in monitoring their behaviour. (Vicinus & Nergaard 1989 p.314)

Nightingale was already clear about the different types of work and future these groups would have. She was anxious that her 'Specials' would emerge to become Training Matrons, who were to have 'some power of organisation and authority'. She considered that 'a higher calibre of woman is needed for a Training Matron ... I will not say higher, but a finer and larger sort of calibre' (Vicinus & Nergaard 1989 p.260). Although she believed that cleaning should be the prerogative of nurses, she does not seem to have envisaged that all nurses would clean.

It is all very well to put the Lady Prob'rs to exactly the same work as the others, viz. housemaids work, making beds, dusting & c. But after 6 months (say) surely they ought to be relieved of all this—i.e. of all housemaid's work. I would not relieve them of emptying slops and the like: for this is strictly Nurse's work. But of the rest I would. The more so because the less physically able who are by no means the less fit for Sisters like Miss Williams are actually tired before 9 in the morning for the day—and worn out before their year's training is over. (Letter to Sir Henry Bonham Carter, Vicinus & Nergaard 1989 p.340)

However, the rest of the probationers were expected to do this work. Sir Joshua Jebbs, chairman of the Nightingale Fund, had clear ideas about what sorts of recruits were required.

Persons of superior manners and education, ladies in fact are not as a rule required, but rather women of somewhat more ordinary intelligence belonging to classes in which women are more habitually employed in earning their own livelihood. (Abel-Smith 1960 p.41)

However, Nightingale was adamant that all nurses should be trained (Vicinus & Nergaard 1989 p.277). Possibly class was a factor in Nightingale's reluctance to introduce state registration, which led to all nurses being treated as professional equals. Certainly by the turn of the last century, all nurses were expected to undertake cleaning duties regardless of their class, but class consciousness was still very strong in England. It may have been an anathema to their Lordships in Hillyer to accord full professional status to a group whose ranks included the working classes.

The significant impact of the domestic worker image and the consequences of its acceptance

For over forty years after Hillyer, in common law jurisdictions all over the world, judges tried to follow precedent by splitting nursing work into professional and non-professional activities. To achieve this, they scrutinised the particular task which the nurse was undertaking in order to determine whether the task: was routine or administrative; was supervised or under the control of a doctor; or could be deemed to be a professional one. This approach was described in Logan v Waitaki Hospital Board (1935), one of a sequence of 'burns cases' which are discussed later. Johnston J observed somewhat scathingly that if liability was to be dependent 'on the nature of the particular service rendered' then 'an adequate classification of duties must be supplied and in each case the exact nature of the negligent act alleged sought' (1935 p.247). His Lordship did not follow this approach, as he found it difficult to equate anything a nurse might do with the work of a doctor.

So far as ... I can see, there is no suggestion that the nurse has per se any duties at all that can be classed as professional, if the significance of that term is the same as when applied to the acts of a surgeon. (1935 p.442)

Notwithstanding such criticism, much deliberation occurred about the nature and designation of each particular nursing task. Fragmentation preoccupied the courts until a new approach to the vicarious liability of hospitals rendered it unnecessary in tort cases (Gold v Essex County Council 1942).

The attempts to follow Hillyer and the designation of the application of heat as domestic work

After the decision in Hillyer, there followed a series of civil negligence cases arising from patients sustaining burns due to the alleged acts or omissions of nurses in the provision of heat to the patients. I have called these cases the 'sagas' because of the long and often tortuous attempts to apply the reasoning in Hillyer to the facts of the case.

An early 'burns saga' was the Canadian case of Lavere v Smith's Falls Public Hospital (1915a). The plaintiff, a woman who had undergone surgery for a prolapsed uterus, sustained burns postoperatively due to a heated brick being positioned, allegedly by the nursing staff, too closely to her leg during recovery. At trial the judge held that a hospital is only obligated to select its nursing staff with due care. On appeal (1915b), the judges found an express contract to provide nursing services, and therefore the defendants were liable for the nurse's negligence.

The judges differentiated this case from Farwell LJ's judgment in Hillyer, stating variously that: because the nurse was not physically in the operating theatre she was not under the control of the surgeon, that she was not at this time acting as an agent of the surgeon, and that the nurse was not obeying doctor's orders at that time and was therefore under the control of someone other than the doctor (1915b pp.364–70). Riddell J also distinguished Kennedy LJ on the facts, stating that in Hillyer the plaintiff came to hospital specifically for an examination, whereas in this case there was an express contract to nurse (1915b p.354), for which the plaintiff had paid the sum of £9 per week. In effect, although the situation could be said to be similar to that in Hillyer, and their Lordships felt obligated to follow precedent, they managed to find a number of ways to differentiate the case from it, in order to fix the hospital with liability.

The changing status of the application of heat (but no change to the status of nurses)

Heat was an accepted aspect of patient care, and took a number of different methods, several of which came under the scrutiny of the courts. These included heated bricks (Lavere v Smith's Falls Public Hospital 1915a & 1915b), rubber hot water bottles (Nyberg v Provost Municipal Hospital Board 1927, Davis v Colchester County Hospital 1933, Bernier v Sisters of Service 1948), radiant heat cradles (Logan v Waitaki Hospital Board 1935, Vuchar v Trustees of Toronto General Hospital 1937), and diathermy machines (Fleming v Sisters of St Joseph 1937). Provision of a heated brick was a routine or administrative duty (Lavere 1915a, 1915b).

Initially, hot water bottles were also used as a matter of routine to keep the patient warm, but their status in practice changed as the number of legal problems associated with them increased. However, in Davis v Colchester County Hospital (1933), Mellish J found (p.71) that the purpose of putting a hot water bottle in the bed was for 'warming the bed, not the patient'. By 1948, having a hot water bottle in the bed 'was negligence ... unless with the express orders of Dr Tiffin' (Bernier v Sisters of Service 1948 p.447).

By the late 1930s other methods of applying heat to the patient had appeared. Two methods, which had quite different status, were the use of radiant heat cradles and the diathermy machine. Radiant heat cradles were viewed as being a form of prescribed treatment, and were therefore classified as professional activities. However, diathermy was identified as a form of comfort provision and was therefore classified as routine.

Electric cradles

In Vuchar v Trustees of Toronto General Hospital (1937) the administration of heat via electric cradles was a specific treatment, specifically distinguished from the use of hot water bottles which were routine or domestic work.

It appears to me there is a very clear distinction between the use of the electric cradle as a method of applying heat to the affected part of the patient's body, being an essential part of the prescribed treatment for curing the patient of her disease, and keeping the bed of the patient properly warmed by the use of hot water bottles or other appropriate method. (1937 p.322)

Notwithstanding this distinction, a nurse had a certain amount of discretion in the management of the heat cradle after it had been prescribed, as here the nurse was instructed by the doctor to administer 'as much as a patient can stand'. It was also reported that 'in the absence of instructions from [a doctor] ... it was the duty of the nurse to exercise her own judgment as to the amount of heat to be applied to the patient' (1937 p.323).

The management of an electrical cradle therefore appeared to have two components in terms of apportioning tortious liability. The decision to administer the heat was a professional nursing activity but under the control of the doctor, whereas the act of regulating the heat was a professional nursing activity over which the nurse had control, and in which the doctor could not be implicated. However, since the activity was one in which the nurse was exercising her special skill, then neither could the hospital. Masten JA summed this up rather succinctly stating that 'the term to nurse includes two different classes of acts, viz, acts which are of an administrative or routine character and acts which involve the exercise of professional nursing skill' (1937 p.328).

In Logan v Waitaki Hospital Board (1935) the application of heat via radiant electrical cradle was also held to be a professional nursing activity. Myers CJ in the New Zealand Court of Appeal (1935 p.421) held that 'the application to a patient of the electrical radiant heat cradle ... cannot, it seems to me, be regarded as a mere routine, ministerial or administrative duty. ... she was either carrying out the orders of the doctor or exercising her own discretion in a professional matter. In either case, I think that she was acting professionally'.

Diathermy

Perhaps because the use of the electric cradle was perceived as being a prescribed treatment, this application of heat was differentiated from other new methods, such as diathermy, which were intended to provide comfort and relief from pain. Thus, by contrast, in Fleming v Sisters of St Joseph (1937) the use of a diathermy machine was held to be 'a matter of routine, and ... the giving of this treatment was assumed by the hospital as part of its duty to nurse the patient' (p.128). However, the nurses had a considerable degree of autonomy as to how the diathermy was applied, as the doctor in question did not know anything about its functions.

The diathermy, it was stated, was used only to see if it might relieve the pain. Whether the nurse would have instigated the diathermy treatment had it not been requested by the doctor is not explored in the case, but there is the sense of a nurse clinician with a fairly wide degree of autonomy. In the light of its 'routine' nature, it seems incongruous that the diathermy activity was billed as 'an extra' with a charge for the diathermy of £1 per treatment (1937 p.124). If the activity formed part of the routine activities of the hospital, why was it not included in the standard nursing fee?

This case provides another example of the devaluation of a nursing activity by classifying it as routine or domestic, rather than professional. This classification seems to relate directly to the fact that the activity was nurse- rather than doctor-generated. However, Masten JA hinted at a greater awareness of the extent of the nurses' responsibility than had been acknowledged in the past. He asked the question: 'is the hospital immune from liability for the negligence of its servant, a nurse acting in the exercise of her professional skill but not under the supervision of a surgeon or physician? I have found no case where that state of facts has arisen for determination' (1937 p.130).

Fragmentation of the nursing role, discrediting of nursing stories and the 'false consciousness' problem

The contemporaneous nursing literature on heat application reveals that nurses would have considered that they were acting professionally and autonomously. In fact, the application of heat to the patient was a well-established therapeutic principle for nurses. Nightingale herself had this to say on the matter:

For the sick, warming is a necessary part of ventilation. A careful nurse will keep a constant watch over her sick, especially her weak cases, to guard against the loss of vital heat by the patient himself. In certain diseased states much less heat is produced than in health; and there is a constant tendency to the decline and death of the vital powers by the call made upon them to sustain the heat of the body. Cases where this occurs should be watched with the greatest care from hour to hour and I had almost said from minute to minute. (1952 pp.26–7)

Many different methods of heat application were used. Heat was considered particularly important postoperatively, as many patients were in a shocked condition following surgery (Jamer 1938). A nurse writing in UNA, the journal of the Royal Victorian College of Nursing, in 1938 described the application of warmth as one of the most effective treatments for shock and stated that '[t]he first and most urgent duty of a nurse is to apply carefully protected warmth to a victim suffering from shock' (Anon p.134).

There is no sense in these writings that the application of heat was purely a domestic task, or one which was differentiated from a professional task. It was indeed a routine task, as nurses would have incorporated it into their everyday nursing knowledge and practice. But its routine nature does not prevent it from being a professional task. Taking a routine medical history it is not discounted as non-professional just because in any other environment it might be described as mere conversation; the doctor performs the activity for a particular purpose and brings to it a specific body of knowledge.

The application of heat provides a striking example of the fragmentation of the nursing role. According to the judgments discussed it could either be a routine/domestic activity or a professional activity. There was even a tentative suggestion that it might be a professional activity which nurses performed and controlled. The status of the activity varied from decision to decision over the years, and the determination of its status depended not only on the evidence presented, but on the presenter of the evidence. However, the provision of heat as a prescribed medical 'treatment' was usually found to be a professional act, whereas the provision of heat as a form of nursing 'comfort' was usually held to be routine or domestic. This fits the recognisable stock story—warming beds is domestic work, providing comfort is routine/non-professional, but treating patients is professional.

The provision of comfort as a professional nursing activity

The idea that activities which provided patient comfort were domestic, menial or administrative would also have met with considerable opposition, since nurses have always prided themselves on their ability to make the intolerable tolerable and the unbearable bearable by the provision of comfort.

At the beginning of the 20th century medicine was not always expected to find a cure for people. It was accepted that infectious diseases were rife and mortality rates were high. The reality was that, in cases such as pneumonia, the nurses provided comfort while the disease ran its course. They did not cure the patient, yet the provision of comfort was undoubtedly the pinnacle of nursing skill.

Pneumonias, who now recover in the twinkling of an eye ... with a few doses of penicillin, once required intensive nursing, and nurses prided themselves on the relief they brought and the recoveries they secured. (Even the doctors conceded credit for recoveries to the nurses!) (Armstrong 1965 p.160)

Patients who were injured or sick were nursed carefully in the hope that they would be as strong and as safe as possible to recover by themselves. Nightingale wrote:

What is sickness? Sickness or disease is Nature's way of getting rid of the effects of conditions which have interfered with health. It is Nature's attempt to cure.

We have to help her ... What is Nursing? Both kinds of nursing are to put us in the best possible conditions for Nature to restore or to preserve health—to prevent or to cure disease or injury. Upon nursing proper, under scientific heads, physicians or surgeons, must depend partly, perhaps mainly, whether Nature succeeds or fails in her attempts to cure by sickness. Nursing proper is therefore to help the person suffering from disease to live. (In Seymer 1949 p.357)

Yet the fragmentation of the nursing role persisted in civil negligence cases, with many acts which nurses considered central to their role being devalued as domestic or routine. This produced perhaps the greatest problem: that the story which is not accepted by the court becomes devalued, and the person who told that story loses credibility. As Scheppele states: 'There are few things more disempowering in law than having one's own believed story rejected ... when legal judgments proceed from a description of one's own world that one does not recognise' (1989 p.2090).

Mainstream medical and judicial thought was in contradiction to the way in which nurses perceived their work. Furthermore, these mainstream views became significant for nurses, both in the way they began to view themselves and the way in which they were treated in relation to their pay and conditions. The fragmentation of the nursing role has also had long-term industrial and professional ramifications.

False consciousness and the nature of outsider responses

If this fragmentation had simply occurred in a handful of court decisions relevant only to a number of specific negligence cases, then the effect on nursing might have been minimal. But, as in many other instances, the stories which judges adopted in court were representative of the mainstream stories recognised by society in general. Thus the view that much of nursing work was considered to be lowly or menial was not isolated to the decisions in the courts or tribunals, but reflected 'the way the world is' (Probert 1989 pp.80–81). Nurses, as outsiders, found it difficult to have their professional persona accepted in court, because it was not congruent with the dominant knowledge or viewpoint of the day.

The difficulty for nurses was to decide what to do about their exclusion. To maintain the stance that the entire gamut of nursing work was professional work offered little hope of improved remuneration or status. Carrie Menkel-Meadow argues that women lawyers deal with their exclusion by being 'forced to assimilate into the culture in order to succeed ... In the parlance of feminist scholarship, women must learn to speak in many voices—in other words, to be bilingual in order to be heard' (1987 p.42).

However, being bilingual can create problems of cognitive dissonance (Festinger 1957) particularly if, in order to communicate with the dominant group, outsiders are required to denounce their own beliefs. This causes them to internalise these views and feel ashamed, which can lead to what Matsuda describes as 'false consciousness', a state where 'subordination can obscure as well as illuminate self-knowledge' (Matsuda 1990 p.1777). But it is called 'false consciousness' because outsiders also know that these feelings are wrong. Critical race theorists also use the notion of 'double consciousness' (Du Bois 1903, cited in Delgado 1995 p.7) as a mechanism to explain the way that people of colour view themselves both from their oppressors' perspective as an underclass, and from their own as normal. Similarly, when nurses are caring for patients they are confident of their worth.

Tragically, false consciousness can lead outsiders to despise and devalue themselves, and to subordinate those in their own outsider group who exercise less power. Matsuda explains that 'the long, cold history of subordinated status generating subordinating impulses is well known to both scholars and targets of recycled hate' (1990 p.1777). Certainly the stock storys' denigration of the value of the domestic component of nursing work led to different grades of nurses, with the 'lower orders' or trainees doing much of the denigrated 'domestic' work.

Recycled hate—the phenomenon of bullying

These trainees and 'lower orders' were subject to extreme discipline, to the extent of being bullied. There is evidence to suggest that bullying still occurs, with more senior nurses picking on their staff and making their lives difficult (NSWNA 1999 p.12). Examples of this behaviour include: 'humiliations, put-downs, devaluing of my work within patients' earshot and even, at times, downright insults which I have suffered whilst caring for the sick' (Name & address supplied 1998 p.3).

Such behaviour was originally considered to be character-building for nurses. Gladwin, writing in a text entitled (remarkably) *Ethics: talks to nurses*, expounds the value of a form of ritual humiliation in a chapter on discipline. She cites with approval an example from Kipling of how boys at a great (sic) English public school had to stand on a chair or table and have 'the most outrageous statements and objectionable expressions ... hurled at him'. The idea was that the child who could withstand such insults without showing distress for the longest was the winner. Her opinion on this ritual was that 'the boy or man who comes out of such a contest with credit has obtained freedom from the power of similar happenings to hamper him and has gained something which will help him all his life in anything he may undertake' (1930 pp.157–8).

There seems to have been an ideology within nursing that such humiliation was also necessary for nurses. Certainly nurses need to learn to cope with abuse and harassment from the medical profession, and some older nurses definitely believe that such 'discipline' was in some way good for them or, at the very least, didn't do them any harm (Legge 1998, McKenzie 1998). Perversely, Gladwin's comparison with the English public school system implies that such ritual humiliation is a preparation for some form of elitist future. But for nurses there is no expectation of huge income as a reward.

Cruelty is not uncommon amongst outsider groups, and relates to their lack of self worth, which in turn leads to a lack of self care. Such oppressive behaviour has been described as 'horizontal (or lateral) violence', a term originally used by Fanon (1963) to describe inter-group conflict in colonised Africans as a result of oppression. This behaviour has only recently been made explicit within nursing. It is believed to stem from the experiences of nurses as an oppressed and marginalised group, whose self worth has been damaged by the knowledge and recognition of their lack of control (Duffy, 1995).

In addition, the difficulty with the devaluation of the domestic aspects of nursing work was that it was not congruent with the way in which nurses had (until then) perceived the work which they did. Nurses perceived that it needed to be done, arduous or not. Nurses did not (and do not) find it difficult practically to identify the scope of nursing. When nurses are at the bedside they know what they need to do to nurse, and that is to do whatever is necessary to make the patient's lived experience as tolerable as possible at that moment in time. To this end they may (still) carry out basic bodily care, delegated medical tasks, physiotherapy, massage, counselling or cleaning. This is because nursing, as the term suggests, requires nurses to focus on the needs of the individual, rather than on the tasks needing to be done. This approach was, of course, first described by Florence Nightingale, but came into popular articulation with the introduction of the nursing process in the 1970s (e.g. Marriner 1975).

The difficulties have arisen for nurses when their work has come under scrutiny in a legal or industrial construct. Then they have discovered that on the occasions when they spoke, their voice was not only different (Gilligan 1982), it simply did not fit any of the dominant constructs of professional or industrial knowing. They have had to learn other 'languages' to explain the work that they did for the purposes of recognition or remuneration. In trying to find a 'language' which might describe the nursing role, the nurse leaders had to comply with the 'stock stories' which existed in society, namely that there were professionals (who didn't get their hands dirty) and there were menials (who did). Thus, they had to divide the nursing role into a collection of tasks, which might be recognisable to the courts and tribunals as either professional (because doctors might do them) or domestic (because servants or housemaids might do them).

Nurses' adaptation to the fragmentation of their role

Emphasising the medical and discarding the para-nursing work

To a certain extent, nurses took their lead from the early court decisions and attempted to align their work with changes in medical practice, in order to achieve professional recognition and remuneration. Numerous tasks, initially undertaken by nurses but held not to be professional, such as managing food and diets (Hillyer 1909, Reidford v Magistrates of Aberdeen 1933), providing comfort via diathermy machines (Fleming v Sisters of St Joseph 1937), and performing X-rays (Abel v Cooke 1938) were relegated to other staff. The people who adopted them became known as dietitians, physiotherapists and radiographers respectively, and most achieved the 'holy grail' of professional status long before nurses. These professions were described as para-medical professions (e.g. Gardner 1995), but it is suggested that they were actually para-nursing professions, because their roles developed from aspects of nursing care.

Trying to deal with the domestic aspects of nursing work

As the century progressed, the nursing leaders employed different strategies in relation to the 'domestic' aspects of their work to increase their remuneration through the industrial courts and tribunals. First they claimed such work as nursing work, and sought to have its arduous nature acknowledged and rewarded (In re Hospital Nurses (State) Award 1936b p.252). As these strategies were unsuccessful, those leaders came to denounce as domestic work those aspects of nursing care they had previously so zealously guarded, and distanced themselves from it.

In reality nurses still undertake work which could be classified as domestic work in the name of patient care (St Basil's Nursing Home v Eliza Duff-Tytler 1993). But because many have internalised the belief that such work is non-professional, this only adds to their feelings of lack of self worth.

The introduction of the second level nurse in the United Kingdom (UK)

Another response to the 'problem' of domestic work was to adopt the notion of a second level nurse. By the mid-1930s the nature of nursing work was beginning to change dramatically, with the introduction of antibiotics and increasing technology used by the medical profession. This led to a concomitant increase in the technology which nurses were using (Armstrong 1965, Bernier v Sisters of Service 1948). There was a shortage of nurses at this time (Abel-Smith 1960) and entrants to nursing were becoming increasingly better educated (Abel-Smith 1960 p.152). These well educated entrants were now the majority and, perhaps because of their own world views, were not as willing to undertake the domestic duties as their working class predecessors had been (Abel-Smith 1960).

Thus, throughout the 1920s and 1930s, there were changes to the work of nurses, with some of the cleaning duties being transferred to other staff (Abel-Smith 1960). In the UK the Athlone Committee proposed that a new grade of staff should be introduced to take on these activities and basic nursing care in chronic and long-stay environments, due to the nursing shortage and the expansion of nursing work (Ministry of Health 1939). Representatives of the nursing profession, especially the College of Nursing, initially resisted the notion of a second grade of nurse, since 'one portal of entry to nursing' was almost sacrosanct (Abel-Smith 1960 p.148). However, fearing a shortfall in the nursing workforce, the College insisted that these new staff should have their training and assessment adminis-tered by nursing (Abel-Smith 1960 pp.157–9). Thus, there was now a second grade of nurse to do, amongst other things, the cleaning. To many this move was heresy, but in my view the reality was that Nightingale's attitude to her 'Lady Probationers' created a second grade of nurse from the outset.

The use of student nurses and assistants in nursing for domestic work in Australia

Another response by nurses was to delegate domestic work to student nurses and unqualified nursing assistants. In Australia the introduction of enrolled nurse training did not occur concurrently with events in England. Instead, registered nurse training was extended to four or even five years, thus providing a lengthy training period where cheap labour was available. In addition, unqualified assistant nursing staff, who had always been repre-sented unofficially by the New South Wales Nurses' Association (NSWNA), were included in the 1936 NSW State Award. By 1942 the membership eligi-bility rule of the NSWNA was amended to include these unqualified staff, who were (and still are) known as assistants in nursing (AINs) (Dickenson 1993). Enrolled (second level) nurses were not introduced into Australia until the 1980s following the recommendations of the Truskett and Sax Reports (Dickenson 1993).

In 1953 in NSW, the NSWNA sought specific exemptions for nurses from 'domestic duties' in the Hospital Nurses (State) Award 'unless the work was necessary for the prevention of infection or required in an isolation ward'. The exception to this was to be first year student nurses, and other nurses when no domestic staff were available (1953 p.328). Notwithstanding this development, cleaning duties were still included in the role of pre-registration students until well into the 1970s in both Australia (Dickenson 1993) and the United Kingdom (Sadler 1990), and even after the concept of supernumerary status had been introduced for student nurses in Australia.

The retention of cleaning duties for nursing students in Australia is illustrated in an industrial case (Re Hedley Gordon Rowe and Capital Territory Health Commission, Re Judith Adella Cooney and Capital Territory Health Commission ACT 1982). The case was brought on behalf of two students in nursing who were undertaking the first two-year programme for 'supernumerary' students leading to registration as a first level graduate. Instead of being paid as student nurses under the local nursing award they were paid a stipend, which was considered to be a scholarship based on their supernumerary status but was considerably less than the award rate.

Keely J held that the students, regardless of any supernumerary status, worked on the wards in exactly the same manner as any other staff member, and were entitled to remuneration under the award. The types of tasks they regularly performed included 'cleaning bedside tables and lockers, scrubbing bed frames after the discharge of patients, participating in dusting rounds and bed making rounds throughout the ward … washing bed pans (as distinct from making necessary observations)' (1981 p.397). The nurse educator defended the practice of students undertaking this work, arguing that 'provided a function is related to the care of a patient or patients it is part of the learning experience'. This 'patient-centred' view is one that prevails today, although now it is generally used to defend the practice of skilled nurses undertaking advanced practice tasks. This case also indicates how deeply entrenched was the belief amongst senior nurses that cleaning ought to be part of a nurse's education because, if it was related to the patient, it was part of patient care.

The introduction of other 'caring' staff

This routine or domestic work has since been picked up by other grades of health workers—originally assistants in nursing and domestic staff but more recently patient care attendants, community care workers, home helps, home care attendants and others. Nurses are now trying to engage in a relationship with these workers to ensure that nurses retain a position of control over the basic nursing care which many of the non-nurses now deliver (Home Care Services (NSW), ACCNS (NSW) & NSWNA 1991, Nurses Board of South Australia 1993, QNC 1998).

This continued erosion of the patient-focused nursing role has been detrimental to the nursing profession. Because so many non-nurses were undertaking work which was originally part of the focus of nursing care, nurses were at risk of losing their identity. As specialisation occurred in the para-professions, so registered nurses in charge of wards found themselves increasingly becoming the coordinators and managers, rather than the deliverers, of care (Keatinge 1995 p.415). A further irony has been that when these para-(nursing) professionals are either not present or not available, nurses still undertake these particular skills, for the very reason that it is in the best interests of the patients that they do. Examples of these include physiotherapy (Ministerial Reference Case 1986), radiography (In re Public Hospital Nurses (State) Award 1971), and pharmacy (The Poisons and Therapeutic Goods Regulations 1994 (NSW) s.63). Nurses also still undertake cleaning and domestic duties when it is in the patient's best interests that they do (Anon 1998b).

The long-term consequences of the fragmentation of the nursing role

A further problem has arisen, indicating that, as in 1909, the desire to protect dwindling health care budgets continues to plague nurses today. Long after nursing's struggle for professional recognition and portability, even today nursing care is allocated to non-nurses because they are cheaper to employ than nurses, and more plentiful (Serghis 1998).

The acceptance of a task-centred approach to patient care in compensation cases

The most significant contemporary legal settings where fragmentation of nursing care occurs are the compensation cases, where the objective has been to limit the financial liability of insurance companies. These decisions exemplify the way in which the nursing role is devalued. There is no concept of a 'professional relationship' between the nurse and the patient, as there is with medicine. There is only the concept of a number of tasks which have to be performed for the patient, and then an allocation of those tasks to either qualified or unqualified staff.

These cases are significant because rarely are nurses called to give evidence on the victim's nursing requirements. It is irrelevant that the injured parties are seeking funding for nursing care, some of which is specifically requested to be delivered by a registered nurse. Many of the cases are concerned with ascertaining whether the nursing care required fits within a particular statutory definition. The nature of nursing is often acknowledged in its breadth and then restricted in its interpretation, usually either due to financial implications or on the basis of medical evidence.

Defining nursing work when the work under scrutiny is not even to be performed by a nurse

In Thomas v Ferguson Transformers P/L (1979) the delineation between domestic work and nursing work was explored to determine a Worker's Compensation award. Significantly none of the work in question was being performed by a nurse. The case was heard on appeal from a decision of the

Worker's Compensation Commission, which made a compensation award to a spastic paraplegic woman who lived with her husband. Her medical adviser had recommended that it would be better for her long-term health if she could remain at home. The judge had made a number of orders including that 'the cost of household assistance to the [woman]' be met by the respondent (1979 p.218).

The question was whether the 'household assistance provided by the carer Mrs Walters fell within the definition of "nursing care"' under the relevant statute, as this was the only way that her employment expenses could be recovered. At the original hearing, the judge held that, because of the intent behind the assistance, it fell within the ambit of nursing work. He explained:

There is a very strong element, here, of two people working together, on numerous single factors, directly related to the prescription of Dr Yeo that the applicant herself should do as much of her former domestic tasks as is humanly possible for her. The view that I have formed is that, even with Mrs Walters being present and standing by, it would be highly unlikely that the applicant, totally unaided, could do any significant part of the domestic work at all. On that basis, in my view, the sort of assistance that has been rendered by Mrs Walters should be classified as nursing. (1979 p.221)

This decision was overturned in the NSW Court of Appeal. Two judges relied on a 1977 decision where it was held that 'it would ... be a misuse of language to call a person who did housework for an incapacitated person a nurse, or to describe the work done as nursing, merely because of the state of health of the employer' (Pennant Hills Restaurants Pty Ltd v Barrell Insurances Pty Ltd 1977 p.841).

The majority of the Court of Appeal held that it was not the recipient's status that determined whether an activity constituted nursing. 'The fact that the incapacitated person is better because she can perform domestic tasks with the domestic working with her does not turn the domestic servant into a nurse' (Thomas v Ferguson Transformers P/L 1979 p.221).

One judge (Mahoney JA) disagreed with the majority decision not to identify the work as nursing. However, neither did he accept that 'aid in the doing of domestic work is nursing, merely because [it] will have a therapeutic effect on the applicant, and she cannot do that work without help' (1979 p.223).

However, he considered that if the work performed by Mrs Walters had been analysed, the applicant might have successfully claimed for that portion of the work which was nursing. Despite the fact that he referred to a dictionary for a definition of nursing, rather than any nursing literature, his process for defining nursing could be construed as a patient-focused approach. He went into some detail about his reasoning for the reference of any future claims and devised a two-fold test for the identification of nursing work.

The question is, in my opinion, not to be solved merely by determining whether acts are 'domestic assistance': there is no rigid determination between domestic assistance and nursing. In determining whether acts that are done are nursing, it will normally be necessary to look to at least two things; the nature of the acts done and the purpose for which or the context in which they are done. There may, no doubt, be some acts which, whatever their purpose, cannot constitute nursing. But there are, in my opinion, acts which take on the character of nursing, according to whether they are done for the appropriate purpose. Thus, I do not doubt that a person who, by injury, has been rendered grossly defective mentally, may be seen to receive nursing from one who prepares his meals, cleans his home, and generally attends to those personal needs which, because of his condition, he cannot properly attend to himself. (1979 p.224)

The judge's definition of nursing has similarities with that of the famous nurse scholar Virginia Henderson (1969) in that he looked to the intent of the act undertaken rather than to the nature of the specific task in question. This case raises several issues for nursing as a profession, however, despite the fact (or perhaps because of the fact) that no nurses were involved.

Defining nursing as a medical prescription

In the first instance decision the judge suggested that it was the medical prescription of the domestic assistance which turned the act into nursing (1979 p.221). The assumption that nursing is something which doctors pre-scribe for patients was not new to this case (In re Public Hospital Nurses (State) Award 1967). However, the judgment highlighted the fact that ther-apy is a broad concept, and that if it proved difficult to determine what might be therapeutic for a patient, the act of prescription might legitimise it. Such a view could create a reliance on the presence or sanction of a doctor to determine whether an act is nursing. This bears some similarity to the early decisions in Hillyer and the 'burns sagas' where an act of a nurse was deemed to be professional if it were performed under the control of a doctor.

Finding the nursing in the work

On appeal it was suggested that the way to determine whether an act con-stituted nursing was to examine the work of the carer and to 'dissect what she does, so that the cost of the nursing can be ascertained' (1979 p.224). Fragmenting nursing work was not a new concept. The civil negligence courts had done so previously in the early 20th century, and nurses had distanced themselves professionally and industrially from the domestic aspects of their role in their aspirations to better status and remuneration. This dissection into nursing and non-nursing duties was consistent with the dominant mind set of the day.

Sanctioning the practice of nursing by non-nurses

But the most critical consequence of the fragmentation in this case is the explicit sanctioning of the practice of nursing by a non-nurse. Under the existing registration statute it was an offence for anyone to hold themselves out or otherwise infer that they were a registered or enrolled nurse. If its purpose was to protect the public from unskilled people practising nursing, such legislation becomes farcical in the light of this judgment.

Nursing defined by the intent to nurse

Why has the accepted methodology for identifying when a nurse is required been a form of task hierarchy, rather than an adoption of patient-centred care? Perhaps it is because there has never been any clear public understanding of what nursing entails. There is no doubt that this case identifies the difficulty in confining nursing to the domain of nurses, since caring cannot be the exclusive prerogative of one group, professional or otherwise. But professional nursing is far more than just good-hearted kindness or domestic duties. It is both an art and a science, and an amalgam of skilled care and technical expertise.

Here Mahony JA and Virginia Henderson diverge for one reason. Mrs Walters was not a nurse. Henderson argued that to turn nursing care over to relatively unqualified personnel carried two dangers. The unqualified person may not be able to assess the patient's needs properly; and the qualified nurse, being unable to have the same regular access to the patient, may not have a chance to make a proper assessment (Henderson 1969 p.13).

Even if nurses might have had concerns about an unqualified carer undertaking tasks the courts identified as nursing, there were none present to express them. A medical practitioner gave the evidence about the nursing care required.

The definition of nursing by its association with medicine

In the later High Court decision in Pennant Hills Restaurants Pty Ltd v Barrell Insurances Pty Ltd (1979–80) the question arose again, namely whether domestic assistance constituted 'nursing' within the meaning of the relevant statute. The High Court of Australia held that 'domestic assistance' in the form of 'bed making, cleaning, laundering and cooking' required by the injured worker was not 'nursing' within the meaning of the Act (1979–80 p.626).

Mason J held that because nursing was included under the definition of medical treatment, the term related only to 'care and attention to a patient which is designed to relieve or remedy the illness from which he suffers' (1979–80 p.682). Murphy J also held that the domestic assistance in question did not fall within the definition of medical treatment within the act, but conceded that it was 'not to state that the activities now in question could not form part of "nursing" in a different context. Some of them may be capable of falling within that term if they were incidental to or directly associated with "nursing" in the strict sense' (1979–80 p.686).

Although there was no further elaboration on the meaning of nursing 'in the strict sense', there was again the propensity to align 'real' nursing to medicine, rather than to care, although an alignment to care does not seem to fall outside the statutory definition. This concept that nursing care is legitimised only by the sanction or presence of a doctor is a recurrent problem for the professional identity of nurses.

Nursing qualifications: not necessarily a guide to competence

A recent compensation case which brings the problems of progressive fragmentation and professional non-recognition to a climax is the unreported NSW Supreme Court decision in Lee v McLennan (1995). The plaintiff was claiming damages for quadriplegia and other injuries sustained during a motor vehicle accident in 1990. Liability was admitted. The major component of the claim was for future domestic care, being a claim of $3 774 430, and for future nursing care, being a claim of $1 044 390. The plaintiff was claiming that he required the assistance of a live-in couple, but also 'nursing assistance morning and night' (1995 p.13).

There were a number of activities which the plaintiff claimed should be performed by a registered nurse, including monitoring of skin integrity, bladder and catheter care, and bowel management. No nurses were reported as having given evidence on nursing care. However, two doctors, Dr B and Dr Y, gave evidence on the relative merits of a registered nurse or an unregistered 'carer' undertaking these activities.

Dr B gave evidence that the development of pressure sores would not necessarily be obvious to a non-registered nurse. Dr Y conceded on cross-examination that a properly trained lay person could recognise their onset. Dr Y suggested that a registered nurse needed to empty the bladder properly at night in order to avoid autonomic dysreflexia, but also acknowledged that such consequences did not often occur because of the level of patient and carer education. Concerning the management of bowel care, Dr B gave evidence that the risks of enemas were much reduced if a professional person administered them because of that person's greater knowledge of anatomy, physiology and pharmacology. However, in cross-examination he conceded that some patients had been taught to administer their own enemas. It was also suggested that it might be less embarrassing for Mr Lee if the person who undertook such care were not the person who prepared his meals and looked after him generally. However, Hulme J noted in his judgment that not all the evidence provided by the medical experts supported the need for qualified nurses.

Dr Y accepted that in some situations, not I think infrequent, care by persons not qualified can be carried out very adequately and that at times registered nurses were deficient. When I take all the evidence on this topic into consideration, it seems to me that providing there exists an appropriate level of training in the matters of concern, the competence and care of the person looking after the patient in the respects mentioned is more important than the formal qualifications of the person. (1995 p.16)

His Honour proffered some gratuitous remarks of his own on the question of nursing qualifications.

Furthermore, the evidence does not satisfy me that the fact of formal qualifications is either a strong indication of greater care or competence in the respects important here or such an indication that the extra cost of the course proposed on the plaintiff's behalf is justified. It seems to be that too much emphasis was placed on the proposition that registered nurses were 'professionals'. (1995 p.16)

The desire to limit the liability of insurance companies

A readiness to substitute unqualified staff for registered nurses is not confined to this case (see also Burford v Allan 1997). There can be no doubt that the argument to use unqualified personnel would stem from the desire to reduce the burden to the insurance company. In these cases, the evidence against using registered nurses has not been led by the plaintiffs, who have sought registered nurse care, presumably because that was what they wished to receive. Rather it has been led by the defendants, whose insurance companies would have been seeking to limit their costs. Some eighty-six years after the judgment in Hillyer, it can be seen that nursing care still falls subject to fragmentation and dissection for the express purpose of limiting liability or the quantum of payable damages.

The disregard of professional nursing qualifications

The readiness of courts and tribunals to devalue and dissect nursing work, and their apparent disregard for the professional education and training of nurses are extraordinary. One cannot imagine lawyers or doctors accepting the same argument about the portability of their skills to another unskilled group of workers. A proposition that, because the quality of service delivered by some doctors or lawyers might not be very good, it would be acceptable to substitute lay people would hardly be supported by either of these professions. (The resistance, in Australia, from lawyers to unqualified conveyancers provides an example of this.) It would be viewed as impertinence, as an affront. Furthermore, neither profession would take kindly to a member of another profession making such a pronouncement about them. Finally, the absence of a registered nurse witness meant that some important areas of nursing care, such as prevention, rather than detection of pressure sores, and patient counselling and education (two critical issues for the chronically handicapped) were not addressed at all; yet they would have been significant aspects of skilled nursing care.

The influence of medical voices and the absence of nursing voices

One cannot help but wonder why Hulme J in Lee v McLennan (1995) chose to adopt such a strident and unsympathetic approach. It is acknowledged that the cross-examination of both doctors by the defendant counsel would be aimed at reducing the award of damages and would focus on the minimisation of the cost of the care. His Honour had also expressed a degree of dissatisfaction with the truthfulness of the plaintiff, and did not describe him in particularly sympathetic terms. But the care under scrutiny was central to the plaintiff's long-term well-being, and the poor management of this care would have dire physical consequences for the plaintiff—such as diarrhoea, pressure sores, severe sweating and headaches, and faecal incontinence. Dr B appeared committed to such care being delivered by a registered nurse, and was described as only 'conceding' some of the points put to him on cross-examination.

Dr Y gave evidence to the effect that he was actively involved in the training of carers, and that they were able to give excellent care. His concessions and evidence about the care requirements of the patient may have influenced the judge in his determinations.

Why were nurses not called to give evidence on what appears to be a strictly nursing matter? The matter under review by the court was the amount of money to be allocated for an express claim for nursing care to be delivered by a registered nurse. Yet medical witnesses were called to advise on the matter, rather than nursing witnesses. Was it felt, perhaps, that nurses would be unable to be objective about whether this patient required care by a nurse or a carer? If so, then that is a harsh indictment of the ability of nurses to be objective; it is not a criticism that would be sustained against other professionals, who are called upon regularly to give evidence about their own profession's work.

Such an expectation of bias is recognised as being one of the difficulties which outsider groups encounter when they are asked to give evidence about members of their own group. In the essay, 'The rules of racial standing', in his book *Faces at the Bottom of the Well* Derrick Bell describes this expectation in the second rule:

This phenomenon reflects a widespread assumption that blacks, unlike whites, cannot be objective on racial issues and will favor (sic) their own no matter what. This deep-seated belief fuels a continuing effort—despite all manner of Supreme Court decisions intended to curb the practice—to keep black people off juries in cases involving race. Black judges hearing racial cases are eyed suspiciously and sometimes asked to recuse themselves in favor of a white judge—without those making the request even being aware of the paradox in their motions. (1992 p.113)

Perhaps the decision to use a doctor to give evidence about a patient's need for nursing care was tacit acceptance of the belief that doctors know all about medicine and nursing—that nursing is simply an arm of medicine.

The failure to seek a professional opinion from a nurse is based on a lack of knowledge about the nursing role and on the silence and invisibility of nurses. The stock story remains that nursing work is not skilled; and that anyone who has a kind heart, who is receptive to instruction, and can perform domestic tasks, can undertake nursing work. Hulme J made this explicit when he stated that 'the competence and care of the person looking after the patient in the respects mentioned is more important than the formal qualifications of the person'. Despite many changes to nursing education and practice over this century, it is clear that the stock story identified at the beginning of this chapter still prevails, and that nursing is still not accepted as a professional role with a patient-focused approach to care.

POOR PAYMENT AND WORKING CONDITIONS: THE INFLUENCE OF THE DOMESTIC WORKER IMAGE?

Having examined the consequences of the fragmentation of the nursing role, this chapter finally explores the effect of the domestic worker designation on the nurses' pay and living conditions. The specific context of this exploration is the NSW industrial awards between 1936, the year of the first NSW nurses' award, and 1967, the year when nursing militancy first became apparent in NSW. This analysis would nevertheless be applicable to many other countries of the Nightingale nursing tradition.

Poor incomes for nurses in the early part of this century

One hundred years ago, the earning potential of nurses working in hospitals was limited. Nightingale's nurses took charge of the Infirmaries, established under the Poor Laws (Seymer 1949 p.129), which cared for indigent patients (Russell 1990 p.7). Hospitals, despite Nightingale's interventions, were not places in which the wealthy would choose to be treated and nursed.

Even after training, nurses had little control over their wage-fixing ability. Many worked privately, obtaining placements through an agency, and a few either worked independently in the community or established small private nursing homes (Wilson & Pearn 1988 pp.221–230). Usually the training hospitals also functioned as the agencies which provided domiciliary nurses, charging the client a fee, but paying the nurses a fixed salary

(Seymer 1949 pp.226–7). Nurses usually worked in and were paid by the hospitals, although unusually patients might bring a private nurse in with them, or a doctor might seek a specialist nurse to care for a patient. Doctors also practised privately, and their appointments to hospitals were either as Visiting Medical Officers to private patients, or as Honorary doctors undertaking *pro bono* work for the indigent.

Despite the potential for nurses to work as private professional practitioners, they did not achieve significant salaries. The income of such a nurse was only 109 per cent of the average earnings (Haralambos & Heald 1985 p.70), whereas a doctor earned 230 per cent of the average earnings. During the Depression, private nursing decreased significantly (Seymer 1949 p.228).

The beginning of the award system: poor pay and conditions remain

When the first NSW nurses' pay award (In re Hospital Nurses' (State) & c (State) Conciliation Committee 1936a) (which was actually reduced on appeal) was handed down, a fourth year student nurse, who would have delivered most of the skilled nursing care, was awarded £60 a year. The working hours for all nurses were accepted as necessarily much longer; no allowance was made for weekend work, night shifts or overtime; and £2 per week was deducted for board and lodgings. A typist, a laundress and a hospital telephonist all earned similar wages, but these staff would have worked a standard 44 hour week, and their responsibilities were incomparable (Dickenson 1993 p.59).

Clearly the vocational nature of nursing work significantly influenced the first award decisions of Webb J at first instance and the New South Wales Industrial Commission on appeal. The references to sacrifice and devotion have been discussed in Chapter 3, as has the 'guilt factor' in wage fixing. However, other factors in the award-fixing principles related to the type of work undertaken.

Reasons for poor pay and conditions: women's work?

Notwithstanding any concept of market forces, the most likely reason that nurses were so poorly paid was, as Ethel Bedford Fenwick said in 1913, because 'the nurse question is the woman question' (Dock & Stewart 1938 p.254). Despite the express judicial opinion (discussed in Chapter 3) that caring for the sick was a privilege in itself which required no greater reward, the real reason why nursing work continued to be undervalued was gender discrimination. 'Domestic work' has long been undervalued at law, particularly in the home, since housework was only recently accepted as a head of economic loss. Previously it was held that housework was voluntary work, and thus not compensable per se (Chesterman 1983, Graycar 1985). Much of the work described in the case law, such as cleaning, feeding patients, preparing meals and providing heat as a form of comfort, would also be recognisable as work a wife or domestic servant would perform.

Reasons for poor pay and conditions: student nurses as 'professionals in waiting'?

The NSW 1936 award was nursing's first attempt to address remuneration for their domestic work. Nurses seemed to have acknowledged its stigma, and its relegation to the 'lower orders' in nursing. But at this stage they sought to reward those, especially students, who undertook it, not to remove it from the nursing role.

It seemed initially that Webb J might be sympathetic to these claims for students. He acknowledged the reasons why higher rates of pay might be awarded (e.g. climatic conditions, the risk of infections, 'the arduous nature of the work') but then determined that the awards should be fixed at an amount closest to the lowest rates currently being paid across the state. Remarkably, he based his decision on his opinion that student nurses were 'receiving free to themselves a necessary course of training which will enable them to enter the profession of nursing' (1936a p.92). The implication is that student nurses, the mainstay of the hospital workforce, contributed nothing.

This finding was upheld on appeal. The NSWNA appealed that these trainee rates were too low, given the 'arduous physical nature of their work, much of which involved cleaning and feeding', particularly in first and second years. They recommended that the work should be assessed at its commercial value as laborious work, and then provision made for the fact that they were receiving a training whilst undertaking the work. But the Full Bench did not accept this, and expressed its view on the good fortune of the trainees.

In our opinion trainees in this calling should be regarded as pupils in a profession rather than employees in an industry. The evidence shows us that at many of the larger hospitals there are extensive waiting lists of women anxious to become trainees in hospitals in which women receive no payment at all. We are satisfied that the work which the trainees are required to do is not more than is proper and necessary for them to do in order to qualify as nurses. There is no evidence that any hospital has exploited these young women by requiring them to perform arduous work under the guise of training but unnecessary therefore, or that any system exists of using trainees as a cheap method of getting the necessary work of the hospitals done. Indeed, it was not suggested by anyone that such a state of things existed. (Hospital Nurses State Award 1936b pp.252–3)

If no evidence of exploitation had been put to their Honours, why did they need to deny its existence so vehemently? The decision to treat trainees as 'professionals in waiting' might have been defensible if the award for trained nurses had reflected this professional remuneration. But the appeal decision was equally miserly for trained nurses. It reduced their annual leave allowances, and did not regularise the differences in hours worked between hospitals, even though in some hospitals nurses worked up to 84 hours per week.

This award and its rationale must have presented the NSWNA with a dilemma. They were aware that to obtain professional status, they needed a different approach to the domestic aspects of their work. They had been told that they were a profession, not an industry. However, as professionals, they could not claim just remuneration for the domestic, arduous work their trainees did, as it was part of the required training for 'professionals in waiting'. Further, they could not claim substantial remuneration on gradu-ation because this might have diverted funds away from the very services they were trained to give, which might in turn cause patients to die. The nurses' arguments, regardless of whether the nurses were 'bilingual', were simply disregarded (Menkel-Meadow 1987 p.42).

Reasons for poor pay and conditions: the family wage-fixing system?

Industrially, nurses' problems were further compounded by the fact that the wage-fixing system was based on the concept of the 'family wage.' The pay for an average worker was determined on the needs of a man, his wife and his three children (Ex parte H v McKay 1907, Rural Workers' Union v Mildura Branch of the Australian Dried Fruits Association 1912). Female general nurses did not receive equal pay status with men until 1973 (Dickenson 1993 p.123). This was despite the fact that trainee nurses were not allowed to marry or become engaged until the 1970s, and thus could not possibly be supported.

Short-lived post-war improvements

Until the award of Kinsella J (In re Public Hospital Nurses (State) Award 1947), nurses' awards in NSW were predicated on the premise that the male was the family breadwinner. The basic wage for women was fixed at 54 per cent of the male rate because men alone were assumed to have family responsibilities. A change of attitude occurred, however, in 1947. It was con-sistent with a general recognition at the end of World War II of the working roles which women had played in wartime. Patsy Adam-Smith explained that women had 'worked long hours in factories, on farms and in a hun-dred more jobs that had not been available to women before this war. Never before had Australia's women been so emancipated from the tyranny of the home, family and conventional society' (1996 p.270).

In the post-war period there was considerable unrest amongst the nursing profession, fuelled in part by the first unsatisfactory pay award in 1936. The 1947 award decision took heed of the nurses and made an award decision which improved pay and conditions, gave nurses a career structure and relieved them of some of the routine or domestic duties. Kinsella J applied to the nurses 'exactly the same principles as would be applied in the making of any other award' (1947 p.256). He expressed his inability to understand why: 'the fact that the work in hospitals is not industry in the ordinary sense, but … the provision of healing services to the sick, has any bearing on the rates proper to be paid to the persons who render these services' (1947 p.285).

Medical concern over nursing industrialism

Some doctors expressed concern that seeking improved pay and conditions might herald an undesirable change in attitude amongst nurses. An impassioned plea to resist this, which makes reference to the domestic nature of nurses as 'home-makers', was made in a popular nursing journal. The text is included here because of its relationship to nursing industrialism, but it is also relevant to the ministering angel image and its potential as a subordinating influence is clear. Paradoxically at the time the plea was made the average earnings of doctors had risen to 220 per cent of the average wage, whereas that of nurses had fallen below the average wage (Haralambos & Heald 1985 p.70).

[A] great attempt has been made in this age to assert the importance of material values as against moral and spiritual values. Deep down it is the sense of spiritual values which makes people so important as distinct from things. But today, pressure is exerted to make things more important than people … Today the nursing profession is, at long last, being offered the means to illuminate its difficult path—shorter hours, less restrictions, better salary, more relief from domestic duties, and, we hope, more nurses soon. All these things are absolutely right and absolutely necessary. But in winning the lesser, do not lose the greater! You must not for one moment underestimate your place in the nation's life. You can bring a great illumination into a dark age. The old lamp which lit the way for the early nursing pioneers—that is the only lamp which works miracles. It needs rubbing hard. It needs to be kept fresh and clean. It needs to be replenished daily with new spirit. In its light men and women see that people come before things. Only by its light can your profession fulfil its great destiny—to be pathfinders and peacemakers in making the world a home for mankind. (Luxton 1947 pp.29–30)

The 1950s: the awards of Richards J

After the war, because of the imperative to make jobs available for returning soldiers, the emancipation of nurses and the recognition of the value of their work was short-lived. Careers in nursing became secondary to careers as wives and mothers, and women in general were relegated to the private sphere again. The Australian army chaplain advised thus:

The vocation of the majority of young women is that of HOME BUILDER and their share in the spreading of God's Kingdom. The girl of today is the BRIDE, the WIFE and the MOTHER of tomorrow. She may type for 2, 3, 4 years, but children and work in the home is her LIFE'S WORK. (In Adam-Smith 1996 p.272)

In such an environment the material gains made by the nurses in the 1947 award were not to 'threaten' their moral fibre for long. The 1950s were significantly less successful for nurses in the industrial arena.

In the 1953 award Richards J reverted to the view expressed in the original nurses award (Hospital Nurses State Award 1936b), that nurses were unique because they dealt with the lives of sick people, and considered their conditions and prospects already favourable and privileged.

Throughout the 1950s nurses' pay status decreased again. There was a demonstration of dissatisfaction by the NSWNA members about the 1953 award, in which the rates of pay increased less than the deductions for board and lodging, effecting an overall reduction in pay (Dickenson 1993 p.128). Richards J also refused to pay nurses for attending lectures in their pre-clinical block, because 'they were not employees for whom the Commission would have jurisdiction to make an award' (Hospital Nurses (State) Award 1953 p.312). He believed the trainees were fortunate to be receiving the lectures free of charge.

Student nurses, as the name implies, are nurses undergoing a course of study and training to qualify them for a career as trained nurses. Their qualifications, once obtained, will endure for life-time, the opportunities of advancement offered by the profession are great, and the industry may be correctly described as a career industry. (Hospital Nurses (State) Award 1953 p.393)

Admittedly most students are not paid during their undergraduate years and so, arguably, to expect trainees to be paid during lectures was not commensurate with their aspirations to professional status. But the recurrent problem for nurses has been the desire to be treated as professionals, and the concomitant failure to achieve corresponding professional rewards on graduation.

Although medical students were not paid to attend their lectures, neither were they expected to be an integral part of the workforce. Miller, writing of his undergraduate experiences in the 1920s, explained that assisting with the dressings was regarded as an opportunity, rather than an obligation, and observed that '[m]any students never did such things' (1985 p.17). In contrast, he noted that when he became a resident medical officer, nurse trainees were integral to the workforce, although then unpaid (1985 p.31).

By 1959, student nurses received a salary and were the mainstay of the nursing workforce. In the 1959 award, Richards J acknowledged that student nurses undertook 'important and valuable work at the hospital' (p.393) but considered that their conditions were favourable. Even despite this value, once they finished training they had no security of employment (Willis v Townsville Hospitals Board 1966). Mass resignations were threatened in December 1959 on the receipt of another unfavourable award decision and ultimately a crisis was averted when the Industrial Commission granted a 28 per cent salary increase following a meeting between the NSWNA and the Labor Premier, R J Heffron (Dickenson 1993 p.129).

Even if similar pay and conditions had prevailed for medical students and interns at the same time, a significant difference lies not in the treatment of students in terms of their study conditions, but in the career expectations of the graduates. By 1955/56 the average pay for a doctor or 'higher professional' was 191 per cent of the simple average for all men (sic), whereas the average pay for a nurse or 'lower professional' was 75 per cent of the average pay (Haralambos & Heald 1985 p.70). Riach, writing in 1969, in the early days of the feminist movement, suggested that the only reason women still entered nursing was because it was one of a small number of careers open to them, and this limitation of careers meant that women became a captive workforce.

The consequence of this limited range of employment opportunities is that females can be retained in many jobs at rates of pay which are lower than those necessary to attract and/or retain males, who have higher alternative earnings available to them in jobs which are either difficult or impossible for females to enter. If females were free to enter and progress in all areas of the labour market with the same ease as males we would expect that at current relative salary levels many potential nurses, social workers, etc would switch towards such male-dominated professions as architecture, law, etc. (Riach 1969 p.100)

A possible positive consequence of poor pay: the futility of suing nurses directly

Significantly, in the early 20th century, despite dicta which stated that hospitals were not liable for the professional acts of nurses (Hillyer 1909, Vuchar v Trustees of Toronto General Hospital 1937), nurses were rarely held personally liable for their professional acts. Although there may have been a reluctance to sue an 'angel', the most probable reason was the relatively shallow pocket of the nurse. If nurses had been held to be personally liable, it is unlikely they would have had the means to pay. In the early days of nurse training, those probationers who were destined for management positions paid for the privilege of learning how to nurse (Seymer 1949 p.94). Those paid out of the Nightingale Fund received a meagre payment plus board and lodging, and were destined for the lower 'ranks' in nursing. Even when award rates of pay were introduced, these did not generate significant financial rewards.

Living conditions of nurses

Early justification for the strict and harsh conditions

Despite nurses being described as professionals, they were treated far more like domestic servants than professionals. They were required to wear uniforms and caps, were housed in cramped, unattractive conditions, and were subjected to excessive scrutiny in their limited personal lives. The uniforms at that time and in the early 20th century were very similar to those of a domestic maid (MacLennan 1996). Nurses training in Nightingale schools were treated very strictly, even harshly, and their living environments were comparable to those of domestic workers. Mrs Wardroper, who was the Superintendent of the Nightingale Training School from 1854 to 1887, was reported to be a strict disciplinarian, severe at times, and the lives of the probationers were far from comfortable. Lucy Osburn's personnel management style seems to have been somewhat similar (Godden 1996). When Unison voted at their 1999 annual conference to request the ICN to stop celebrating International Nurses Day on Florence Nightingale's birthday (12 May), her somewhat oppressive management style seems to have figured significantly. One nurse is quoted as saying, 'She was a woman who not so much kept her nurses under her thumb, as under her boot', and it was agreed that she represented 'some of the most negative and backward thinking elements in nursing' (Brindle 1999).

Such behaviour has been excused by Seymer on the grounds that training for women was revolutionary, unless they were in holy orders, particularly training for women by women (Seymer 1949). The Nightingale schools were in the nature of an experiment and still open to much criticism, as the general public were far from convinced that such a role for respectable women, rich or poor, was actually a good idea.

Overcrowded living conditions

These poor conditions continued long after registration had been achieved, and various wars had validated the nursing role and increased the popularity of nurses. In the early 20th century nurses experienced dreadful living conditions and until the late 1960s strict controls were imposed over their public and private lives. The living conditions for nurses varied greatly in the 1930s, with nurses sleeping on crowded verandahs, in old sheds and garages, and in one instance a nurse slept in a store room which she had to get into by climbing up a ladder. Beds were sometimes so close together that they touched and nurses had to climb over one another to get in and out of bed (Russell, 1990 pp.60–1).

These conditions were acknowledged in the 1936 NSW Award, and were described as 'far below what might be regarded as a proper standard' (Hospital Nurses (State) Award 1936b p.103). However, because the necessary improvements were reported to be unattainably expensive, no provision was made to improve accommodation. Instead, if the accommodation was too bad, the employer could not charge for it. Kinsella J made some attempt to redress the problem by identifying minimum standards for accommodation in his 1947 award. Nothing was done to implement them, and by 1953 Richards J made reference to a list of hospitals which either fell 'short of compliance substantially but not gravely' or which fell 'short of compliance gravely and irreparably'. However, he declined to 'award conditions with which it is impossible for the parties generally affected by the award to comply' (Hospital Nurses (State) Award 1953 p.323).

Living conditions for the matrons

Sometimes even the matron, the most senior nurse in the hospital, was not considered to require her own bathroom or toilet. Matrons' living conditions were raised in the 1967 award, where a claim was made to allow them to have their own laundry. This was refused on the grounds either that their laundry could be performed by the hospital domestic staff or that alternatively they could use 'either a basin in the bathroom or in a laboratory sink in the kitchenette where they prepared light refreshments' (Public Hospital Nurses (State) Award 1967 p.365).

Such conditions are more akin to those expected for the domestic staff than for a professional. Such a solution would never have been proposed for medical staff, who would probably have had their own housekeepers. Richards J also considered it impractical for matrons to have their own entrance to their residence. Many appointments required the matron to live on the premises. The lack of a private entrance would have meant that the matron had to go through the hospital or Nurses' Home even when she was off-duty, which would have given her little or no privacy.

Supervision and constraints in the Nurses' Home: little change from the days of Miss Wardroper

For many nurses, there was often no alternative to living in the Nurses' Homes because other accommodation was too expensive for their salaries. Even in the late 1960s and early 1970s both student nurses and many trained nurses still lived in cloistered environments in Australia (McCormick v Ballarat and District Base Hospital Inc 1967) and England (personal experience). Their rooms were checked for tidiness, their comings and goings were monitored and sometimes restricted, and they were required to obtain late and weekend passes. For many student nurses this may have been in part because they were still minors, being under 21. But for trained nurses living in the Nurses' Home there were similar restrictions.

Thus the messages which student nurses were receiving about their status were very mixed. They learnt that nursing was a wonderful career and that they were very fortunate to be able to train as nurses, a message reinforced by the industrial courts and tribunals who considered it a 'privilege to nurse' and viewed nursing as a 'career industry'. However, they received poor pay, worked long hours and lived in uncomfortable, over-crowded conditions. In addition, whilst living in the Nurses' Home and working on the wards, they were treated by other nurses, who would all have suffered the same treatment, in a restrictive and often oppressive manner not much different from Florence Nightingale's day.

CONCLUSION

This and the previous chapter have explored the stock story of the nurse as a domestic worker, a story which suggests that nursing is not really a profession in the way that, for example, medicine or law are professions. This is because nursing work involves many tasks which could be identified as domestic or women's caring work; and which traditionally have not been perceived to have sufficient status to be described as professional work. Nonetheless, because nursing is closely linked to medicine in many ways, certain aspects of nursing work have been accorded professional status, leading to confusion and ambivalence over the status of nursing as a profession. This ambivalence has led to a dissection or fragmentation of the nursing role when the courts or tribunals have found it expedient to do so. The expediency has usually been of a financial nature, due to a reluctance to fix a party with liability.

From the case law analysed in this chapter it can be seen that the courts and tribunals accorded differing status to different aspects of nursing work. There is no concept of an overall professional role called 'nursing' which is accepted without question, due in part to a lack of coherent public definition of the role of the nurse. There has been a general reluctance on the part of the civil and industrial courts and tribunals to accord professional status to all aspects of nursing work. This reluctance led to a fragmentation of the nursing role into a series of tasks. These tasks were classified as routine, menial or domestic or, alternatively, as professional. The fragmentation had little to do with the evidence presented to the court by nurses, but was in part a reflection of the way in which society viewed women's caring work in general and domestic work in particular.

As nurses came to believe that these tasks were hindering their quest for professional status, they explicitly aligned their bids for better pay and working conditions to medical tasks. Publicly they denied performing those tasks which were judicially devalued, despite the fact that unofficially they perform many of them to this day. This has led to further role frag-mentation and the rise of both the allied health professions and unqualified health workers, who have taken what were initially aspects of the nursing role and adopted them as their own.

Nursing has of late recognised the problems which role fragmentation has caused, and has attempted to articulate its professional focus more precisely. But one of the recurrent difficulties for nurses has been that they have not often been invited to give their own accounts in the courts and tribunals. Instead, doctors have given evidence about nursing and nursing work, which has often corroborated the stock story. Recent compensation cases confirm that this stock story has not changed, and that there is little more respect for the holistic and complex nature of nursing care today than there was at the beginning of the 20th century.

Finally, it is argued that this ambivalent status initially also led to the living and working conditions of nurses—even very senior nurses—being far more akin to those of domestic servants than to those of professional staff.

PART 3

Medical domination

PART CONTENTS

6

The nurse as the doctor's handmaiden

Elements of the image

- Nursing is an extension or component part of medicine;
  - Nurses are physical extensions of doctors;
  - Nursing work is solely delegated medical work under the close control of a doctor;
  - Nursing is a part of medicine's business, and doctors can speak for nurses.
- Because the nurse is no more than a participant in medical care, the nurse is expected to obey the doctor.
- Nurses are not expected to challenge doctors even if they believe the doctor to be making mistakes which are endangering the patient's life.
- If the nurse carries out the orders of the doctor without question the nurse will not be at fault even if (s)he believes on reasonable grounds that the doctor's orders are incorrect or immoral and may endanger the patient.
  - Even if the nurse performs activities which s(he) knows to be morally wrong the nurse can be exonerated if s(he) were ordered to do so by a doctor.

INTRODUCTION

The nursing profession is the handmaiden of medicine and the final success of the treatment of disease is often bound up with the efficiency of both. (Hon. Dr Parr, Hansard 9 September 1953 p.488)

This chapter addresses the stock story of the nurse as the doctor's handmaiden. This story is based on the premise that nursing is no more than a subordinated subset of medicine, and thus it is acceptable for doctors (and the courts and tribunals) to treat nurses as extensions of doctors. The implication of the story is that nurses have a primary duty to the doctor, rather than to the patient; or, alternatively, nurses owe a duty to the patient through their obedience to the doctor. Nurses are less than subordinates of doctors, they are subsumed within doctors' professional personae.

It is a compelling argument running just below the surface of many judicial decisions—but it is almost always subliminal. For instance, in case law, it rarely forms what is known as the *ratio decidendi* (the reasoning for the decision) of a judgment, but instead it is mentioned as an aside (what is known as *obiter dicta*, that which was also said). In fact, I found no substantive law which determines that doctors are responsible for nurses' acts, but much was contained within the dicta to imply that they control them.

Many of the acknowledgements of medical control or nursing subordination are 'thrown' into a sentence as commonplace observations. Such allusions are pervasive, in that they both form part of the existing world view, and provide a mechanism to reinforce it. For nurses, such comments do not address the reality of their subordination in any meaningful way. However, they do act to maintain the status quo of medical domination without adding to the burden of medical liability.

The most disturbing endorsement of the 'doctor's handmaiden' stock story is the one which manifests, not as a result of some throwaway comment by a judge, but where a nurse's unacceptable behaviour fails to elicit comment. There are a number of cases where nurses have behaved abominably or, at the very least, ineffectually. In several of these cases, little criticism has been made of their behaviour because the implication was that, since they were under the control of the doctor, they could not control themselves.

Chronologically, the elements of this story (detailed at the opening to this chapter) have all been present from the early case law and all continue to manifest in the recent case law, although they are less dominant than they were in the first half of the last century.

NURSING IS AN EXTENSION OR COMPONENT PART OF MEDICINE

Nurses are physical extension of doctors

A measure of society's internalisation of this stock story is that nurses are sometimes described as various body parts of doctors. One use of this analogy has been for lawyers to refer to a nurse as the 'doctor's hands', particularly in an attempt to fix a doctor with liability for her actions (Logan v Waitaki Hospital Board 1935 p.442). Nurses have also been described less frequently as other body parts. For example, in the Royal Commission into Matters affecting Callan Park Hospital (hereafter the Callan Park Report), McClemens J described the doctor as working 'through the nurse' and referred to the nurses as the 'doctor's eyes and ears' (1961 p.118). Working 'through the nurse' is a similar metaphor to the 'doctor's hands', as it also seems to imply that the doctor controls the nurse, that the nurse is in some way an instrument of the doctor's brain.

The eyes and ears analogy introduces a new dimension, though, which will be explored in some detail in the discussion of the nurse as a subordinate professional. For example, the relationship between the hands and the brain could be likened to a 'motor' relationship, one where the information flows from the brain to the hands and tells them what to do. By contrast, the relationship between the brain and the eyes and ears also has the element of a 'sensory' relationship. Eyes and ears bring information back to the brain—they keep the brain informed of what is going on around it. Most 'brains' are reliant on good sight and hearing to be able to function, and if eyes and ears fail we describe these people as 'handicapped' or 'impaired'— they cannot be expected to function as well as those who are fully sighted or hearing. The ability to rely on the nurse for information, the natural inference of the eyes and ears analogy, is used by the medical profession as a defence.

Nurses as 'doctor extenders' for abortions?

One of the few cases which directly addressed the control of nurses by doctors was the House of Lords decision in Royal College of Nursing (UK) v Department of Health and Social Security (1981). The Royal College of Nursing (RCN) sought a declaration from the court that a circular sent out by the Department of Health and Social Security (DHSS) was wrong in law. The declaration was refused at first instant, and RCN appealed. The Court of Appeal granted the declaration but the DHSS appealed to the House of Lords, who allowed the appeal by a 3:2 majority. Their decision was based on a variety of fairly pragmatic policy arguments.

The circular in question sought to clarify s 1 (1) of the Abortion Act 1967 (UK), which provides that 'a person shall not be guilty of an offence under the law relating to abortion when a pregnancy is terminated by a registered medical practitioner'. The concern of the RCN arose because they believed when abortion was induced by prostaglandin infusion, known as 'extra-amniotic induction', it was the nurse, not the doctor who performed the termination.

The DHSS circular stated that an abortion which used the extra-amniotic induction could be described as terminated by a registered medical practitioner provided 'it was decided on and initiated by him and provided he remained throughout responsible for its overall conduct and control in the sense that acts needed to bring it to its conclusion were done by appropriately skilled staff acting on his specific instructions, but not necessarily in his presence' (1981 p.800). The RCN claimed that this was wrong in law.

Lawyers for the DHSS argued that it was 'usual practice' for doctors to give instructions to nurses, and for the nurses to act as extensions of the doctor. Counsel used the doctor's hands analogy rather graphically.

S 1 (1) ... covers ... cases when the doctor supervising allows the nurse to do some of the mechanical acts ... His [the doctor's] decisions and his instructions constitute treatment by him. A prescription issued by a doctor is a medical treatment. A doctor is treating the disease if he directs the patient to be treated by his nurse. If a highly skilled gynaecologist, having cut his hand, watched a highly skilled nurse perform an operation, the act would be his act. It does not matter who does what so long as the direction and supervision is by the doctor and what is done is according to normal recognised medical practice. (1981 pp.815–16)

This line of argument raises several issues. First, the delegation of medical tasks to nurses is described as the doctor 'allowing' the nurse to do some of the mechanical acts. This seems to imply that the doctor is benefiting the nurse in the delegation and not vice versa. This was a particularly inappropriate choice of language in this case since the RCN contention was that nurses did not want to do the 'mechanical acts' of prostaglandin infusion. Second, DHSS counsel also referred to a doctor directing the patient to be treated by 'his' nurse. By 1980, since nurses and most doctors were employees of the National Health Service, the use of the possessive pronoun did not describe the employment relationship, but is symbolic of the stock story.

Third, the argument that 'it does not matter who does what so long as the direction and supervision is by the doctor' insinuates that the 'highly skilled nurse', performing the operation supervised by the gynaecologist with the injured hand, brings nothing to the equation. If this analogy holds good, and an operation performed in this way is akin to an operation performed by the gynaecologist himself, there is no requirement for a 'highly skilled nurse's' hands. They could just as easily be those of a postman. The implication is that the nurse's hands are a substitute for the gynaecologist's hands, under the control of the gynaecologist's brain. But the reality is that it would be crucial that these were the hands of a highly skilled nurse, controlled by a highly skilled nurse's brain.

Fourth, a submission was made that the Act must be construed in the light of medical progress, in that doctors could not undertake every specific detail of every medical act (1981 p.819). This is a form of the 'floodgates' argument (e.g. McLoughlin v O'Brian 1983), along the lines of 'if doctors had to supervise personally every instruction they gave to a nurse, they would be with the patient all the time'.

In the House of Lords, it was held by a majority of 3:2 that assistance of this sort by nurses in prostaglandin terminations was legal. A number of disparate reasons were given. One was that the phrase 'when a pregnancy is terminated by a registered medical practitioner' should be construed in a much broader context. All it meant was that 'a registered medical practitioner ... should accept responsibility for all stages of the treatment for the termination of the pregnancy' (1981 p.828).

Another was that the procedure could be properly regarded as having been performed by a medical practitioner because, '[t]he doctor has responsibility for the whole process and is in charge of it throughout. It is he (sic) who decides that it is to be carried out. He personally performs essential parts of it which are such as to necessitate the application of his particular skill. The nurses' actions are done under his direct written instructions' (1981 p.835).

A third reason was that the nurse's role was, 'fully protected provided that the entirety of the treatment for the termination of the pregnancy and her participation in it is at all times under the control of the doctor even though the doctor is not present throughout the entirety of the treatment' (1981 p.838).

Nurses as mere participants in medical activities

This case is particularly interesting for this book. It goes to the heart of one of the key problems faced by nurses in the doctor–nurse relationship, particularly where there is concern or disagreement over a clinical management issue. The concept of nurses merely as obedient participants in a medical act denies them an independent role, and seems to suggest that they have no legal or moral agency. This status (or non-status) should protect them from any legal repercussions, since it suggests (as does this chapter) that they should have no individual decision making role or responsibility. The argument presented by DHSS, and accepted to some extent in all of the majority House of Lords judgments, is that doctors make the decision(s) and nurses merely carry out those activities required to implement them. This implies that decision(s) of doctors induce a series of events in which nurses are inexorably carried along because they exist merely to carry out the doctor's instructions. As you will read later, where nurses have been 'inexorably carried along' and have demonstrated reluctance to intervene, the outcomes for both nurses and patients can be tragic.

Nursing work is solely delegated medical work
under the close control of a doctor

Nurses deserve to be financially rewarded for taking on delegated medical work

In several NSW award decisions, nurses themselves have successfully used the argument that nursing is an extension of medicine in terms of workload, and forms a part of what is really medical work (In re Public Hospitals

Nurses (State) Award 1976, In re Public Hospital Nurses (State) Award 1986). There is a sense that these medical tasks are exceptional for nurses and thus deserving of reward. But if such an argument is followed to its (il)logical conclusion, the norm must be that nursing is relatively unskilled, because nurses usually do only what the doctors order.

An example of this is seen in a 1967 award decision, where one of the few gains of the award was the recognition of some of the changes in the duties and responsibilities of nurses. The claim was that the way in which patients were nursed had altered, in that they were now nursed in specialised units, such as intensive care units and burns units (In re Public Hospital Nurses (State) Award 1967). Richards J conceded these changes and acknowledged the introduction of specialised units, such as intensive care units and recovery wards; and the introduction of new machinery: monitoring, respiratory type and other equipment. He based his (small) wage increase on the changes to nursing work which were related to the use of these new technologies in workplace practice.

A number of the machines in the above list are used under fairly close supervision of medical practitioners, but once the machines have been connected up to the patient by the medical practitioner, nurses are required to keep a close watch on the patient's condition and report any change to the medical practitioner. In the case of an emergency, some of the machines would be used directly on the patient by the nurse until a medical practitioner could be summoned. The artificial kidney machines, which are at present only to be found at Sydney Hospital and Prince Henry Hospital, are used by trained nurses under medical supervision to treat patients suffering from renal failure. Previously the whole of this treatment would have been carried out by the medical practitioner himself. (1967 p.337)

Nurses do not deserve to receive further rewards merely for nursing activities

In contrast, acknowledged changes in drug administration did not achieve increased remuneration, as it was held that drug administration was not a new part of the nurses' role. He found that the changes to drug administration were no more than a modernisation of existing nursing practices.

It has always been a basic part of the nurses' duty to accurately administer drugs to patients in accordance with the orders of a medical practitioner and to keep the patient under surveillance so as to detect any change in his condition. It must be remembered that in the public hospitals of New South Wales, particularly the large University Teaching Hospitals, the treatment of the sick is carried out in accordance with the latest advances in medical knowledge. Members of the medical profession are in charge of the patient's treatment and the nurses provide nursing care in accordance with the doctor's directions. Medical knowledge and methods of treating illnesses are in a constant state of change, but these changes only occur gradually. New drugs take the place of old ones, new methods of treatment and new operative procedures are developed and the nurses in public hospitals become familiar with these in the course of doing their daily work. The salaries fixed under the nursing award are designed to remunerate nurses for nursing the sick by applying up to date nursing procedures. The calling of nursing, by its very nature, is one which requires the nurse to keep herself up to date with new drugs, new methods of treatment and new operative procedures. (1967 p.338)

Note the apparent inconsistency between His Honour's attitude to drug administration and his attitude to machinery. He justified the refusal to take account of the changes in drug administration because keeping 'the patient under surveillance so as to detect any change in his condition' and 'keeping up to date with new drugs, new methods of treatment and new operative procedures' were part of the 'basic duties of the nurse'. However, the introduction of new machinery was included in the changes to nursing practice he agreed to take into account. When reviewing the list of machinery, a group described as 'monitoring equipment' contained items such as cardiac monitors, fetal heart monitors and venous pressure manometers. This equipment is designed specifically 'to keep the patient under surveillance so as to detect any change in his condition' (1967 p.338). Similarly the group described as 'respiratory type equipment and other equipment' contained items such as artificial kidney machines, nebulisers and respirators, which would fall into the categories of 'new methods of treatment and new operative procedures'. If Richards J were consistent, he ought to have refused the inclusion of these machines in his deliberations on the same grounds as he refused to allow drug administration. Thus it would seem that his Honour was influenced by other factors in his determination, the most significant of which would appear to be the close relationship of these tasks to the work of medical practitioners.

Nursing is a part of medicine's business and
doctors can speak for nurses

Substitution of doctors for nurses—in their governance

The conception of nurses as extensions of doctors has meant that, in addition to nurses substituting for doctors in performing tasks, doctors can speak/act on behalf of nurses in exercises of power. The acceptance of this phenomenon is demonstrated in the NSW Parliamentary debate on the Nurses Registration Bill 1953 (NSW Hansard 2nd September 1953). The requirements for the registration of nurses were to be amended to reflect the changes in the practice of nursing, and it was also proposed to give nurses greater self regulation by increasing the number of nurses on the Nurses Registration Board to seven out of the thirteen members. There was debate about the extent of medical representation on this newly formed Board. The Honourable Member for Temora, Mr Dickson, expressed surprise that four of the Board's members should be doctors. But the Honourable Member for

Burwood, Dr Parr, quoted at the beginning of this chapter, viewed this composition as most advantageous to nursing:

The nursing profession is the handmaiden of medicine and the final success of the treatment of disease is often bound up with the efficiency of both ... The number of members (of the Board) is being raised from seven to thirteen. The fact that eleven of them are medical men or registered nurses augurs well for the future. The predominance given to these two great professions should ensure a high standard of training in all sections of nursing. (NSW Hansard 2 September 1953 p.488)

... and later:

Research is fundamental to progress and we can regard this aspect of the Board's activities with satisfaction. Medicine and nursing are dynamic, not static; a flowing stream, not a still pond, and a review of nursing must take place from time to time. Alternate schemes of training and examination may subsequently be found to be desirable, and the Board should have the courage to adopt them. The members of the Board, with their intimate knowledge of nursing and medicine, inspire in us the hope that both nursing and the community will benefit. We can leave the future of nursing in the hands of two professions; my own and nursing—two hands well equipped for progress. (NSW Hansard 2 September 1953 p.492)

Linguistically, although both medicine and nursing are the subjects of the sentences, only nursing is present as an object within the sentences. Thus, medicine and nursing (one and the same anyway?) comprise the Board; medicine and nursing are dynamic; medicine and nursing have knowledge; and medicine's and nursing's hands are well equipped for progress. Conversely, only nursing's training standards are ensured by the two of them; only nursing will require a review from time to time; and only nursing (and the community) will benefit from medicine's and nursing's interventions. Mr Dickson was correct in his observation that there were no nurses adding their hands (however well equipped they might be for progress) to any reviews of medical education and training. Catharine MacKinnon would not be surprised by such language. She has observed that '[a]nyone who is the least bit attentive to gender since reading Simone de Beauvoir knows that it is men socially who are subjects, women socially who are other, objects' (MacKinnon 1987 p.55).

Mr Freeman, the Honourable Member for Blacktown, perceived the presence of the doctors to be a positive attribute to the Board, 'a fine tribute to the nursing profession' (NSW Hansard 1953 p.497). The implication here is that the professional status of nursing is validated, or at the very least, enhanced, by the proximity of medicine. However, such a belief did not originate solely from the medical profession. The all-nursing consultative committee originally suggested a Board of twenty-seven members, which included five Professors from Sydney University Faculty of Medicine.

Thornton uses Teresa de Lauretis's construct of the 'technology of gender' to provide an explanation for why women have often felt the need to have men to legitimise or add value to a position of authority.

The result is that the 'best person' to occupy a position of authority has tended to be unproblematically defined in masculine terms, which reflect the values of the public sphere ... the niggling suspicion that women cannot be quite trusted in unsupervised positions of authority demonstrates how residual notions of disorder remain significant, albeit at a subliminal level. (Thornton 1996 p.35)

Thornton goes on to explain that the technology operates subliminally, and 'seduces women, no less than men, into believing that men really are intellectually superior, more rational, and more authoritative. Indeed, many women choose to identify with men who, they believe, confer the imprimatur of legitimacy by their presence' (1996 p.37). There is no doubt that nurses have long used doctors to confer the 'imprimatur of legitimacy' (see for example, Bendall & Raybould 1969 p.69).

Substitution of doctors for nurses—in health care legislation and policy

It is not unusual for doctors to speak with universality about medical and nursing care. And there are a number of significant situations where nurses are not even mentioned in health care legislation or policy. The 1993 NSW Health Department Interim Guidelines for dying with dignity made no mention of the role of nurses whatsoever, despite the central role that nurses play in the care of the dying (Chiarella 2000 pp.140–156).

This substitution is also evident in representation on many major health-related committees (Re Karen Ann Pullinger v Secretary to the Department of Community Services and Health & Ors 1990). If there were proportional representation on such committees, nurses would be in the majority. The usual format over many years is that there are several doctors from varying specialties and perhaps one nurse.[1] The nurse is generally considered to be there to present a 'nursing perspective' whereas doctors are generally considered to be there to inform about their specialist areas of knowledge. Since nursing varies quite considerably from aged care to critical care, presumably the doctors are expected to give input into specialty nursing as well as specialty medicine, as one nurse would not be able to provide valuable and informed input into all areas of debate. A 'nursing perspective' is viewed in the same way as an 'ethical perspective'—something which might assist in the 'real' deliberations, but which is not central to them.

There are certain health committees of considerable relevance to nurses which now boast an economist, but no nurse. For example, the Australian Health Technology Advisory Committee (AHTAC) has no nurses, but at least four doctors and an economist. Yet nurses would be using new

---

[1] It should be noted that most of the committees established under the NSW Government Action Plan for Health do have nurse co-chairs and nursing representation, which is a most welcome development, but until now this has been the exception, rather than the rule.

technology equally as much as doctors (Brewer 1983). The membership of the Working Party on Minimal Access Surgery (1996) out of nine members had six doctors, one economist, but no nurse. Yet the impact of minimal access surgery is being experienced acutely by operating room nurses in the management and care of patients in the operating room and in recovery, and specifically by surgical and community nurses who care for these patients postoperatively and on early discharge.

Substitution of doctors for nurses—as expert nursing witnesses

In a number of cases involving questions of nursing negligence, medical practitioners, rather than nurses, have given expert and factual evidence about nursing. Although this was the norm in the early part of the 20th century, it still occurs today.

This is noteworthy, as there are recognised limitations on the ability of expert witnesses to comment on 'matters requiring other expertise' (Gillies 1991 p.379). For example, in R v McKenney (1981) it was held that a psychologist, as distinct from a psychiatrist, should not be permitted to express an opinion in evidence as to whether a particular person was suffering from a specific disease of the mind. However, while such a limitation might act to proscribe the scope of medical practice from comment by non-medical practitioners, it does not appear to act to protect non-medical practitioners from comment by medical practitioners.

In Le Page v Kingston & Richmond Health Authority (1997) the four midwives (three of whom were named) were not called as witnesses nor were their witness statements tendered to supply their accounts of the events under scrutiny. However, it was held that they had contributed to the 'catalogue of errors' which led to the 22-year-old plaintiff having to undergo hysterectomy due to post-partum haemorrhage. The judge noted that none of the midwives had given evidence, but drew the conclusion from a charting omission that the midwife did not routinely palpate the uterus. All of the seven doctors involved either gave evidence or provided witness statements, and provided factual accounts of the activities of the midwives, which supplemented the written midwifery records.

The complaint was lodged at the hospital only four months after the incident occurred, thus it is unlikely that all four midwives were unavailable to give their accounts of what happened. By not calling any of the midwives as witnesses or tendering witness statements from them, the parties and the court seemed to accept that the doctors' evidence was sufficient to establish the behaviour of the midwives. Their evidence may have made no difference or may have been withheld for forensic reasons, because they were advised that it was more damning for them to tender it than to remain silent. Nevertheless, one cannot imagine that the seven doctors would ever have agreed to the midwives giving factual evidence in their stead, or have allowed only the midwives' accounts of what transpired to go on record. This is one of several cases where factual medical evidence has been the only account of nursing activity (other than the plaintiff's) to be presented and where the outcome has been either equally unfavourable or less favourable for the nurses involved than the doctors (Karderas v Clow 1972, MacDonald v York County Hospital & Dr Vail 1973, Farrell v Cant et al 1992, Lee v McLennan 1992).

In cases where nurses have presented their own evidence, their perspective on a particular matter has been qualitatively different from that of the doctor (Savoie v Bouchard 1982, Hay v Grampian Health Board 1995). However, despite the demonstrated relevance of a nursing perspective, it is still commonplace for a medical practitioner to give expert or factual evidence about nursing, yet unimaginable that a nurse might be called as an expert medical witness.

BECAUSE THE NURSE IS NO MORE THAN A PARTICIPANT IN MEDICAL CARE, THE NURSE IS EXPECTED TO OBEY THE DOCTOR

The expectation that self-employed nurses will obey the instructions of a doctor

Hall v Lees (1904), an early vicarious liability case, highlighted the requirement for a nurse to obey the instructions of a doctor, even though she was an independent contractor. In this case, the plaintiff was badly burned as a result of the negligence of a nurse obtained on the plaintiff's behalf through a nursing agency by her surgeon. Despite the fact she was held to be an independent contractor, the nurse was also required under her contract with the agency to 'be subject to the control of the medical man attending the patient'. The agency undertook only to supply nurses 'in cases which are attended by a medical man', and stipulated that 'the nurse shall implicitly follow his instructions' (1904 p.613). Thus the situation was that the nurse, although labelled as an 'independent contractor', was not independent, being controlled by a person who was not vicariously liable for her actions.

The expectation that hospital nurses will obey the instructions of a doctor even if the nurse is employed by the hospital

At the beginning of the last century there were a series of cases where plaintiffs attempted to fix hospitals with liability for the negligence of their nursing staff. Most of these cases have been discussed in some detail in

Chapter 5, and are mentioned here only in terms of the judicial references to the expectation that the nurse will obey the surgeon. The facts are not reiterated unless they are of particular significance.

In the landmark case of Hillyer v Governors of St Bartholomew's Hospital, Farwell J described the nurses as being 'at the disposal and under the sole orders of the operating surgeon until the operation has been completely finished' (1909 p.826). This assumption of the supremacy of the surgeon in the operating room went unchallenged in later cases because it was not material to the case. The matter did not come under review until attempts were made, as a result of what was later described as a 'transmutation of employment' (Gold v Essex County Council 1942 p.300), to fix a surgeon with liability for the acts of a nurse in the operating room. In Lavere v Smith's Falls Public Hospital (1915b), one of the first of the 'burns sagas', the judge stated that it was 'the duty of the nurse' to obey 'the express orders of the surgeon' (1915 p.348). He added that the doctor 'may give the orders as he sees fit, and these orders must be obeyed' (1915 p.349). Ingram v Fitzgerald (1936) was one of the few cases that specifically dealt with the doctor's liability for the negligent acts of a nurse. The Court found that the doctor should not be held liable for the nurse's acts as it would impose an 'intolerable burden on the surgeon, even though he himself had exercised all possible care and even though it was wholly impossible for him to guard against or prevent the damage' (1936 p.913). Nevertheless, it was held that the surgeon 'had the right and the duty to intervene and he could do so'. In Paton v Parker (1941) it was held that the staff were neither the servants nor the agents of the surgeon, but that it was 'true enough that the operating surgeon ... could give directions to the[m]' (p.195).

These cases propound that doctors control nurses but are not vicariously liable for their actions. Such subordination was the norm at that time. An early medical instructor informed the nurses that 'criticism on your part of the treatment by the doctor only renders you ridiculous, since you talk about matters of which you do not know—and cannot know—anything whatever' (Pearn 1988 p.225).

NURSES ARE NOT EXPECTED TO CHALLENGE
DOCTORS EVEN IF THEY BELIEVE THE DOCTOR TO
BE MAKING MISTAKES WHICH ARE ENDANGERING
THE PATIENT'S LIFE

'Not part of a nurse's duty ...'

If nurses are no more than obedient extensions of doctors, it may be inferred that they have no legal obligation to challenge doctors should the doctors do anything wrong.

This inference is borne out to some extent in Pillai v Messiter (No.2) (1989), an appeal by a medical practitioner against a finding of professional misconduct. The finding was based on a prescription error made by the appellant which had caused the death of a patient. The appellant's ground for appeal was that, since several other medical practitioners had also transcribed the error without comment or query, the act was not one which 'incurred the strong reprobation of professional brethren of good repute and competence', the prevailing test for misconduct (Qidwai v Brown 1984). The argument was accepted on appeal, but Samuels J. commented in passing on the nursing staff's role in the error.

I might add that no member of the nursing staff expressed any concern about the dosage that had been ordered. I make that comment in the full appreciation that it is not part of a nurse's duty to question the medication ordered by a doctor. (Pillai v Messiter 1989 p.206)

This quote reinforces the proposition that nurses have no duty to challenge doctors. However, it also emphasises the ambiguity nurses face so regularly in their clinical practice. For example, if it were not part of the nurses' duty to question doctors, why did his Honour mention their failure to do so at all? Were they supposed to 'wonder aloud' conspicuously about such a dosage, whilst taking care not to usurp medical authority? It seems his Honour was suggesting that nurses might do more than their duty required, and draw the doctor's attention to the error—perhaps as a favour, or as an optional extra. Thus, no legal obligation or authority is stipulated, but some moral, or at least collegial, expectation is suggested.

'Commendable courage' required to challenge a doctor

The following cases provide examples of the way in which the absence of any legal obligation to intervene is acknowledged in default. In two tragic operating theatre cases, there was medical mismanagement of the patients and arrogance on the part of the medical practitioners. One, an appeal against the decision of a medical tribunal, had no direct relevance to nursing, whereas the other, a coronial decision, did. In both cases, the nurses directly involved in the operation made rather weak attempts to alert the surgeons to their concerns, but in neither case was the nurse sufficiently assertive to intervene actively on behalf of the patient. The interventions that were made by the senior nurses occurred post hoc. In both cases, the interventions were too little, too late.

In the first case, the fact that the theatre superintendent challenged the authority of the doctors was described obiter as being an act of 'commendable courage'. Re Anderson and Re Johnson (1967) comprised a joint appeal against a decision of the Medical Tribunal that found two medical practitioners guilty of infamous conduct in a professional respect. Anderson was suspended from practice for twelve months and Johnson for six months. The suspension related to the death of a patient during a surgical procedure for the removal of a thyroglossal cyst by her surgeon, a partner of Dr Anderson. Dr Johnson was an employee of the partnership. Dr Anderson was to give the anaesthetic to the patient.

It was found at the inquest that the patient had been clinically dead for the duration of the operation, having suffered a cardiac arrest during a difficult intubation. The senior nurse in charge of the operating theatres was present at the end of the operation and requested another doctor to attend the patient.

It is clear from the evidence that the nursing staff were concerned about the patient from the beginning of the operation. At the incision, the darkness of the blood brought comment from the scrub nurse, who also remarked on the lack of bleeding. In addition, the circulating nurse queried the speed of the operation. The operation was conducted in a tense atmosphere, with three changes of anaesthetist, and the nursing staff commenting cryptically to the surgeon on the patient's cardiovascular status.

Herron CJ, commenting obiter on the fact that the charge nurse sought a second opinion, observed that she did so 'with commendable courage' (1967 p.565). His Honour could hardly imagine that a senior nurse would require courage merely to act in the best interests of a patient who was pale, pulseless, and had dilated pupils. Thus, it can be inferred that he was allowing that a nurse, even a senior charge nurse, would require courage to seek a second opinion from a doctor other than the one who was managing the case. That such an act should be described as courageous, even in passing, is an indication of the power which doctors, even doctors who were seen to be putting patients at risk, are judicially acknowledged to possess.

Failure to intervene until it is too late constitutes 'efficient and appropriate' nursing practice

In the second case, the Inquest touching the death of PDP (1994), the patient died of haemorrhage due to perforation of the aorta during surgery. Following laparoscopy, during which profuse bleeding was observed, the surgeon proceeded to laparotomy, revealing a large amount of blood in the abdominal cavity. The scrub nurse testified that she advised the surgeon that the abdominal cavity was still moist when he pronounced it quite dry, and that when she offered him a choice of drain, he refused it, and closed the cavity.

Before the patient's transfer to recovery, the scrub nurse instructed the scout nurse to warn the recovery room staff that the patient might still be bleeding internally, and to keep him under very close observation. On arrival in recovery the patient collapsed. The theatre manager, a senior and experienced nurse, was called. She examined the patient, and insisted that the surgeon return the patient to the operating theatre.

During the second operation, the surgeon again disregarded the observations of the scrub nurse who was assisting him, that she was 'sucking up bright red blood from deeper in the abdomen'. He announced his intention to close the wound. The scrub nurse gave evidence to the effect that even at this stage 'the abdomen was moist and appeared to still have a lot of fluid in it' (1994 p.11). The post mortem examination revealed an unsutured 6 mm penetration of the aorta. By the time that the wound was closed the patient's pupils were fixed and dilated and the anaesthetist announced generally that further efforts were useless.

The Coroner acknowledged the fact that the surgeon did not take up the offer of the scrub nurse to insert a drain, observing that although it would not have stopped the bleeding, it might have indicated its presence. In his conclusions, the Coroner made positive comments about the behaviour of the nursing staff. He made some criticism of the surgeon, stating that he should have realised in the recovery room 'that the condition of his patient was deteriorating, that it was highly likely that there was significant haemorrhage continuing and that further surgery was necessary'. He accepted that '[t]his situation was recognised by experienced nursing staff' and that it was the theatre manager who initiated the patient's return to theatre. He described the way in which the nursing staff collectively carried out their duties as being 'in an efficient and appropriate manner' (1994 p.20).

Did the doctor suffer from too little or too much authority?

These two cases provide examples of ineffectual nursing behaviour when they are concerned about the medical management of a patient. In Re Anderson and Re Johnson, the scrub nurse mentioned the darkness of the blood; the lack of bleeding, the small number of artery forceps used; and the speed of the operation. Why did she not plainly state that the patient was hypoxic, and ask the anaesthetist what was happening?

In the Inquest touching the death of PDP, during the initial surgery, the scrub nurse was obviously concerned that the patient was still bleeding and made observations to the surgeon to that effect. She was sufficiently concerned about the patient's condition to send the scout nurse out in advance to warn the recovery room staff to expect a patient who 'may still be bleeding internally' (1994 p.4).

In PDP, the Coroner stated that the surgeon 'did not exercise that degree of authority in the delivery of care to his patient that might reasonably be expected of a consultant surgeon' (1994 p.4). This criticism followed his finding that the theatre manager organised the return of the patient to theatre, a responsibility which the Coroner believed should properly rest with the surgeon. The use of language is telling: the surgeon is criticised for his lack of authority in the delivery of care, not for his refusal to take notice of or even discuss the concerns and/or suggestions of the scrub nurse. Surely, he exercised too much, rather than too little, authority?

When the surgeon came before the WA Medical Board he was found guilty of causing the death of Mr PDP, banned from performing particular kinds of surgery and ordered to undertake a Royal Australian College of Surgeons retraining programme. The Board did not suspend or fine him as 'he had restricted his laparoscopic surgery since the death'. Although he was found guilty on eight counts, none of them mentioned his failure to heed the concerns of the nurses. Remarkably, the surgeon claimed in his defence that 'there was no indication a major blood vessel had been penetrated as the bleeding was not heavy'. The impression is that there were no nurses present, offering drains and commenting on the fact that the bleeding had not ceased (Information Australia 1998 p.3).

Should patient safety be personality dependent?

The PDP case was a Coronial inquest. The purpose of the inquest was to determine the manner and cause of death. The Coroner made no criticism of the nursing staff, despite the fact that they made no attempt to prevent a surgeon from closing a patient's abdomen when they had strong grounds to suspect that the patient was still haemorrhaging. Rather the Coroner praised them for carrying out their duties in an 'efficient and appropriate' (1994 p.20) way. The implication is that it was 'appropriate' for the nurses not to confront the surgeon about their concern for the patient in the operating theatre, that it would only be 'appropriate' for the theatre manager to intervene post hoc in an assertive way as a form of damage control. If their behaviour was 'appropriate', this condones a form of institutionalised powerlessness whereby it is more important to comply with the established etiquette of the operating theatre hierarchy than it is to intervene actively when the patient is at risk. In addition, the description of 'efficient' seems odd, since two operations were performed when only one might have sufficed, if the scrub nurse's belief that the patient was still bleeding internally had been heeded and investigated.

A more receptive surgeon might have heeded the scrub nurse. A more confident scrub nurse may have been more assertive (Brennan 1994). But personality is no basis for ensuring patient safety. There should be no doubt in the mind of the most timid nurse faced with the most objectionable surgeon that the primary duty is to ensure patient safety. But no scrub nurse is an island. Such clarity of purpose would exist only in a system where concerns expressed by nurses were encouraged and supported by management even if they proved to be incorrect, and where domineering or overbearing behaviour by surgeons was not countenanced. People who are afraid of other people's moods and tempers learn ways of avoiding them, methods of evading confrontation. If it is 'not part of a nurses' duty to question' the doctor (Pillai v Messiter 1989) then, in a situation such as this, there would be no collegial inclination to go beyond one's duty in order to assist a surgeon who did not heed one's concerns. Even in a major teaching hospital in 1994, the culture of the hospital, accepted as the norm by the courts, condoned the fact that a nurse did not forcefully intercede even when she suspected the patient's life to be in danger.

The impact on the nurses

It would be easy to argue that these were medical mistakes, the nurses were not held responsible for them and that was only fair. But the anguish of the theatre nurses after the deaths in these two cases, and the unresolved anger and guilt that they would have felt about the fact that they did not do more at the time, can only be imagined. The Coroner's lack of criticism undoubtedly reflected this. But such anguish is a recurrent theme in nursing stories, which used only to be told orally in the 'wee small hours of night duty and over numerous cups of coffee at our friends' houses' (Walker 2000 p.87). Of late, these stories have started to take a written form. The tragedy is that many of the stories are told in research papers examining why nurses leave nursing (NSW Health Department 2001). Zwickler recounts an horrific incident in which she failed to intervene when a patient had his head of femur, which was protruding through a pressure sore, amputated under local anaesthetic on the ward. She describes herself as follows:

Standing by, the silent staff nurse is taking no part in the contretemps, but is embarrassed, and would like to take sides against the doctor. It is not her place to do so. Her conditioning has made her compliant. She is there to serve doctors, to carry out commands, a handmaiden, a vestal to the priests of medicine. But she looks uncomfortable, even a little rebellious.

In the final line of this harrowing true story she apologises to Smithy, the patient.

It was such a long time ago, in my staff nursing days, and I remember, I remember— we did not defend you, Smithy, and this is your memorial. (Zwickler 1997 p.11)

Judicial tolerance of nursing stupidity: an exercise in believing the patient and obeying the doctor

Gregory v Ferro & others (1995) highlights the ridiculous extent of judicial acceptance of the nurse's duty to obey the doctor. Although the negligence of the nurses in the emergency department was not fully addressed due to procedural issues, the behaviour of the nurses in this case is sufficiently schizophrenic (metaphorically speaking) to warrant comment.

The plaintiff, having injured her right ankle in a fall at work, went to see her general practitioner (GP), who (erroneously) wrote out an order for an

X-ray of the left ankle, and sent her to emergency. She was seen by nursing staff, and explained to them that it was her right, not left, ankle that was injured. The nurses obviously believed her, as they bandaged her right ankle. However, they X-rayed the left ankle as they were ordered to do, and sent the patient home. It was later shown that she had been suffering from a partial tear of her right Achilles tendon, which would have shown up had the correct ankle been X-rayed. She sued for damages in negligence. All claims were held by the judge to be time-barred. Her appeal was dismissed.

The trial judge did not criticise the nursing staff's bizarre behaviour, but only observed that '[n]ot surprisingly, the hospital X-rayed the left ankle' (1995 p.325). In the Court of Appeal, it was also stated without criticism that, although the plaintiff explained that it was actually her right ankle that was injured, the nurses 'preferred to go by the doctor's letter and X-rayed the left ankle' (1995 p.332). Why was it 'not surprising' that a nurse would accept that a patient had pain in her right ankle and bandage that ankle, but disregard that knowledge in favour of the doctor's instruction and X-ray an ankle which she had not even bandaged? It can only be 'not surprising' because the judge would expect the nurse to obey the doctor, even if she actually believed the patient. A simple telephone call could have clarified the situation. The social pathology that must exist for such dissonant behaviour to occur is staggering.

Judicial tolerance of nursing's loyalty to doctors

Judges recognise and tolerate the fact that nurses feel bound by loyalty (or a sense of duty?) to doctors, even though it may be misguided. In Strelic v Nelson & Ors (1996) the defendant doctor was accused (inter alia) of negligently causing spinal damage to the plaintiff's baby during delivery.

A midwife was caring for the plaintiff before and during the doctor's intervention. She was called as a factual witness as she was present throughout the delivery. The judge found that she believed that the doctor had applied excessive force at the wrong time during the delivery. Smart J was exquisitely sensitive to her predicament. He stated that if taken 'gently and sequentially' (1996 p.20) she did know what had happened. He observed that she was 'a gentle lady who was far from robust' and that she was 'no match for counsel' and 'not suited to adversarial litigation'. He recognised that she 'did not wish to give evidence against [the doctor]' (1996 p.21).

She was nervous and embarrassed but not untruthful. She was conscious of her duty to tell the truth when giving evidence. When various people spoke with her over the years she did not want to be involved. She wished that she had not seen what had happened. She was torn between the allegiance which she believed she owed as a nursing sister towards the medical profession and telling what had happened. As she added, 'you are torn to perhaps tell what you saw and to keep that in silence'. (1996 p.20)

The midwife's situation must have been extremely difficult. The plaintiff, an influential figure in the town, was very distressed ('frantic'), the delivery was a difficult undiagnosed footling breech, the obstetrician was 'angry', 'abrupt' and 'cross', and the plaintiff was his private patient. The midwife's evidence suggests that she felt at the time that the doctor was mismanaging the delivery. As a qualified midwife, she would have understood the consequences for the baby of pulling too much, too hard, and too soon.

This situation is qualitatively different from a situation in an operating room, where the patient would usually be unconscious. If the midwife wished to challenge the doctor she would need to comment in front of the patient and her husband, as neither she nor the doctor would have been able to leave the delivery room. Clearly she did not feel able to do this. So there she must have remained; feeling powerless to intervene, but knowing nevertheless that things were going dreadfully wrong, and that the baby might be damaged permanently.

A more assertive midwife might have intervened even given the surroundings; but she was not assertive, she was 'far from robust'. It was hardly surprising that, after the delivery, when the obstetrician was called back to the hospital, she did not want to speak to him. No criticism was levelled at her in the judgment, instead there was a genuine note of sympathy. But whilst such situations arouse our sympathy, they can be intolerable for the nurses and calamitous for the patients involved. As long as the courts and tribunals accept the doctor's handmaiden story, they condemn the nursing staff to re-enact such dilemmas and enhance the risks for patients in such situations. Loyalty to the doctor and loyalty to the patient would not normally contradict one another, but when they do, the courts and tribunals should make it unequivocal to nurses exactly where their duty lies.

IF THE NURSE CARRIES OUT THE ORDERS OF THE DOCTOR WITHOUT QUESTION, THE NURSE WILL NOT BE AT FAULT EVEN IF (S)HE BELIEVES ON REASONABLE GROUNDS THAT THE DOCTOR'S ORDERS ARE INCORRECT OR IMMORAL AND MAY ENDANGER THE PATIENT

Will nurses be at fault if, rather than passively observing a doctor doing something wrong and failing to intervene, they obey an order from the doctor to do something that they clearly know to be wrong? The implication from the doctor's handmaiden story is that they could escape blame because their primary obligation is to obey the doctor passively, not to intervene actively.

Early cases: a nurse is not negligent if (s)he accurately carries out an incorrect clinical medical instruction

In some of the pre-1960 cases, this proposition is quite clearly enunciated, although invariably obiter, and sometimes with qualifications. Some statements of Riddell J in Lavere v Smith's Falls provide good examples. His Honour observed that '[i]f the nurse obeyed the express order of the surgeon, she was not guilty of negligence at all. That is the duty of a nurse' (1915b p.348). He continued with some requirements for checking the accuracy and authority of the order, suggesting that she must not obey what she should know to be 'a slip of the tongue'. He concluded by stating: '"he is the doctor", and it is not negligence for a nurse to act on the belief that he is the more competent' (1915 p.348). The nurse would follow the orders with due care, and the doctor would be entitled to rely on the nurse to execute the order efficiently and in accordance with the standards of reasonably competent nurses.

In Petite v MacLeod and St Mary's Hospital (1955), in discussing the relationship between doctors and nurses, Doull J elaborated on this situation.

[I]t follows that although if a nurse executes the doctor's actual orders, her act in that respect cannot be negligence on the part of the nurse, yet if there actually is negligence in the carrying out of the duties which are properly routine nursing duties, her employer will be responsible. (1955 p.153)

This seems to indicate that nurses would not be held responsible if they carried out a wrong order accurately (e.g. if they gave an excessive dose of a prescribed drug exactly as it was prescribed), but would be at fault if they gave a correctly prescribed dose inaccurately.

Much of this rather convoluted reasoning came about because of the need to ascertain a hospital's tortious liability for its nursing staff, but persisted even when the issue was about to be settled. For example, in Gold v Essex County Council, Lord Greene MR differentiated between nurses acting in their capacity as nurses, and nurses carrying out the orders of doctors.

I should myself have thought that the true ground on which the hospital escapes liability for the act of a nurse who, whether in the operating theatre or elsewhere, is acting under the instructions of a surgeon or doctor, is not pro hac vice she ceases to be the servant of the hospital, but that she is not guilty of negligence if she carries out the orders of the surgeon or doctor, however negligent those orders may be. (1942 p.299)

Goddard LJ concurred with His Lordship.

It is part of the nurses' duty, as servants of the hospital, to attend the surgeons and physicians and carry out their orders. If the surgeon gives a direction to the nurse, which she carries out, she is not guilty of negligence, even if the order is improper. (1942 p.310)

These observations are consistent with the image of nurses as extensions of doctors, and the concomitant implication that blame should therefore rest with doctors. However, Chapter 7 demonstrates that there is some considerable ambiguity as to the accuracy of these dicta when attempts are made to hold doctors liable for the acts of nurses.

> *Even if the nurse performs activities which s(he) knows*
> *to be morally wrong the nurse can be exonerated if s(he)*
> *were ordered to do so by a doctor*

This willingness to exonerate nurses has also extended to situations where nurses have been involved in behaviour which was obviously morally wrong (Lahey v St Joseph's Hospital 1992, Inquest touching the death of BRC 1989, Inquest touching the death of LB 1989). In two Royal Commission Reports, the Callan Park Report (1961) and The Report of the Royal Commission into Deep Sleep Therapy (1990), the nurses were treated leniently despite the fact that they were accused of (and found to have committed) quite extraordinary acts of cruelty and neglect.

The Report of the Royal Commission into Callan Park Mental Hospital

Following Dr Harry Bailey's appointment in 1960 as Medical Superintendent of Callan Park Mental Hospital, he submitted a critical report on the living conditions and treatment of patients at the hospital. He made serious allegations of theft, cruelty and neglect against the nursing and other staff of the institution and a Royal Commission was appointed.

The lengthy Report of the Royal Commissioner was published in 1961. McClemens J was critical of the custodial nature of the care but was reluctant throughout to criticise the nursing staff, preferring to blame the environment and financial constraints. Whilst he found some, although not all, of the allegations of theft, cruelty, neglect and drunkenness to be substantiated, he was careful not to apply them to the majority of the nursing staff.

The Commissioner stated that the nurses were the 'central figures' in the care of the mentally ill. He suggested that the medical staff may be unable to 'share [the] sorrows and [the] problems' of the patients and relatives, because of 'elements of time, educational and social differences and other factors, including sometimes even the personality problems of the doctor himself' (1961 p.118).

The Report of the Royal Commission into Deep Sleep Therapy

Perhaps the Commissioner was making reference to the personality of Dr Harry Bailey, who became the subject, rather than the instigator, of the subsequent Report of the Royal Commission into Deep Sleep Therapy (Chelmsford Report 1990). His personality has been described (inter alia) as paradoxical, arrogant, charismatic, powerful, generous, foul-mouthed, authoritative and charming (Chelmsford Report 1990, Bromberger & Fife-Yeomans 1991). Here again the issue was the care and treatment of psychiatric patients.

The ambit of the Chelmsford inquiry is beyond the scope of this book, and only the evidence of the Matrons will be discussed. The Matrons were all registered nurses and were the subject of extensive scrutiny within the Commission. The term 'nursing staff' in this Report includes non-nurses, itself a sad indictment on the authority of nursing qualifications.

The Commissioner was cognisant of the fact that, although the Royal Commission sat in 1988 and 1990, the events under scrutiny occurred in the 1960s and 1970s. From mid-1963 Dr Harry Bailey admitted patients into Chelmsford Private Hospital to receive an unusual form of treatment, which he claimed to have developed and researched himself, known as 'Deep Sleep Therapy' (DST). This consisted of a barbiturate-induced coma maintained over a long period of time, sometimes up to 14 days. In addition, many patients were given electroconvulsive therapy (ECT).

Over the ensuing 16 years until 1979, at least 24 people died as a direct result of the DST. During the course of the Commission, nursing notes were received for 1127 DST patients. In general hospitals, death rates of 1.5 per year would be considered low, but the majority of patients treated at Chelmsford were psychiatric patients, whose conditions are not usually life-threatening. The Commissioner expressed concern and surprise at the lack of whistle-blowing by the nursing staff. Over the 16 years in question the dosage of barbiturates given to patients undergoing DST approximately doubled, and the visits of Dr Bailey reduced from daily to approximately once a week. An enormous amount of latitude was given to the nursing staff, who appeared to have been ill-prepared for their role.

The events of Chelmsford have been the subject of much media attention, and the character of Harry Bailey, which is central to the tragedy, has been the subject of separate analysis (Bromberger & Fife-Yeomans 1991). For the purposes of this book, the complaints levelled against the 'nursing staff', and the findings of the Royal Commission in relation to those complaints, are the relevant matters. The complaints regarding the administration, treatment and nursing care of patients were numerous and horrific, and included the following allegations:

- there was a lack of informed consent or any consent at all,
- ECT treatment was given when patients had specifically refused it,
- patients were nursed naked, shackled, and with nasogastric tubes inserted,
- ECT was given without an anaesthetic,

- female patients feared they may have been sexually molested whilst sedated heavily,
- there was a blanket prohibition against visits during the treatment; and patients suffered pain and adverse effects from ECT.

In relation to information giving and consent, the Commissioner found that the 'nursing staff' had colluded with the lack of information regarding the nature of the patients' treatments, despite the fact that by the 1970s they knew that the treatment was dangerous. Entries in the nursing notes confirmed that patients were being lied to and deceived about their treatment with Deep Sleep Therapy. The Commissioner described this as 'a policy of deception' (1990 Vol 6 p.76). Matron Smith, probably one of the more assertive of the matrons at Chelmsford during that period, and certainly the one who tried hardest to get Dr Bailey to conform with legal requirements for medications, explained that these deceptions occurred on Dr Bailey's orders. In addition, patients who expressly refused ECT and DST were also given the treatments. Two matrons described what they would do in these situations:

Some who did know, if they refused to sign the consent form, then the instruction was that you gave them some medication to quieten them down; that's what you would say, 'I'll give you this little injection now, it will calm you down. You will feel a lot better after it'. But of course that little injection was Sodium Amytal and I think some Valium as well and then of course they were off on the sedation. (Matron Smith) (1990 Vol 6 p.76)

Then the patient had said subsequent to their admission 'I don't want sedation' and you think, 'Oh dear, here we go again'. So we rang up Dr Bailey and you would say, 'Did you explain to the patient that they were going to have sedation?' He would say either yes or no but either way he would say they have to have it, get them into sedation the best way you can. I don't suppose—we were deceitful without actually lying to them. We would say that they were having an injection to put them to sleep and they would have a nice rest. It was awful. I mean, that didn't happen a lot, but it happened. (Matron Fawdry) (1990 Vol 6 p.77)

Signatures for consent forms were obtained from patients when they were semi-conscious, and many were treated without any consent at all. The Commissioner was critical of the nursing staff and visiting medical officers in this regard.

The quality and intensity of the nursing care which patients received featured in many of the complaints. The Commissioner found that patients had been nursed naked, shackled, and had nasogastric tubes inserted. Some expert nursing witnesses expressed sympathy for the difficulties under which the nurses worked, and considered that they had performed satisfactorily under such circumstances.

Considerable criticism was made about the degree of latitude that the 'nurses' had (or took) in the administration of the DST medications, and the lack of preparation which they had for the task. The Commissioner acknowledged the stress which this may have placed upon the 'ill-prepared staff' (1990 Vol 1 p.159). He also found that 'the standard of nursing care fell short of the high standard which was necessary for patients who were undertaking a dangerous treatment like DST'; he concluded that he was 'satisfied that the nursing care which was given to DST patients at Chelmsford over the relevant period did not measure up to the standards of nursing care which were then practised in hospitals where patients were in a long term unconscious condition' (1990 Vol 1 pp.162–3).

The defence of obedience

The failure of the registered nurses to challenge the doctors' authority was held to be a reflection of the relationships between doctors and nurses generally at that time. It was the nurses themselves who introduced the subsumed nature of their relationships with the doctors as a defence against their morally unpardonable behaviour.

Miss Moroney (matron) drew attention to a change in attitude in and towards the nursing profession on the mid 1970s. When she began her training in 1965 it was 'an era where nurses walked with their hands behind their back behind the doctor, never spoke unless spoken to, and it goes downhill from there' ... 'you did not get in the same lift with the doctor'. In her words, 'nurses were allowed to think, around about 1976'. She thought this process was more rapid in the public hospitals, probably relative to staff turnover. (1990 Vol 1 p.148)

Matron Robson described the power which doctors exercised over decision making. The expert nurse witnesses supported this. One defended the nurses by stating that even in 1978 he doubted that 'nurses would have been in any position to go and question the medical staff regarding their treatments and instructions' (1990 Vol 5 p.105).

Another expert witness described the changes in the way doctors gave instructions to nurses and the way nurses responded to practices that they believed to be questionable. She explained that relationships between doctors and nurses had changed a great deal since the 1960s, when nursing was still very much a 'medic-dominated profession', and nurses were 'intimidated by doctors'. She further explained that 'nurses were taught to literally have doctors on a pedestal. They were seen as all-powerful and all-knowing'. She referred to the personality of the nurse as being the only factor in controlling poor medical practice: 'Except where a tough ward sister had won the respect and fear of the medical profession, nurses had no other option but to accept the practice of the treating doctor and remain silent' (1990 Vol 5 p.113).

However, she felt that nurses were currently more concerned about their legal responsibilities and less prepared to be the 'patsies' should things go wrong. She described the avenues available in the 1960s and 1970s for nurses who were critical of a doctor, stating that they would need to go to 'the director of nursing or the senior nurse and she in turn might have approached the treating doctor'. However, she also testified that it was very difficult for nurses to challenge the hierarchy. Often the only option was to leave. She attested that the changes in nurse education had improved the situation, although there was still 'a reluctance to take steps critical of the hospital or the treating doctor' (1990 Vol 5 p.114).

A third witness described doctors in the 1960s and early 1970s as being 'so all-powerful' that nurses would 'generally do as the doctor prescribed'. He suggested that a refusal to carry out a doctor's instruction would be very unlikely 'except in an ethical or perceived life threatening situation' (1990 Vol 5 p.113). However, the situation at Chelmsford would seem unequivocally to fall into both of those categories, simultaneously rendering this comment somewhat redundant and bringing into relief his own view of what might be expected of a nurse.

There is in fact substantial evidence to suggest that the nurses were deeply concerned by the events at Chelmsford. After the death of Mary Isobel Rodgers in 1964, Dr Bailey ripped up the notes made by Sr Edwards and told her to mind her own business. In 1974 Sr Crozier expressed her concerns about the management of Mr Peter Clarke both to Dr Bailey by telephone and to Dr Herron immediately before he administered ECT to the patient. This was to no avail, as he died about 10 minutes after its administration. She left the hospital one week after his death. In 1974 Matron Fawdry expressed her concerns about the suitability of Stavroula Leousis for sedation at all, but she died of pneumonia. Matron Fawdry was attacked personally by Dr Gill during the Royal Commission.

After the death of Miriam Podio in 1977, the 'nurses' gave evidence to the effect that the place was 'a buzz' (1990 Vol 4 p.206). Sr Switzer telephoned Matron Fawdry on three occasions to express her concern about the patient's condition, and was then telephoned herself by Dr Gill, telling her not to bother the matron any more and that there was nothing wrong with Miss Podio. She noted this in the nursing records, and the relevant pages went missing from the notes after the patient's death. She eventually expressed her concerns in an interview by the police in 1986, but she had left the hospital in November 1978, some 15 months after the death of Miss Podio and 14 months after the death of John Adams, both of which she remembered vividly.

In addition to these 'life-threatening situations', there were Dr Bailey's sexual relations with some of his patients, which would undoubtedly fall into the category of 'ethical' concerns for the nursing staff. Matron Fawdry recalls on at least one occasion arguing with Dr Bailey about his relationship with Sharon Hamilton, and the way in which she was treated at the hospital. There was also evidence given by the nursing staff 'that late at night or in the early morning Dr Bailey would sometimes telephone the hospital and direct that particular female patients be sent in to see him by taxi' (1990 Vol 2 p.99). At least one of these patients was known to be having sexual relations with him.

Dr Herron described the nursing staff's questioning of DST as 'hysteria' (1990 Vol 2 p.155) and Dr Gill suggested that all the nurses who had complained had 'colluded with the Scientologists' (1990 Vol 2 p.218). Matron Nelson explained that in her time as Matron between 1971 and 1972 there was a rumour that a complaint was made to the Department of Health about DST in 1970 which had been investigated by the Department leading to the treatment being approved. The Commissioner held that if this was the case, it was asking too much of the nursing staff 'to vigorously oppose the treatment' (1990, Vol 1 p.120). However, the DST went on for some considerable time after 1971, and 15 more people died unexpectedly at Chelmsford during the next six years.

The Commissioner was unable to totally excuse the lack of intervention by the nursing staff, despite the descriptions of the expert witnesses and the doctors. But he was far less critical than might have been expected, given the outcomes for the patients. He acknowledged that 'many were undoubtedly embarrassed by the nature of the DST and ECT treatments' and that while some resigned, others had to remain for 'the lack of employment opportunities, for financial reasons'. Still others, he suggested, tolerated the DST 'believing that as it was prescribed by specialist doctors and the hospital had been visited and inspected by officers of Health, there was little that could be done'. He described their dilemma as 'understandable' but was moved to observe that it was 'a little surprising that only two nurses during the period 1963 to 1979 were known to have complained to Health about events at Chelmsford' (1990 Vol 1 pp.163–64).

Dealing with moral dissonance: to leave or to rationalise?

This was a most generous exoneration by the Commissioner, but it left unresolved the question of the nurses' morality and professionalism. That the nurses felt powerless to change the situation is obvious. Yet they certainly had the industrial might to have simply refused to perform the requested illegal activities. Their failure to act speaks volumes for their perception of the doctors' power. The Commissioner accepted the evidence of the expert nurse witnesses and the matrons that the instructions of the doctor would have been very difficult to contradict. But, difficult as the position of these senior nurses may have been, the fact remains that they knew that what was happening was morally wrong (Johnstone 1995). They would certainly also have known that the unqualified staff were practising well beyond their scope of responsibility with regards to the medication administration. Yet, they continued to allow the patients to suffer and, in many cases, to die.

It is difficult to see how their conduct might have been condoned, yet the Commissioner specifically stated that the nurses in the sedation ward 'made every effort to uphold the traditions of the nursing profession' (1990 Vol 1 pp.163–64). This says little for the traditions of the nursing profession but illustrates the reluctance of the Commissioner to deal too harshly with the nursing staff. But sympathy of this nature does not benefit the nursing profession; it helps to perpetuate the stock story of the nurse as the doctor's handmaiden, to the ultimate detriment of future nurses involved in such situations.

Madjar's work (1997) on the dissonance nurses experience when inflicting pain on patients may provide some insight into the behaviour of the Chelmsford nurses. Madjar found that nurses view such treatments solely as delegated medical work and, in this way, distance themselves from their effects. Many of the nurses involved did what nurses who find themselves powerless usually do. They left (NSW Health Department 1996a). In a study undertaken by Millette, based on the work of Carol Gilligan (1982), 50 per cent of the nurses in the study who felt unable to act on their moral convictions or provide care which they felt would benefit their patients 'left nursing or changed their practice site' (Millette 1994 p.670).

When nurses encounter such difficulties, they do not often raise the issues publicly—perhaps because they do not feel very proud of themselves (Johnstone 1995). The dilemma for nurses is that, in order for this moral paralysis to be addressed judicially, the nurses under scrutiny would have to admit that they were morally (and legally) culpable when they stood back and allowed such incidents to occur. They would have to acknowledge that they should have taken the initiative (and the risk) of challenging medical authority. When nurses find themselves under the judicial gaze in this way, it is understandable that they revert to the handmaiden defence, and seek to show that they did their best within their area of limited autonomy—that they meant well, but were powerless to intervene. Their role was to obey, and that was what they did. Since the stock story is so widely accepted, their lawyers exploit it and the judges accept it.

There are undoubtedly situations where it is perfectly reasonable for the nurse to claim reliance on the doctor. The purpose of this book is not to argue that nurses alone should take responsibility for the well-being and safety of patients. They are entitled to expect that doctors will normally be knowledgeable and skilled, just as doctors are entitled to expect the same of nurses. For example, in Moore v Castlegar & District Hospital (1996) Gill J held that: 'it is thus surely the case that a nurse is entitled to rely upon the diagnosis of a physician who has examined a patient, and is not required to repeat the examination' (p.187).

CONCLUSION

The image of the nurse as the doctor's handmaiden is embedded within the psyche of the society in which we live and in which nurses and doctors work. The phrase has been used by parliamentarians, doctors, and nurses, and has as its pivot the concept that nurses are no more than extensions of doctors, and that the nurses' actions and thoughts are congruent with those of the doctors whom they serve. Such a concept means that nurses are appropriate people to perform delegated medical tasks and for it to be as though such tasks were performed by a doctor. The emphasis however, is on the doctor's authority to make the delegation.

The image also means that doctors are able to advise and comment on nursing as a part of medicine, and to substitute their views for the views of nurses. Furthermore, because there is no expectation of nurses having independent moral agency, they are not criticised when they fail to intervene if doctors are putting patients at risk. They do not even receive substantial criticism if they follow the orders of doctors which are clinically incorrect or morally wrong. Nurses have been known to rely successfully on this story as a defence to potential opprobrium. The problem for nurses is that, because the courts and tribunals condone this subsumed position, the nurse has no legitimate separate right of intervention on behalf of the patient. The implication of this story is that the nurse owes a duty to the doctor, and the doctor owes a duty to the patient. The nurses' duty to the patient is exercised via obedience to the doctor.

7

The nurse as subordinate professional

Elements of the image

- Nurses are acknowledged to possess specialised skills, although much of the nursing work which is regarded as specialised is delegated medical work.

- Nurses are expected to be able to perform these specialised skills without direct supervision by a doctor.

- However, nurses are still under the control of doctors; BUT

- Nurses are expected to be able to bring specific problems to the attention of the doctor; AND

- Nurses are expected to challenge doctors when the doctor appears to be wrong.

- Nurses may only substitute for doctors with the doctor's permission.

INTRODUCTION

The image of the nurse as a 'subordinate professional' is, to some degree, a different point on the same continuum as the doctor's handmaiden image. The nurse is still controlled and dominated by the doctor, but to a lesser extent. Chronologically, the elements of this image appear more frequently later in the last century than those of the 'doctor's handmaiden' image. The major difference in the subordinate professional image is that nursing work is accorded some professional status, albeit a subclass of professionalism. Nursing has some professional attributes, but not equal professional status to other established professions, such as medicine or law. The image suggests that much of the professional status which is ascribed to nursing is 'extrinsically professional' status, i.e. it occurs because of nursing's association with medicine.

The subordinate professional image is a stock story. The elements of this image (detailed at the opening to this chapter) are of great significance for this book. They highlight a major dilemma nurses face in their everyday practice; namely, which of the images ought they to depict? Ought they to behave as doctors' handmaidens and dutifully carry out the doctors' orders without question? Alternatively, ought they to act as subordinate professionals which, it will be demonstrated, creates considerably greater responsibility without concomitantly giving them considerably greater power? If the doctor's handmaiden image suggested an abdication of moral agency on the part of nurses, the subordinate professional image is more complex. It gives them a degree of moral (and clinical) responsibility, but no promise of power.

This is not to suggest that doctors are never held to be tortiously liable or professionally responsible for their mistakes when nursing staff are also involved. The previous chapter described situations where nurses were not blamed at all, and, indeed, where they were not expected to exercise any moral agency. Nor is it suggested that doctors never accept tortious or professional responsibility for their mistakes, but instead always try to shift the blame from themselves to the nursing staff. The recent case of Raji-Abu-Shkara v Hillingdon HA (1997) featured a consultant who 'never ... [sought] to off-load the responsibilities which remained his throughout, on to the shoulders of others, nor ... to place upon any of them the blame for the misfortune which befell the plaintiff' (p.121). In addition, medicolegal textbooks provide abundant examples of successful medical negligence suits.

The point is that, when reading these textbooks, one could be forgiven for imagining that only medical practitioners are held to be responsible, and that they alone shoulder all the responsibility. Such cases, in which the nurse is not mentioned at all, are not helpful to this research as they offer no indication of what role the nurse might have played (although if the facts were played out in a hospital there would almost certainly have been nurses present). The purpose of this book is to address the status of the nurse at law, and thus the case law which has been collected provides specific insight into that question. Much has been written about the legal status of doctors. The intent here was to redress the balance—to "find" the nurse in the law.

NURSES ARE ACKNOWLEDGED TO BE
PROFESSIONALS WITH SPECIALIST SKILLS,
ALTHOUGH MUCH OF THE NURSING WORK WHICH
IS REGARDED AS SPECIALIST IS DELEGATED
MEDICAL WORK

The professional status of nursing: profession or vocation?

Florence Nightingale herself was opposed to the notion of nursing as a profession, preferring to use the term vocation or calling (Vicinus & Nergaard 1989 p.425). However, other powerful nursing leaders at the beginning of the 20th century wanted nursing to be recognised as a profession. Organisations such as the Australasian Trained Nurses Association, founded in 1899 (Russell 1990), and the College of Nursing in England, founded in 1916, were open in their use of the term 'nursing profession'. The College of Nursing even used the term in its objects (Abel-Smith 1960). Anne-Marie Rafferty, tracing the tensions between the mid-Victorian Nightingale ideologists and the suffragettes of the early 20th century, points out that: 'the new nurses that emerged from the first wave of nursing reform strove for freedom and mobility in the health care market. They were not satisfied with the place allotted to them by the statesmen and stakeholders in health care; they strove to define their own occupational turf and territory' (1996 pp.40–41).

The professional status of nursing: Flexner's criteria for a profession

Whether nursing fulfilled the criteria for a profession in those early days is debatable. Abraham Flexner, well known for his early work on the characteristics of professions, identified eight criteria for a profession (1915). Flexner was an educator with a Bachelor's degree from Johns Hopkins University, and a Rhodes scholar. His views on professions are particularly appropriate to this book as they were representative of the white male majority. They were as follows:

1. Professions involve essentially intellectual operations accompanied by significant individual responsibility.
2. They are learned in nature, and their members are constantly resorting to the laboratory and seminar for a fresh supply of facts.
3. They are not merely academic and theoretical, however, but are definitely practical in their aims.
4. They possess a technique capable of communication through a highly specialised educational discipline.
5. They are self-organised, with activities, duties and responsibilities that completely engage their participants and develop group consciousness.
6. They are likely to be more responsive to [the] public interest than are unorganised and isolated individuals, and they tend to become increasingly concerned with the achievement of social ends.
7. They abide by a code of ethics whose ambiguities have been clarified and interpreted, rendering it completely understandable.
8. They receive a high level of compensation in terms of both money and satisfaction. (1915 pp.576–81)

The professional status of nursing: in the early part of the 20th century

When these criteria are applied to the nursing profession, it is clear that, although nursing met some of them, it was deficient in others. In the first half of the 20th century, nursing only partially fulfilled Flexner's criteria. Significantly, it was not entirely self-organised, either in its working sphere or its professional sphere, as there was considerable medical direction in nursing work, and equally considerable medical dominance over professional aspects of nursing such as the nurse registering authorities. In addition, although nurses may have gained considerable personal satisfaction from their work, there was little or no financial reward.

The professional status of nursing: in the second half of the 20th century

The quest for professional status in the second half of the 20th century became something of a crusade, and forms the content of Chapters 8, 9 & 10. There has been a recent proliferation of literature analysing both the nature of professions and the place which nursing holds in any professional hierarchy (Partlett 1985, Davis & George 1988, Willis 1994, Lupton 1995, Rafferty 1996, Field & Taylor 1998, Petersen & Wadell 1998). Daniel, for example describes the characteristics of a profession in the late 20th century as follows:

Autonomy, based on knowledge claims, definitively expresses the power of a profession to control its field of work and its own reproduction. Professions control the criteria for entry, the lengthy educational training, registration, and standards of practice and conduct within the profession. The socialisation of a professional is a subtly pervasive process that continues throughout a lifetime of practice.
  Related to professional autonomy, controlling conditions and standards of practice, is the authority which the professional assumes; the professional is sole arbiter in her domain of work and that work is usually in critical, dangerous areas of human activity. (1990 p.62)

Daniel is clearly undecided and guarded about the professional status of nursing, and uses terms such as 'calling' and 'occupation' rather than 'profession'. She acknowledges the fact that Australian nurses are seeking greater professional status, but considers that they are still subordinate to doctors. She observes that 'the critical factor rests on whether the break with the traditional apprenticeship-style training and adoption of more intensive college-based education will be accompanied by more enhanced authority and responsibility in patient care. Without any concomitant increase in autonomy of practice, the enlargement of education and upgrading of qualifications will make for further frustration and job dissatisfaction' (1990 pp.76–77).

Mike Saks contends that, since the medical profession still holds a monopoly over specific aspects of diagnosis and treatment, it is not surprising that nursing is still viewed as a semi-profession. He suggests that nursing can be viewed as an example of 'dual closure'. He explains that 'having failed to secure full professional closure, they are seen to combine the exclusionary device of credentialism with the usurpationary tactics of organised labour against employers and the state' (1998 p.181).

This chapter demonstrates that the improvements in education and the upgrading of clinical and academic qualifications have resulted in an increased expectation of responsibility. However, to date these changes do not appear to have led to an overall enhancement of authority or an increase in autonomy of practice.

The professional status of nursing: in courts and tribunals

In the first half of the 20th century, the need to determine liability for the acts of nurses was the genesis of many of the pronouncements on their professional status. This is seen in Strangeways-Lesmere v Clayton (1936), a case in which two nurses were (unusually) found personally liable for the death of a patient due to their failure to check properly the written instructions for a dose of paraldehyde. Here the judge held that '[t]he administration of the paraldehyde is a skilled operation...I do not think this is a matter of a nurse's routine, but one in which she is to use professional skill, and the only duty of the hospital is to see that the nurses they engage are duly qualified persons' (pp.486–87).

However, on some occasions the courts did make broader comments, usually obiter, which suggested that nursing was itself a profession. Kennedy LJ in Hillyer v Governors of St Bartholomew's Hospital acknowledged that 'in matters of professional skill' nurses were 'experts' with 'professional competence' (1909 p.829) although he did not accord this status to all aspects of nursing work. In Ingram v Fitzgerald (1936), the judge held that nurses were 'members of an allied profession and have duties of their own to perform' (p.915). Somervell LJ supported this view some fifteen years later in Cassidy v Ministry of Health and stated that 'it is important to bear in mind that nurses are qualified professional persons' (1951 p.351). The desirability of maintaining this professional status was used as a 'carrot' by Boyd McBride J in Bernier v Sisters of Service (1948) to encourage nurses to persevere with their professional studies.

In the second half of the century, the term 'professional' was sometimes used to describe nurses in the industrial courts and tribunals, although not necessarily to the benefit of those student nurses whose case was under scrutiny (In re Public Hospital Nurses (State) Award (No.1) 1959). In more recent appeals against decisions of disciplinary tribunals, nursing has been routinely referred to as a profession properly capable of self regulation (Re Cabrera 1980, Slater v UKCC 1988). On occasion it seems to have been elevated to a 'super-group', along the lines of the ministering angel theme (Re Crandell v Manitoba Association of Registered Nurses 1976).

The expert skills of nurses have been recognised in industrial courts and tribunals for most of the second half of the 20th century (Public Hospital Nurses (State) Award 1967, Public Hospital Nurses (State) Award 1971, Public Hospital Nurses (State) Award 1973, Ministerial Reference Case 1986). A significant number of judges have held that the increase in educational standards and a search for improved practice has achieved greater professionalism in nursing. By way of example, Wells C stated that the pursuit of accreditation under the Australian Council on Health Care Standards Accreditation Scheme had achieved for nurses: 'a higher professional plane ... generally' (Ministerial Reference Case 1986 p.23).

However, the professional role of nurses is consistently diminished by the courts and tribunals when it is examined alongside the professional authority of doctors. Much, although not all, of the work that has contributed to improving the pay and conditions of nurses has been delegated medical work (Public Hospital Nurses (State) Award 1973, Public Hospital Nurses (State) Award 1976, Ministerial Reference Case 1986). However, the medical profession has not been held responsible when its performance has come under judicial scrutiny. Doctors have been able to argue successfully that they were entitled to rely on the nursing staff to perform such work thoroughly. Yet despite this apparent shift in/revocation of responsibility, there has been little concomitant loss of power and control over the clinical environment.

NURSES WILL UNDERTAKE THE WORK THEY ARE ASSIGNED OR REQUIRED TO PERFORM WITHOUT FURTHER SUPERVISION BY OR ADVICE FROM THE DOCTOR

Judicial examination of nursing responsibility as an ancillary issue

In the second half of the 20th century litigating patients have often sought to make hospitals liable for the negligence of hospital personnel. This often arises when a plaintiff is trying to fix a hospital or a doctor with liability for a situation which also involves the activities of a nurse. On such occasions, the courts have held that the doctor was not liable for the nurse's behaviour and have conceded that nurses can and do organise their own workloads. Thus, although the work under scrutiny may have been doctor generated or delegated, the expectation of a certain level of professional skill and competence from the nurses involved has served to absolve at least the doctor, if not the hospital, from civil liability. This phenomenon will be termed 'the defence of reliance'. It presupposes a degree of independent moral agency and autonomy of action by the nurse.

For this reason it has often been difficult to identify cases which actually addressed either questions of professional status, or the standard of care/level of skill which might be expected of the 'reasonable registered nurse'. But it is inherent in the nature of outsider scholarship that nurses (as outsiders) would be ancillary to many examinations of health care practice in the courts—which is a reflection of their perceived ancillary role in health care practice in general. Questions about nurses are rarely addressed as matters of importance because they are not considered to be matters of importance to anyone except nurses. Graycar and Morgan elucidate the point when discussing the place of women in the law:

For women, these artificial classifications [tort, crime, family law etc] are especially problematic since women have played no part in defining these categories. It is because of this exclusion of women from traditional legal scholarship that taking women's lives as a starting point for any legal analysis requires a fundamental rethinking of those categories. (Footnotes omitted, 1990 p.3)

There have been a number of recent British midwifery cases which have focused directly on midwifery practice and the standard of reasonable midwifery care (e.g. Corley (by Wendy Jane Corley her mother and next friend) v North West Hertfordshire Health Authority 1997, Gaughan v Bedfordshire Health Authority 1997). However, midwifery has a much wider scope of practice within the public health system in the UK than it does in Australia, and the hospital medical staff would play a much smaller role in public patient, well-women deliveries.

Doctors are entitled to rely on the expertise of nurses and have no responsibility to intervene

The proposition that doctors need not involve themselves in the performance of nursing work is one with which most nurses (especially those in pursuit of professional autonomy) would concur. It would go to the heart of another proposition, long held by many nurses, that nurses and doctors are part of a team of equal, but different players. However this second proposition is not necessarily the natural consequence of the first. Doctors may not necessarily be held legally responsible, but may still be treated as maintaining control. Hence the notion of a subordinate, as opposed to autonomous, professional.

This principle, that doctors are entitled to rely on the expertise of nurses and are not required to supervise nursing work, was clearly enunciated in 1955 in the Canadian case of Petite v MacLeod and St Mary's Hospital.

It seems quite clear that there can be negligence on the part of the doctor and also on the part of the nurse. One is a check against the other in such cases but each has his or her own duty which must be done with the care which a reasonable and competent person would exercise in a matter of such importance ... It is also clear that a doctor may rely upon the work of a competent and qualified nurse. If a nurse takes a patient's temperature and reports it to the doctor or marks it on a chart, the doctor is not required to check this by himself taking the temperature, nor if the nurse is told to obtain a harmless preparation by a written or even an oral order, the doctor is not ordinarily put upon his inquiry as to whether what is brought to him is a harmful substance. (1955 p.154)

Over time, the level of expected competence has increased and there have been numerous instances of judicial acceptance of a doctor's entitlement to rely completely upon the assurances of the nurse. For example, it has been accepted that doctors were entitled to assume, in the absence of any contrary statement, that a nurse would be able to manage her workload, even when the nurse was alone in a busy post-anaesthetic (or recovery) room (PAR) (Laidlaw v Lion's Gate Hospital 1969 p.739). This was reconfirmed in Krujelis v Esdale (1971), where it was held that 'Dr Esdale had no control or jurisdiction over the PAR and no vestige of reasonable anticipation that [the child] would receive anything but the best of care in it'. He was further absolved from responsibility for the draping and positioning of the child because 'the PAR nursing staff, all specially trained for their exacting task, have complete jurisdiction, without consulting with anyone, to change the draping of a patient, if they consider such to be desirable' (1971 pp.559–60).

It has been repeatedly determined that surgeons are entitled to rely on the nurses' sponge count, and only have to feel around in the abdomen to see that all sponges were removed (Karderas v Clow 1972, Langley & Anor v Glandore Pty Ltd (in liq) 1997, Elliott v Bickerstaff 1999). In MacDonald v York (1973), doctors were absolved from giving specific instructions regarding pain management or circulatory observations on a patient's foot because 'the nursing staff, in whose charge the patient was, was (sic) competent in such matters' (p.323). In the Inquest touching the death of TJB (1989), it was held that that a paediatrician could leave the determination of appropriate oral fluids for a child with gastroenteritis to the discretion of the nursing staff.

The way in which such a right of reliance can advantage the medical staff

Decisions such as these, which have delineated areas of unique nursing responsibility, have led to inconsistencies between the expectations of the practices of doctors and nurses. For example, an identical lack of care has been construed differently when exercised by a doctor and a nurse in the same case.

In Bugden v Harbour View Hospital (1947) it was held that the patient died as a result of wrongly administered medication. The action was brought by the deceased's widow against the hospital, the two nurses, and the visiting surgeon. Doull J acknowledged that all three defendants involved in the incident might have prevented the incident if only one of them had looked at the label on the bottle.

If either Nurse Spriggs or Nurse Bonnar or Doctor McKeough had looked at the label on the bottle they could have seen that what it contained was not novocaine or procaine ... If it is the duty of several persons to guard against danger, one who fails to take precautions cannot escape by saying that another should have been careful enough to have caught his error. (1947 p.340)

It was held that Nurse Spriggs and particularly Nurse Bonnar were two of those persons 'under a duty to guard against danger'. The judge stated 'whatever the duty of Miss Spriggs ... I think that it was Miss Bonnar's duty when she received a labelled bottle to see that it was the proper bottle' (p.342). Both nurses were held to be negligent because, 'in the case of drugs where the consequences of a mistake may be so grave, I think anyone who is procuring a drug should use whatever means are within his (sic) power to prevent a mistake'. This seems perfectly reasonable. As Doull J said, 'It was only a matter of looking at the label in this case and I must hold that she was negligent in not doing so' (p.343).

However, what seems unreasonable is that, despite the judge's opinion that no one who failed to take precautions should 'escape', an exception was made for the doctor. Doull J held that the doctor was not under the same duty to guard against danger, although he admitted he had found it to be a difficult question. Nonetheless, he found that the surgeon was entitled to rely on the expertise of the nursing staff, and this ability to rely on their expertise exonerated him from even taking a cursory look at the bottle. This was despite his assertion that 'a surgeon is in charge of the treatment ... and exercises control and supervision over everything which is going on'; and his acknowledgement that 'in the present case a look at the label would have been sufficient to have avoided the accident'. He moved from the particular to the general, finding that 'in a good many cases of operations it would be difficult to make a personal check'. Further, he suggested that 'in a matter of such simplicity as looking at a label I think he was justified in following what was no doubt the routine' (p.342). He also cited a previous decision where it had been found that 'in the absence of knowledge to the contrary or of facts sufficient to put him on enquiry (sic), a surgeon visiting a hospital ... has a right to assume that its nurses ... are competent'. The hospital was held vicariously liable for the negligence of the two nurses and the action against the doctor was dismissed with costs.

That the nurses were negligent is not challenged, nor is it questioned that they were both wrong in failing to check the medication. But Doull J expressly stated that everyone ought to take precautions in a situation such as this and that an individual ought not to be absolved from responsibility because 'another should have been careful enough to have caught his error' (p.340). Nonetheless, the surgeon escaped liability because he was held to be entitled to rely on the duty of the nurses to take care.

NURSES ARE STILL UNDER THE
CONTROL OF DOCTORS

Doctors—not responsible for the conduct of nurses, but still in control of them

Judicial recognition of (quasi) professional status, specialist clinical skill, and exclusive areas of clinical responsibility has not led to the judicial conclusion that nurses are also clinically self-governing. Instead, the relevant judgments go to extraordinary lengths to ensure that the ability to exercise power and retain control over the nurses is still maintained, even when medical liability for their acts is negated. Judgments which find doctors not liable for the wrongs of nurses invariably contain qualifying comments. Examples of these are: 'they are subordinate to the surgeons, but they are in no way their servants [employees]' (Van Wyk v Lewis 1924 p.454); 'he was in supreme control ... but ... would [not] expect to find it necessary to intervene' (Ingram v Fitzgerald 1936 p.913); 'the operating surgeon was in charge ... and could give directions ... but they were not his servants or agents' (Paton v Parker 1941 p.195); and 'even when they are under the direction of the surgeon ... [he] has not that "entire and absolute control" over them which is necessary to make them his servants, even temporarily' (Cassidy v Ministry of Health 1951 pp.261–62). Even after the decision in Gold v Essex County Council (1942) determined that a hospital would be liable in tort regardless of whether the negligent party was a doctor or a nurse, this affirmation of the exercise of medical power did not cease. In Elliott v Bickerstaff (1999) Giles JA stated that 'the surgeon can be regarded ... as the master of ceremonies, but ... should be able to concentrate on his own skilled task without shouldering the responsibilities of the other members of the team' (p.29).

THE NURSE IS EXPECTED TO BRING SPECIFIC
PROBLEMS TO THE ATTENTION OF THE DOCTOR

Nurses—not in control of doctors, but still potentially accountable for their mistakes?

Accordingly, medical control and dominance over the nursing profession is still very much a stock story, an accepted norm, a 'given' for the courts and tribunals, as it is in the 'doctor's handmaiden' image. However, in the 'subordinate professional' image, it becomes a 'given' with a twist, as doctors are in control of nurses, but not responsible for their conduct. This twist becomes further pronounced on examination of the various arguments advanced by the medical profession and their counsel, when the behaviour of the doctor is under scrutiny, and they are practising either assisted by or in collaboration with a nurse. Sometimes, a defence raised by the allegedly responsible doctor is to argue that, not only can doctors expect to rely on nurses to carry out their own responsibilities unsupervised, but they may also rely on the nurse to assist them to practise more safely. Such 'assistance' might manifest as nurses alerting the doctor to specific problems, which the doctor would not necessarily investigate in the absence of such express notice; or challenging the doctor if they are concerned about the doctors' actions (whether the actions are deliberate or inadvertent).

The particular duty of a nurse to communicate

Nurses spend a great deal of time on the wards with patients when no doctor is present. It is therefore a critical aspect of experienced nursing practice to be able to assess a patient's condition and determine exactly when the patient needs to be seen by a doctor. To call the doctor unnecessarily might take him/her away from a sicker, more needy patient. To call them too late might endanger the patient's health. The ANCI Competencies (1999) specify that a beginning practitioner needs to recognise the limits of their competence and to know when to refer matters of concern to a senior nurse or doctor. Beginning practitioners are expected (except in an emergency) to refer any abnormality to a more experienced nurse, who then makes a decision on referral. In the absence of a more experienced nurse, they should seek advice from the medical practitioner.

The courts have confirmed this obligation for nurses to relay any concerns about abnormalities in a patient's condition to doctors, even if they are unsure what they mean (Gleason (Guardian ad litem of) v Bulkley Valley District Hospital 1996, Granger (litigation guardian of) v Ottawa General Hospital 1997). However the case law seems to suggest that the greater communication duty rests with nurses. Not unreasonably the nurses seem to be expected to give detailed and specific information about their clinical concerns. However, there does not appear to be a reciprocal duty for a doctor actively to seek information of a similar quality. A failure of nurses to communicate information in sufficient detail has been used successfully by doctors as grounds for mitigation. This is in contrast to the stock story of the nurse as doctor's handmaiden, where the nurse is not expected to challenge the doctor at all.

In the 1992 Inquest into the death of HAB, the patient had a bladder irrigation system in situ following prostate surgery. The nurse was concerned because the patient was in pain and in positive fluid balance, which meant that more fluid was going into the bladder than was coming out of it via the catheter. She contacted the duty doctor to communicate her anxiety who gave a verbal order for analgesia. The duty doctor testified that the nurse did not mention the patient's positive fluid balance; thus, when she came to examine the patient, she missed the positive fluid balance because it was not drawn specifically to her attention, and consequently she mismanaged the patient's condition. Later that evening, the patient went into severe shock. He was transferred for laparotomy, but died in the early hours of the morning.

The duty doctor invoked the defence of reliance, testifying that the nurse should have specifically brought the imbalance to her attention. The coroner criticised the failure of the nursing staff to inform the doctor of their concern over the patient's fluid balance status, and held that it was a positive duty of a nurse to relay such information to the doctor (p.8).

There is no argument with this finding. However, it is submitted that the nursing staff's failure to inform the doctor was only one of the mistakes which led to the problem going undetected until it was too late for the surgeon's intervention to be effective. If the duty doctor had examined the fluid balance chart, it would have revealed the same information. The registrar testified that it was one of his first actions when he was called to examine HAB, and so significant did he consider it that he photocopied it. However, the coroner did not suggest that the duty doctor had a positive duty to read the fluid balance chart in the same way that he held that the nurses had a positive duty to communicate the information from the chart to the doctor. He simply observed, mildly and without comment, that the records had been available, but that she not read them, and that if she had looked at them, she would have known about the imbalance at an earlier time (1992 pp.7–8).

The nurses were found to have a positive duty to advise the doctor about what they had observed. The doctor would have 'been wise' to have read the fluid balance chart, but was not criticised openly for failing to do so. The primary duty rested with the nursing staff to relay all their information verbally to the doctor. It seems that the maxim '[i]f it is the duty of several people to guard against danger, one who fails to take precautions cannot escape by saying that another should have been careful enough to have caught his error' is more readily honoured in its breach (Bugden v Harbour View Hospital 1947 p.340). Surely in HAB the duty of nursing and medical staff alike was to 'guard against danger' by reading the available records? Yet, as in Bugden, the maxim does not seem to have the same application to the doctors as it did to the nurses.

An unequal 'interdependence'

In the Inquest touching the death of MAQ (1989) Sr Heathcote was criticised strongly for not giving the doctor all the relevant information over the phone. She was described as 'the doctor's eyes and ears' (p.000741). In contrast, the doctor received less criticism for failing to question further, despite the fact that the nurse had already expressed her uncertainty about the patient's condition. In addition, whilst the official stance of the AMA might be that diagnosis is the 'sine qua non' of the medical profession (AMA 1992), the doctor in MAQ testified that he relied on nurses to make diagnoses and convey clinical impressions (1989 p.000742). The recognition of his reliance on the nurse and their interdependence in matters of patient management effectively absolved him from the level of criticism visited on Sr Heathcote.

The influence of nurses over a doctor's clinical decision making was also acknowledged in an English negligence case, where the court found that a doctor made a decision to prescribe Depo-Provera 'because the [nursing] sister said that it was often used in these circumstances' (Blyth v Bloomsbury HA 1993 p.155).

These cases would seem to imply that a doctor is entitled to rely on the information received from a nurse even when it is not particularly explicit or helpful. The onus seems to be on the nurse to be the active communicator. The doctor does not seem to have a corresponding role of active questioner. If the nurse does not actively provide further, and more accurate, information, the doctor seems to be able to obtain some degree of exoneration from blame. However, the ensuing cases in this chapter demonstrate that nurses are not similarly entitled to rely passively on the information received from a doctor as being correct. They are expected actively to check and clarify it, and they ought not to seek support from the 'casual assurances' of a doctor (Nyberg v Provost Municipal Hospital 1927 p.231).

NURSES ARE EXPECTED TO CHALLENGE DOCTORS WHEN THE DOCTOR APPEARS TO BE WRONG

The nurse will challenge the doctor if concerned about the doctor's actions (whether the actions are deliberate or inadvertent)

The next series of cases takes the defence of reliance one step further. Here, not only are nurses expected to communicate their concerns adequately to doctors, they are also expected, if concerned, to challenge doctors' actions. In several cases, it was found that nurses should have questioned a doctor's behaviour, whether it was deliberate or inadvertent. In some, the nurses' failure to do so has to some extent mitigated the culpability of the doctor. However, a further difficulty for nurses is that, because doctors are considered to be in control, they are under no obligation to act on the concerns brought by nurses to their attention.

Inconsistencies in the early case law

An early example can be found in Lavere v Smith's Falls Public Hospital (1915b). The judge quoted a remark he had heard made by a very eminent surgeon: 'If I cannot trust my nurse, I must give up surgery' (p.349). Riddell J made the somewhat tortuous pronouncement that the nurse's duty was to obey the doctor, but only if she was sure that he was right. His Honour gave fairly detailed instructions as to how this could be achieved.

If the nurse obeyed the express order of the surgeon, she was not guilty of negligence at all. That is the duty of a nurse. Of course she must take some pains to see that she quite understands the doctor's meaning, and she must not act upon what she would know to be a slip of the tongue. To put it in other words, the order she obeys must be a real order, not such as is apparently an order, but so expressed that it cannot be supposed to set out the doctor's real meaning.

A nurse holds herself out to the world as being possessed of competent skill, and undertakes to use reasonable care. If the command of the surgeon is plainly a slip, she should call his attention pointedly to the order. When his attention has been called to the order, and he shews (sic) that the order was made was that intended, she may obey; 'he is the doctor', and it is not negligence for a nurse to act on the belief that he is more competent. (p.348)

He continued 'granted that an order is a real order of a medical man, a nurse is justified in obeying it, unless it is plainly dangerous' (p.349).

However, the case of Nyberg v Provost Municipal Hospital Board (1927) demonstrated that this requirement was more difficult in the execution than in the description. A patient was admitted for surgery following a ruptured appendix and was subsequently burned by the hot water bottles. Postoperatively, the nurses employed by the defendant hospital warmed the bed with two hot water bottles in flannel covers, specifically to 'combat the shock of the operation' (p.226). Nurse Switzer, who assisted in the operation and cared for the patient afterwards on the ward, testified that she was concerned about the heat of the bottles and had checked this with the doctors in the operating room.

The physicians testified that they were afraid that the patient might develop pneumonia, as he was in 'a chilly condition' when brought into hospital (p.239). Nurse Switzer attested that postoperatively she had dressed the patient's wound and covered him with a blanket. She testified that she noticed the skin on his chest was reddening and consequently inquired about the bottles to Dr York, the plaintiff's physician who was present during surgery, who answered: 'Now they are all right'. Dr York, although not asked to corroborate her evidence, testified that he 'left no instructions whatever with the nurse in regard to hot water bottles'. Nurse Switzer averred that she also approached the senior surgeon, Dr Sarvis, in the operating room and asked him, 'How about the bottles'. She testified that he answered, 'They are all right, they have been on the floor long enough to cool off'. Dr Sarvis, when called in rebuttal of this conversation, did not deny that it had taken place, although he had no recollection of it (p.238).

The majority of the court found that the nurse had negligently caused the burns to the patient and described her failure to check on the patient's skin as 'inexcusable'. Her evidence that she had taken the extra step of seeking assurance about the safety of the bottles from the doctors was not rejected, but was described as 'attempts to excuse herself by stating that she had some casual assurance from Dr York, the plaintiff's physician' (p.232).

The advice of Riddell J in Lavere, when tested out against the events in Nyberg, creates a scenario fraught with contradictions. Admittedly, no direct order was originally given to Nurse Switzer about the bottles. Their management was part of her routine work. But the court accepted her evidence that she raised her concerns about the heat of the bottles with the doctors. Seen from an outsider perspective, Nurse Switzer seems to have been in an unenviable position. She knew the hot water bottles were her responsibility, but she was also cognisant of the patient's need to be kept warm. However, she was clearly sufficiently concerned to ask, not one but two of the doctors present, about the bottles. Arguably to ask two doctors for their advice on the bottles could be construed as 'call[ing] their attention pointedly' to the matter.

That the surgeons did not recall the conversations was hardly surprising. Their focus would have been on treating a sick patient. But Nurse Switzer was sufficiently concerned to interrupt twice, yet obviously felt unable to remove or adjust the bottles without their approval, and her evidence that she was 'assured by Dr Sarvis and Dr York that they were all right' was accepted. Yet it would seem that it was wrong for her to rely on those assurances, even though (to quote Riddell J in Lavere) '[they were] the doctor[s], and it is not negligent for a nurse to act on the belief that [they were] the more competent'. In fact, it was found that it was negligent. To describe her behaviour as 'inexcusable' and to suggest that she ought to have treated the doctor's remarks as 'casual assurances', and removed the bottles anyway, is to deny the power differentials in the relationship between nurses and doctors, particularly in 1927.

Criticism of nurses' failures to pursue persistently a concern about medical management

The failure of nurses to challenge persistently has led to some fairly trenchant criticism, even where they were finding it difficult or even useless to approach the doctor to challenge his decisions. In Bergen v Sturgeon General Hospital et al (1984), the defendant hospital and certain of its doctors and nurses were found to have negligently caused the death of a woman from septic shock following a ruptured appendix. The acute appendicitis was not diagnosed, despite her spending five days under observation on the ward. The judge found all three doctors jointly negligent, holding that they had fallen into the trap of 'Tunnel Vision' (p.175).

With regard to the defendant nurses, Hope J was also extremely critical of the behaviour of the two charge nurses. The expert witnesses in this case were all doctors, and they gave evidence that the nurses' performance was poor in not calling the doctor immediately the patient experienced what she had described as a 'snapping sensation'. However, it was also revealed that the doctors had not acted upon information about the patient's deteriorating condition recorded in the nurses' notes by numerous entries over the previous three days. Whilst this does not excuse the failure of the nurses to contact the doctor, it is indicative of the uncertainty and helplessness which they may have felt with regard to their concerns being taken seriously. This was also illustrated when one RN advised the doctor that the patient was 'in need of urgent medical help'. The doctor did not tell the nurse that he had two or three other patients to see, and did not attend until some time later. These facts were not viewed as critical by the judge, and the cause of death was attributed to the failure of the nurses to inform the doctor about the 'snapping' incident.

This inherent paradox of the subordinate professional role is further demonstrated in the Inquest touching the death of TJB (1989), where a 21-month-old boy died due to dehydration caused by gastroenteritis. The mother brought the child to hospital at about 9.30 p.m. and he was admitted for review by the paediatrician, who made a diagnosis of viral gastroenteritis and ordered regular oral fluids and observations by the nursing staff.

During the following day, the child continued to vomit and have diarrhoea. The paediatrician saw the child at about 10–10.30 p.m., but did not examine the child physically at this stage because he testified that he had done so earlier. He testified that he observed evidence of dehydration at this stage and considered a drip. Between 11.00 p.m. and 2.00 a.m. the condition of the child appeared to stabilise and, when reviewed at 2.00 a.m., the paediatrician determined that stabilisation had occurred, because he had ceased to vomit. However, at 4.00 a.m. and 5.15 a.m., the nurses noted changes in his pulse and respiratory rates which they did not report to the doctor. Between 5.40 a.m. and 5.45 a.m. the child had a cardiac arrest. The doctor was notified on two occasions of this event and stated twice that he could not attend. However, he finally decided to attend and arrived at the hospital at 6.45 a.m., by which time the child had died.

The Coroner was critical of a number of matters, particularly the nurses' failure to communicate adequately their concerns about the child's condition to the paediatrician. However, they had communicated their concerns about the child and the paediatrician's management of him to the Director of Nursing, who spoke to the Chief Executive Officer about the matter. The Coroner expressed the view that it was 'perhaps unfortunate, although understandable, in some respects, that not one of the staff expressed their concern directly to [the paediatrician]' (p.3). However, he later acknowledged that one of the staff did suggest intravenous therapy to him that afternoon.

Paradoxically, the Coroner also acknowledged that there was a 'protocol' that nurses ought not to approach a member of the medical staff expressing their concern about a patient, and conceded that some practitioners might resent a 'trained sister' behaving in this way (p.13). Such a paradox is not uncommon. This group of cases seem to suggest that nurses ought to intercede with the medical staff whilst acknowledging that such intercession may well be unwelcome or unorthodox.

I accept the reluctance of staff members to approach a medical practitioner expressing his/her concern about a patient, but there are times when this protocol should be set aside. It is no doubt true that some practitioners may well resent being approached by a trained sister in such circumstances. There is no evidence to suggest that [the paediatrician] falls in this category. Nevertheless, I consider that trained nursing sisters have the requisite experience to express an opinion concerning a particular patient's condition. It is not suggested that they should tell the doctor what treatment should be undertaken. I can recall at least one other inquest where a theatre sister did make comments during the course of a surgical procedure to the anaesthetist. Her comments related to her concern about the patient's condition. As comments and events turned out they were well-founded but unfortunately were not heeded. (p.13)

Thus, it would appear to be acceptable for the nurse to 'express an opinion concerning a particular patient's condition', but not to go so far as to 'tell the doctor what treatment should be undertaken'. The Coroner, whilst debunking one protocol (that nurses ought not to approach a medical practitioner expressing concern about a patient), seems to be substituting another (nurses expressing an opinion concerning a particular patient's condition, whilst not telling the doctor what treatment should be undertaken). Nurses would need to tread very carefully in their communications to ensure that they did not breach this etiquette. The expert medical witness testified that nurses were encouraged to communicate concerns directly to doctors at his hospital, an approach the Coroner described as 'commonsense' (p.10). There does not appear to have been any evidence tendered by expert nursing witnesses—the expert medical witness gave evidence about normal nursing practice. The Coroner expressed confidence that 'most, if not all, medical practitioners would not oppose this practice by trained nursing staff in hospitals generally' (p.13).

It is unclear why the Coroner should have been so confident that this 'commonsense approach' would achieve the requisite changes in medical practice. In this case and another example he used the nurses were ignored, and the patients died anyway. The 'unwritten protocol that a nurse should not challenge the orders of a doctor' was probably the reason why the nurses took the exceptional step of involving the Director of Nursing and the Chief Executive Officer in a clinical matter. Perhaps they did not consider that they had sufficient authority to breach such a 'protocol' a second time.

The Coroner was particularly critical of the nurses' failure to advise the paediatrician of the changes in pulse and blood pressure in the early hours of Friday morning. He accepted the expert medical witness's evidence that the nursing staff were 'not sufficiently experienced with the illness to notify the doctor when a change in the condition of [TJB] occurred' (p.8). He linked the nurses' failure to notify to the doctor's failure to commence intravenous therapy.

It is difficult to predict the doctor's response had he been informed earlier of the changes in the patient's condition. On two later occasions when he was told of the critical condition of a cardiac arrest, he told the nursing staff that he could not come. He later admitted in evidence that this was 'a silly thing to do' (p.4), but explained that he did not finish work until 2.00 a.m. and then had to drive home, and thus at the time of the 'phone calls had only had three hours' sleep. There is no suggestion here that his immediate attendance at the hospital could have saved the child's life. However, neither is there any guarantee that, had he been woken an hour earlier after only two hours' sleep, he would have behaved differently and returned to insert the intravenous infusion.

When everything in one's power is not enough

A case in which the nursing staff actually did everything in their power provides a powerful contrast to these previous cases. In Bolitho v City & Hackney HA (1998) the RN, a 'skilled and experienced nurse' felt that 'something was acutely wrong' with a 2-year-old boy who had been admitted with croup. She was so concerned that she took the unusual step of paging the registrar to visit, instead of the senior house officer. She did this at 12.40 p.m. and, after the nurse had described the child's condition, the registrar promised to attend. However, no-one came to see the child. She called the registrar again at 2.00 p.m. and was told that someone would be coming soon. She advised another nurse to do the same at 2.30 p.m., around which time the child arrested, suffered severe brain damage, and eventually died. Actionable negligence was not established against the medical staff because causation could not be proved. The doctors testified that, even if they had attended, they would not have taken the steps which would have prevented the arrest, namely intubation of the child, because the child had made some improvement between episodes.

Similarly no criticism was made of the nurse's role in the scenario, probably because she did everything within her power to save the child. But therein lies the rub. The power of a 'skilled and experience nurse' to compel the doctor to attend and take action which may well have saved the child's life was non-existent, despite her serious and well-founded concerns. Such predicaments must surely be completely unacceptable, and yet there is little or no alternative for nurses, having alerted the doctor to their concerns, but to trust that the doctor will appear and act in the necessary way.

Learned helplessness: ought nurses to give up when doctors don't listen?

Cases such as those above highlight the difficulties nurses experience when they are concerned about a patient and bring their concerns to the doctor's attention, but experience little success in doing so. From both the courts and the literature, it seems that the subordinate professional 'stock story' is well accepted, and is probably the dominant contemporary stock story.

However, what if the nurse believes the doctor is wrong, and a conflict of authority occurs? If the stock stories of 'doctor's handmaiden' and 'subordinate professional' are correct, and the doctor is in 'supreme control', then is there anything more to be done? Cases such as Bergen and TJB may demonstrate that the nurses conceded that their clinical concerns for the patient were ill-founded and the doctor was right. Alternatively they may indicate that the nurses had just 'given up'. Seligman's research (1975) demonstrated that when a behaviour elicits no response, individuals come to learn that their actions are futile, and thus they stop trying to influence the outcome of that or similar situations.

The difficulty is that when a patient dies, if the nurses have 'given up' and stopped asking they are still blameworthy, and the doctors are, to some extent, exonerated by their failure to persevere. This places the nurses in an invidious position. It would be potentially most unpleasant to challenge repeatedly someone who has the decision making authority about a patient's management, when that person has made it manifestly clear that they do not agree with the concerns being expressed.

It seems that although it is acknowledged that there is a protocol that nurses do not generally question doctors, there is nevertheless an expectation that when necessary they will question them. The fact that doctors may choose to disregard them does not appear to exonerate nurses for failing to persevere. Neither are nurses alleviated of the responsibility to question by the acknowledgement that some doctors may resent it. For nurses to feel able to question there would need to be a clear and legitimate expectation that they would do so. For doctors, there needs to be a clear and legitimate expectation that nurses' authority to question would be respected and heeded.

These cases raise the question: 'But what if nurses are sure that the doctor is wrong and they are right? At what stage ought they to defy the doctor's "supreme control" and refuse to obey the medical instructions?' The two operating theatre cases examined in the previous chapter (Re Anderson and Re Johnson 1969, Inquest touching the death of PDP 1994), illustrate that, if they take the initiative to intervene and override the doctor's control, nurses may be exonerated if the patient dies despite such intervention.

But in both those cases it was 'too little intervention, too late' and the nurses knew long before they actually intervened that the patients were in extreme danger. For nurses this is the 'agony tale'—the tale they take home and cry over to their colleagues, the case that haunts them many years afterwards (Bonnet 1997, Zwickler 1997). It provides little solace to the nurses to know that they were really only subordinate professionals, whose primary duty it was to follow orders. It is also cold comfort to console themselves that they had tried to tell the doctor, but the doctor wouldn't listen. It is cold comfort because, unless the power differential between doctors and nurses is rectified, a similar situation may arise again. By accepting and therefore sanctioning the stock stories of doctor's handmaiden and subordinate professional, the court system effectively renders nurses impotent to act immediately and appropriately. It leaves them in a shadow land of moral and clinical uncertainty, where they can undoubtedly be classed as 'outsiders'.

Challenging the doctor: exemplification of the doctor–nurse game?

Leonard Stein's 1967 description of the 'doctor–nurse game'[1] is familiar to nurses and can be recognised in the cases where nurses have employed less than forthright strategies to express their concern (Re Anderson and Re Johnson 1969, Inquest touching the death of TJB 1989, Inquest touching the death of PDP 1994). The rules of the game are spelt out explicitly in some of the judgments (e.g. express concerns, but do not tell the doctors what to do). In a later paper, Stein suggested that the rules of the doctor–nurse game had changed due to the deteriorating public esteem for doctors, and the changing gender demographics of the medical and nursing professions (Stein et al 1990). However, although there has been some support for Stein's assertion (Hughes 1988), several other studies have shown that the unequal power relationships and covert methods of communication still exist (Heenan 1990, Mackay 1993). The nurses' dilemmas occur when doctors do not comply with the rules of the game by accepting their covert suggestions. Such situations benefit none of the players. The doctors gain nothing from the nurses; the nurses experienced a loss of self-esteem and job satisfaction; and the patients lost their lives.

Clinical implications of the subordinate professional stock story

If, to clarify the position to a practising clinical nurse, the elements of the stock story are integrated with relevant aspects of the nursing literature, the

---

[1] It has been suggested that Stein's description of the 'game' would seem to have been formulated from his personal experience as a doctor rather than from systematic inquiry, but the fact that it has been so well recognised and accepted is one test of its validity (see Sweet S & Norman I (1995) The doctor–nurse relationship: a selective literature review. Journal of Advanced Nursing 22 (1): 165–170).

situation could be summarised thus:

1. You are subordinate in professional status to the doctor, but aspects of your work are regarded as skilled professional work.
2. When you are carrying out skilled nursing duties, the doctor is entitled to rely on you to bring all information relating to the patient to the attention of the doctor without having to question you or seek specific information.
3. If you fail to bring all relevant information to the attention of the doctor, the doctor will be exonerated to some extent from liability if the outcomes of the treatment or management are negative for the patient.
4. You ought to obey the doctor because of your subordinate status, but only if you believe that the doctor is right, as your professional nursing skills and expertise ought to alert you to when the doctor may be wrong.
5. If you suspect or fear that the doctor may not be right, you are expected not only to draw the matter to the doctor's attention, but to do so persistently. You have characteristically done this in a somewhat cryptic way, and nurses have been criticised for a lack of directness. However, it is recognised that a protocol exists that you ought not to challenge doctors, and that doctors may resent it if you do.
6. If you challenge the doctor, and the doctor orders you to continue on the same path of management or treatment, you may well be exonerated to some extent from liability if the outcomes of the treatment or management are negative for the patient.
7. It is clear from narratives of nurses that this form of mitigation, i.e. being excused for collaborating with clinical practice which a nurse believed to be inappropriate or wrong, may be a Pyrrhic victory.

The immense value to the medical profession of the nurse as a subordinate professional

Two significant anomalies arise from this analysis:

1. There is an expectation that the nurse will need to question the doctor if an order seems unclear or incorrect, but no corresponding expectation that the doctor will need to question the nurse, as the doctor is entitled to rely on the nurse to bring concerns to his/her attention.
2. The nurse is expected to obey the doctor, but the doctor is not expected to obey the nurse.

This means that the doctor has the means to exercise unlimited power coupled with an acceptable method of mitigating liability, whereas the nurse has a mechanism for exercising very limited power (the power to question), coupled with an unacceptable means of mitigating liability. The relationship is not egalitarian, but hierarchical. It is not even a collaborative relationship as so expressed.

For nurses, the situation as described above is, at best, extremely distressing and frustrating, leading to significant moral dilemmas (Johnstone 1994). At worst, it is untenable. As Jesse B. Semple, one of Bell's fictitious black characters, rather wryly remarked: 'the law works for the [white] Man most of the time, and only works for us in the short run as a way of working for him in the long run' (1992 p.25). Analogous to that observation is the fact that, for doctors, the existing situation is relatively favourable and positive. Since there has never been any question of self-employed doctors being other than both professionally and civilly liable for their actions, the situation is not worsened for them by the presence of nurses. As has been demonstrated, this presence may provide a source of mitigation, using either the defence of reliance (the doctor was entitled to rely on the nurse) or possibly the defence of handicap (the doctor's 'eyes or ears' failed).

In addition, nursing provides medicine with a skilled workforce over whom they are still able to exercise considerable power and control, particularly in terms of the clinical management of the patients. Further, nursing provides medicine with the infrastructure to practise its discipline at its most complex and physically compromising level. When patients are admitted to hospital it is because they are either already too sick to remain at home to receive treatment or because the treatment they are about to receive will (temporarily) render them too sick to remain at home. The reason that patients need to stay in hospital is because they require assistance 'to perform those activities leading to health or its recovery (or to a peaceful death) that they would normally perform unaided if they had the necessary strength, will or knowledge to do so' (Henderson 1969).

At first glance this would seem to imply a real symbiosis between medicine and nursing. If medicine did not bring its patients to hospitals to be nursed through these times of physical threat, nurses would have considerably fewer patients to nurse; although it is acknowledged that there are some patients who need to be nursed, rather than treated. These are often people who are having difficulties managing new aspects of their lives e.g. nursing mothers, newly diagnosed diabetics, patients learning to live with a colostomy; but there may also be people who simply require nursing, perhaps because they are dying. But doctors bring (refer) their patients to nurses in hospitals because they require the nursing infrastructure to enable them to treat a particular patient. Both know when the need to refer to the other arises, and both use these 'referral' systems constantly.

The lack of equality in the relationship between doctors and nurses

However, the implications of this symbiosis are not recognised in terms of the exercise of power over the clinical care and management of the patient. In order for this to occur, the relationship would need to be viewed as one of equal power and responsibility. Thus, doctors would be expected to treat nurses' concerns with the same legitimacy as those of their peers. In such a relationship the concept of the patient as medical property, signified by the doctor's name above the bed, would be inappropriate, because the care and management of the patient would be a matter of joint concern.

It is indefensible that there is no legitimate system for a nurse to challenge formally the clinical management of a doctor, as it assumes that doctors must always be right. Furthermore, to suggest that nurses, having expressed misgivings, should simply ignore such concerns if doctors choose not to act on them, is to deny nurses any moral agency, and to imply that nurses do not have any moral or clinical duty to the patient. Finally, situations where nurses have repeatedly expressed concerns, yet doctors either ignore them or choose not to act upon them, are absolutely unsatisfactory to experienced clinical nurses. Yet there is very little, if any, redress.

The experience of 'microaggressions'

The repeated failure of the courts (and doctors) to recognise the difficulties nurses might be experiencing in such situations resonates with Grillo's description of a 'microaggression' (1987 p.309). Grillo states that microaggressions 'contain assumptions that diminish us in some way; and they are casually made but far from casual in their impact. The actions that may be taken on the basis of these remarks and the assumptions underlying them affect us quite concretely' (1997 p.749). Microaggressions are as problematic for nurses as they are for minority women law professors. Grillo observes that 'each of [them] saps our energy and raises our unexpressed anger to a dangerous level' (p.749). This is true for nurses, yet until the law recognises these anomalies of power their choices are similar to those described by Grillo—either 'staying and being a victim or walking away'. But, as she rightly observes, 'neither of these is going to advance me much in either my career or my personal growth' (p.754).

Simply bringing this unacceptable situation to the attention of those in power does not mean they will seek to redress it. Systems which oppress or disadvantage one group inevitably bring advantages to another. Even those who recognise the importance of nurses in health care still acknowledge the dominance and power which doctors yield in the Australian health care system (Alexander 2000 pp.161–62). It is also important to remember that the establishment of such a system was assisted (admittedly for self-serving reasons at the time) by some of the founders of modern nursing (Vicinus & Nergaard 1989 p.123). Thus the apparent anomalies of power which emerge from this case law may not be unacceptable to the dominant group, but rather an essential ingredient of the status quo. As Hochschild states 'the apparent anomaly is an actual symbiosis' (1984 p.10). Bell explains this further in relation to racial discrimination:

The permanence of this 'symbiosis' ensures that civil rights gains will be temporary and setbacks inevitable ... We rise and fall less as a result of our efforts than in response to the needs of a white society that condemns all blacks to quasi-citizenship as surely as it segregated our parents and enslaved their forefathers. (1992 p.10)

Nurses are also condemned to a form of 'quasi-citizenship' by the condoning of their institutionalised powerlessness by the courts. The medical profession has actively resisted attempts for nurses to exercise equal power, and has been content to allow a system of dominance and inequity to continue, unless they wished to distance themselves from a particular problem. To quote Bell through the words of Jesse B. Semple again:

Unless there is a crisis, they learn nothing! And if they can get out of a bad situation by messing with our rights, that is what they do, have been doing for [two] hundred years, and likely will continue to do. (1992 p.28)

NURSES MAY ONLY SUBSTITUTE FOR DOCTORS WITH THE DOCTOR'S PERMISSION

In terms of 'messing with [the nurses'] rights', the domain of professional substitution is undoubtedly that which is most fraught with controversy. There can be considerable overlap between the work and domains of doctors and nurses, and substitution often occurs.

As was discussed in the doctor's handmaiden chapter, doctors often see it as completely appropriate that they 'represent' nurses on committees and as expert witnesses. This substitution occurs almost daily at local, State and Federal level, and is difficult for nurses to challenge. It has been in place for so long that to suggest an alternative is seen as somehow ungrateful or untrusting.

Substitution of nurses for doctors: a form of 'affirmative action'?

However, to reverse the position and suggest substitution in the opposite direction, that a nurse might represent both nursing and medicine on a major health care committee, would be as controversial as 'affirmative action' and almost sacrilegious. It is well accepted that doctors can speak for nurses, it is 'the way the world is', and the majority of doctors and nurses do not question it. To turn such stock stories on their head would be to challenge seriously the established order. Those who might seek to do so would be seen as deviant, labelled as troublemakers. As Delgado writes:

Any practice [like affirmative action] that the majority group perceives as favouring minorities to protect racial justice will appear unprincipled and wrong ... Our society has been based on racial privilege since its inception. Formal equality today serves the same purpose as the formal inequality of earlier years. (1995 p.78)

In just this way the health care 'society' or community has been based on medical privilege since its inception, and the similarities in inequality are strong and enduring.

In contrast, when nurses undertake tasks previously the clinical professional domain of doctors, the response from the medical profession has varied according to the status of the task. For example, the administration of medications is now considered to be an activity in which nurses play a primary and pivotal role (Easson 1995 p.11). Many tasks have slipped into nursing usage in this way, and most of this slippage has been welcomed by the medical profession as being more convenient and appropriate to be performed by nurses. However, whilst this has occurred with tacit, if not express, medical permission in the past, the most recent collection of tasks which nurses have begun to undertake has evoked considerable controversy and even animosity nationally and internationally. A brief review of the development of the nurse practitioner role confirms that the substitution of nurses for doctors is 'allowed' only if it conveniences the medical profession. Where nurses have sought legitimation for work that provided a source of funding to doctors, there has been considerable outcry.

Need for medical permission—the legitimation of nurse practitioners

The development of roles akin to those of nurse practitioners in Australia

Tasks which nurses have argued that some are already undertaking clandestinely include the prescribing of certain medications, the ordering of pathology and radiology, and the referral of patients to other practitioners. Nurses who undertake these tasks are considered to be working at an expert level of practice, and are described in other countries as 'nurse practitioners'.

In Australia, the need for nurses to undertake these tasks has usually arisen from expediency. In remote areas, nurses had not only been ordering radiology, but also performing it, for many years (Public Hospital Nurses (State) Award 1971). Nurses, working in Women's Health or Sexual Health centres (NSW Health Department, 1985) with women who would not normally access a General Practitioner (GP), have been initiating diagnostic pathology and sending the samples for processing to hospital laboratories, thereby bypassing the need for a Medicare rebate. It is expedient for these nurses, if for example they are undertaking cervical cytology testing or urinalysis, and they identify a further abnormality, to obtain a specimen at the time, rather than advising the patient to visit a GP—if indeed, they have one. Procedures such as pre-signed pathology order forms, or post-hoc medical signatures are acknowledged to be ways in which nurses have overcome the inconvenience of having to obtain a doctor's signature to authorise the taking of specimens and ordering diagnostic tests (NSW Health Department 1992 pp.13–14). Remote area nurses have prescribed medications for patients who may have travelled long distances and would find it difficult to return in order to see a doctor (NSW Health Department 1992 p.14). They do this in a number of ways, including collusion with medical practitioners in post-hoc prescription writing, various protocols for nurse-initiated medications and by extending and circumventing the 24 hour telephone order regulation.[2]

The outrage of the Australian Medical Association and (some) other medical practitioners

Such activities were acknowledged by industrial organisations such as the Australian Medical Association (AMA 1992 p.2), and privately supported by some doctors. These anomalies were identified in a Discussion Paper and recommendations for legitimation were made (NSW Health Department 1992). However, key factions of the medical profession were outraged. These doctors insisted that their permission must be sought if these activities were to become a formal part of the nursing role. The medical press published comments from doctors who considered that nurses, in seeking this legitimation, were 'out of line', perhaps impertinent, and should stay doing that which they had always done. There is a sense of this in the following quotes:

To claim to be able to work as independent nurse practitioners is certainly a gallant wish from the militant nursing educators to justify their existence and their claim for glory. (Kwong 1992 p.9)

Strong threats to our profession are being mounted by a handful of nurses with a grossly inflated opinion of their abilities. (Buhagiar 1992 p.6)

Nurses do excellent work but they are not doctors—they aren't trained in diagnosis and treatment, and a bridging course won't be enough to cross that gap. There are better ways for the government to spend public money—we need more skilled nurses rather than semi-qualified people acting as de-facto GPs. (Napier 1998a p.11)

---

[2] A verbal order may be issued by telephone under the *Poisons and Therapeutic Goods Regulations 1994* (NSW) s.38 and 100, provided it is written up by a medical practitioner within 24 hours. As already stated, since some doctors visit remote outposts only once or twice a week unless there is an emergency, this is not possible. For the duration of the Nurse Practitioner Pilot Project, Wilcannia, the Deputy Chief Pharmacist, Mr John Lumby, gave permission for facsimiles confirming the medical order to be used, with the doctors confirming the facsimile order in writing on their next attendance (Correspondence from Mr John Lumby to Miss Judith Meppem, Chief Nurse, NSW Health, 13.2.1995, tabled for the Nurse Practitioner Stage Three Steering Committee).

The language used is telling: 'militant nurses', 'claim for glory', 'threats', 'grossly inflated opinion of their abilities'. This is surely the language of domination. An analogy may be drawn with women within the legal profession. Mary Jane Mossman, in the Foreword to Thornton's book on women in the law, quotes Elizabeth Elstob, a self-taught Saxon scholar (1683–1756) who apologised for her own literary achievement in the preface to her book. She argues that Thornton demonstrates that 'women who assert their own claims to legal knowledge—nearly three hundred years after Elizabeth Elstob's words were published—continue to be viewed as "impertinent" and suspected of "neglect of their household affairs"' (Mossman in Thornton 1996 p.viii).

Two medical groups, the AMA and the Royal Australian College of General Practitioners (RACGP), were consulted and included in the Stages 2 and 3 Nurse Practitioner Working Parties. Their concerns were addressed as a result of a significant number of compromises and, although the AMA never really shifted in its opposition to nurse practitioners during the three year consultative process, for a while the RACGP supported the outcomes of the research and the Stage 3 recommendations. Of late the RACGP has been publicly less supportive of nurse practitioners (AMA et al 2000), although its position statement remains sympathetic (RACGP 1999).

The AMA made it clear from the outset that its agenda was more obstructive. The negotiations with the key medical groups effectively transpired to delay the legislative change from its initial proposal in 1989 up until 22 October 1998, when the legislation was passed by the Upper House of the NSW parliament. The AMA nominee on the Stage 2 and Stage 3 working parties openly acknowledged that delay was their intention. He claimed that the AMA representatives on the Stage 2 Working Party, which recommended a series of pilot projects to assess the safety and efficacy of nurse practitioners, had 'put on hold any recommendations to change legislation'. He crowed that 'the projects, which will take some three years to complete and evaluate, have effectively stalled progress on the establishment of fully accredited nurse practitioners' (Nicholson 1993 p.2).

The reaction of some women doctors: the experience of 'intersectionality'

Clearly nurses are seen as 'neglectful' of their routine duties (Napier 1998a) and 'impertinent' in their desire to have these advanced roles legitimised. And some of the most vocal medical opponents of nurse practitioners in NSW are women. Crenshaw (1989) calls this phenomenon 'intersectionality', the meeting of a double layer of prejudice. Thus the nurse problem is not simply a woman problem; since nursing epitomises that caring, domestic ethos from which feminism has tried to free women. Feminists have argued (rightly) that women should be free to work in previously male-dominated professions, such as medicine and law, and ought not be forced to become nurses or teachers, just because these are the archetypal female professions. The difficulty for nurses has been that such arguments have caused other women to believe that there is ipso facto something inherently wrong, even unintelligent, about being a nurse, and thus nursing has remained a 'lower order' profession, unliberated by women's liberation.

Numerous microaggressions towards nurses serve to confirm the existence of this belief (Napier 1998, Phelps cited in AMA et al 2000). The attitude of women doctors to nurses is particularly ambivalent. Pringle observed that '[n]urses do assume that women doctors will be less demanding and more cooperative', but that 'some women doctors experience [this] as taking liberties' (1998 p.187). She found that female nurses were far more positive about female doctors than female doctors were about nurses, as female doctors felt that nurses did not accord to them the respect and deference which they accorded to male doctors. The nurses experienced easier communication and less tension when working with female doctors (1998 p.195). Pringle also observed that female doctors felt uncomfortable about having to change in the nurses' change rooms. She notes, however, that 'the nurses never, ever, mentioned that having the women doctors in their change rooms was a problem and male nurses had no difficulty sharing with male doctors' (1998 p.191). This would suggest that women doctors see their status as superior to nurses, despite any potential gender affiliations. This can be observed in a statement by Kerryn Phelps, President of the AMA, opposing nurse practitioners prescribing medication. She made the (football) analogy that patients would not want to see 'a winger in the forward pack' (AMA et al 2000).

The feminist movement helped nurses to understand the nature of their oppression by (previously predominantly) male doctors. However, it has not helped nursing to deal with the prejudice they receive from other women in (previously predominantly) male professions, many of whom come from middle class backgrounds (Daniel 1990, Thornton 1996). This has increased difficulties in recruitment to the nursing profession (NSW Health Department 1996b), and also raised the numbers of poor and working class students entering nursing (Nurses Registration Board of NSW, University of Newcastle & Central Coast AHS 1997) because nursing is still not perceived, even by women, as an equal professional career. Thus, when nurses try to tell their stories, to seek legal recognition of their position as practitioners, there is a sense in which their views are discredited automatically.

Matsuda cites Rich who, writing of her response to a story told by a poor black woman, expresses this problem most eloquently.

In my white North American world they have tried to tell me that this woman—politicised by intersecting forces—doesn't think and reflect on her life. That her ideas are not real ideas like those of Karl Marx and Simone de Beauvoir. That her calculations, her spiritual philosophy, her gifts for law and ethics, her daily emergency political decisions are merely instinctual or conditioned reactions. That only certain kinds of people can make theory; that the educated mind is capable of formulating everything; that white middle-class feminism can 'know' for all women; that only when a white mind formulates is the formulation to be taken seriously. (1990 p.1767)

This passage not only describes the problems for nurses in this context, it also echoes the problems for nurses in their dealings with the ethical and legal dilemmas discussed earlier in this chapter.

The continuing medical requirement for control

The extent and vehemence of the responses from the medical profession to the legitimation of the nurse practitioner role has been remarkable. It was never suggested that nurses already working in such roles should work without doctors to any greater extent than they already did. They would continue to make medical referrals and to acknowledge the limits of their competence (NSW Health Department 1992 p.5). However, there was medical concern that nurses would no longer be subordinate if these changes to policy and legislation were to occur. The AMA, for example, has continued to mount trenchant opposition to any legislative change unless the government agreed to a number of additional conditions, which entrenched medical domination and nursing subordination (Napier 1998b).

Such conditions imply that the practice of nursing is still seen very much as the business of doctors. The Minister for Health released his framework for Nurse Practitioner Services in New South Wales on 25 August 1998 amid caustic opposition from the AMA (1998). The legislative requirements and implementation framework were approved by the Upper House on 22 October 1998 (Moait 1998). The policy supporting the legislation allows for only 40 positions in rural and remote areas, which brings no relief to nurses in some of the inner city sites caring for homeless men or street kids. Each position is to be determined by an Area of Need Committee on which the AMA has representation. In the meantime, all those nurses who are practising in roles akin to those of nurse practitioners continue to do so either in a legal vacuum, or worse, outside the law. To paraphrase Rich, the 'calculations ... spiritual philosophy ... gifts for law and ethics, and ... daily emergency political decisions' of these nurses are not 'merely instinctual or conditioned reactions'. Rather they are the determinations of highly skilled nurses, whose emergence threatens the stock story of the subordinate professional.

In other countries the opposition to the introduction of nurse practitioners by medical stakeholder organisations has been similarly vehement, even when the 'grass roots' relationship between the doctors and nurses concerned has been completely amicable. Although the nurse practitioner role has been legitimised in America and the United Kingdom, it still has very limited application in parts of Canada (Price 1998). In Alberta a programme to develop nurse practitioners was introduced in the 1970s and existed for about ten years, but the title is not currently in use.

'A case in defense (sic) of privilege disguised as merit'

In Atcheson v College of Physicians and Surgeons (Alta) (1994), the problems of practising as a nurse practitioner outside a legislative framework are illustrated. Here, the plaintiff was employed by a doctor-run Family Medicine Clinic in a position described as that of a nurse practitioner. This work included (inter alia) the activities of assessing and diagnosing patients, prescribing medications and making referrals to other doctors. She was highly qualified and had previously worked as a nurse practitioner in remote outposts, so there was significant evidence to suggest that she was both competent and safe, and no evidence adduced to the contrary. She was advised to bill her services through the Alberta Health Insurance Plan under the physicians' names.

The regulatory authority for doctors, the College of Physicians and Surgeons of Alberta, wrote to the Clinic seeking further information about the nature of her employment. Upon receipt of this information, the College instructed the doctors that she was 'operating too independently' and that she was to stop 'seeing patients as a nurse practitioner and … mak[ing] management decisions consisting only of some discussion at the end of each day with you' (p.399). The nurse was dismissed from her employment. She unsuccessfully brought an action against the College for inducing breach of contract and unlawful interference with her economic interests. Although the judge found (inarguably) that the College was within its rights to give instructions to the physicians, she did acknowledge the nurse's contention that 'the result of the action was the protection of the professional interests of the physicians' (p.399).

It is questionable whether the use of statutory powers for such a purpose fulfils the definition of a public protective jurisdiction, one whose role is to 'supervise physicians and act in the best interests of the public' (p.397). The nurse was both qualified and competent, and had fulfilled such a role before. The 'public' seemed to consider that their interests were being served, as a number of patients joined a meeting of the College, the physicians and the plaintiff to 'express unqualified praise' for her (p.399). The judge also acknowledged that 'where physicians are not available, as in isolated outposts, the responsibility for medical diagnosis and treatment has been delegated to specially trained nurse practitioners such as the plaintiff' (pp.401–2). Her Honour also acknowledged that '[t]here is an overlap in function between nurses and physicians'.

Such comments would suggest that nurse practitioners are allowed to work in locations where there are no doctors available, notwithstanding the scope of the Medical Profession Act to control medical practice. The underlying rationale for the College's objection to the nurse's practice, questionable though the billing methods may have been, would appear to be that 'the Thickwood Clinic in Fort McMurray was not a place where the services of a physician were not available' (p.402). It could be argued that the defendants exercised their statutory powers 'for the advancement of their own trade interests', rather than in the interests of the public. The bottom line is that it is acceptable for the public to have nurses working as nurse practitioners, as long as it does not threaten the provision of services by a medical practitioner. The College did not write the letter to the Thickwood Clinic because they ought to write it, they wrote it because they could. This was an action, to quote Charles R Lawrence III 'in defense (sic) of privilege disguised as merit' (1997 p.759). The case provides a striking example of the medical profession's interference in the work of nurses, even when other doctors and patients are perfectly happy with the arrangement. Significantly, although this nurse was working at an advanced level of practice, she was working collaboratively with doctors, not independently of them.

CONCLUSION

The subordinate professional stock story presents some complex dilemmas for nurses, and begins to weave together the threads of the nursing image, as the various stories jostle for dominance. The fact that the nurse is viewed as a subordinate professional, rather than as an equal, is inextricably linked with the stock stories of the nurse as domestic worker and doctor's handmaiden. In addition, the counter story which Nightingale worked so hard to 'sell' at the end of the 19th century, that of the nurse as a ministering angel, has to some extent now become a stock story. The ministering angel image compounds the 'naturalist' argument—that nursing is the obvious career for women, as it is a natural extension of women's work. The professionalisation of nursing has been supported in the industrial courts and tribunals by reference to delegated medical tasks, and nurses, through capitalising on this, have to some extent perpetuated the subordinate professional stock story.

The subordinate professional role accordingly presents two dilemmas for nurses. First, recognition as professionals exposes nurses to a higher duty of care to the patient, which includes an expectation that they should be able to recognise potential problems in medical management and intercede to prevent harm to the patient. However, the fact that they are subordinate created the second dilemma: they do not have the ultimate authority to act on their concerns, other than in a circuitous manner, via the doctor. Thus there is an expectation that nurses will intercede but no legitimate authority for them to do so, as there are acknowledged protocols and policies which entrench medical dominance. When nurses do try to obtain legitimate authority to act, via mechanisms such as policy or legislative changes which recognise the advanced and complex nature of their work, these changes are vehemently opposed by key factions of the medical profession, who are understandably anxious to maintain the status quo.

To quote MacKinnon (1983 p.35), the resultant situation is almost 'metaphysically perfect' for the medical profession. It retains control, but has a ready means of mitigating its responsibility. For nurses, the results are often untenable, and result in the 'agony tales' which have been referred to in this and preceding chapters.

Towards autonomy

8

Autonomy in regulation and management

Elements of the image

- The nursing profession must be self-regulating;
  - Entry to the nursing profession must be restricted and governed by their own regulatory authority;
  - Nurses must be able to control standards for the practice of nursing, which should be recognised by the courts and tribunals;
  - Nursing must be able to control continuance in the profession.
- Nurses must manage and control the nursing workforce and nursing work on a day-to-day basis.
- Nursing has a unique body of specialist knowledge;
  - Nursing education is the formal theorising of women's work (early argument);
  - Nursing is a scientific discipline with the same characteristics of knowledge as medicine, just different content areas (later argument);
  - Although nursing and medicine are separate and distinct disciplines, there is an overlap of workload, due to the fact that the two operate so closely together;
  - Nursing is a caring discipline based on research, which has created a distinct body of nursing knowledge (current argument);
  - The practice of nursing requires specialised training and education;
  - Nursing as a profession requires proper professional remuneration.
- Clinical nursing knowledge and expertise should be given equal weight to that of medicine in clinical decision making.

INTRODUCTION

The following three chapters examine the last of the five images, the nurse as an autonomous professional. The terms 'autonomous' and 'independent' are frequently used in nursing literature to describe the attribution of full professional status to the nurse.

The previous chapters describing the doctor's handmaiden and subordinate professional images have demonstrated that nurses know and live with professional subordination, particularly in clinical practice. Nurse leaders, wishing to be free of such difficulties, have tried to address them through regulatory, educational, administrative and clinical solutions. From the beginning of the 20th century, they have striven for independence in professional and educational governance. In the past thirty years they have fought to retain hierarchical control over their administration by ensuring that they had direct hierarchical management structures, often referred to as 'line management' structures. In their clinical lives, nurses have not sought to be independent per se, because health care is an interdependent activity. However, in the last twenty years, they have begun to address the vexing areas of medical dominance and nursing invisibility in clinical decision making.

Autonomy: a nurse-driven ideal

The nurse as an autonomous professional is an outsider story; an ideal which many nurses promote actively. These next chapters examine the elements of this outsider story, and consider the extent to which the courts and tribunals have incorporated these elements into their world-view and their decision making. The application of narrative scholarship anticipates that, by hearing nurses' voices and stories and gaining insight into the different way in which nurses view their world, readers will 'vacillate between their own world and that of the storyteller(s)' (Delgado 1989 p.2435). It is hoped that telling these outsider stories will 'attack and subvert the very "institutional logic" of the system' (Delgado 1989 p.2429).

The propagation of an outsider story is not a new tactic for nurses. Florence Nightingale promoted the image of the ministering angel to make nursing a respectable and acceptable career. So successful was she that this has now almost become a stock story. Nurses have been proactive in trying to deal with the problems they encountered in their political, professional and clinical lives. It is important to understand that nurses are more than 'passive victims ... complainers ... unassertive game players and ... power hungry professionalisers' (Wicks 1999 p.174). These chapters explore the extent to which their bid for professional recognition has been successful.

The Nightingale model plus the medical model of professionalism: an uncomfortable fit for nursing?

The autonomous professional image was certainly not promoted by Nightingale. She does not seem to have considered that nurses ought to have autonomy in their clinical relationships with doctors, although she was adamant that nurses should be managed and controlled by nurses—who then answered to doctors (Vicinus & Nergaard 1989 p.123). Her main aims were respectability and effectiveness, and these she pursued through a rigorous regime of discipline and training. Rafferty explains that her preoccupation was with the character of the women who worked as nurses, not their ability to pass examinations (1996 pp.23–41). The exercise of power may not have been an issue for Nightingale, as she was well connected and influential by reason of her birth, and was able to exercise considerable influence on politicians and power brokers. So anxious was Nightingale to practise nursing, and to make that practice respectable, that she was careful not to disturb the status quo or to threaten the male hierarchy in any way. This is not a criticism of Nightingale. She was a product of her time and class, and her achievement in developing a third career path for women (other than marriage or holy orders) was a significant accomplishment.

Nightingale and her contemporaries capitalised on their femininity and docility in order to achieve a desired respectability for themselves. The outsider story which they pursued was that of ministering angel, rather than autonomous professional. It was only when the 'new feminist-inspired nursing elite' (Rafferty 1996 p.42), led by Ethel Bedford Fenwick in England and Lavinia Dock in America, took up the pursuit of professionalism that the notion of a middle class model of professionalism based on a 'sameness' argument of equality emerged. Simplistically, their argument was that nurses are professionals in the same way as doctors are professionals, so they should be able to exercise equal power and have equal status. Such a model was originally viewed as the preferred route to autonomy.

With the wisdom of hindsight, the foundation of this quest for autonomy seems ideologically flawed. Those early nurses had not adequately analysed the nature of their oppression, if indeed they would even have described themselves in that way. Thus they tried to develop a model of professionalism for nursing which mirrored medicine (Goodman-Draper 1995). This was despite the fact that the nursing workforce, unlike that of medicine, was drawn from a wide mix of social classes. This mix had significant implications for the achievement of any concept of a homogenous, middle class professional elite, because the nursing workforce simply did not fit the mould. Not all nurses were educated and/or articulate, but all had been schooled in Nightingale's 'docility and purity' model. Many would not have been used to taking an assertive stance, let alone to entertaining any thoughts of professional autonomy. Rather, they would have known their 'place' in society from an early age. Those who might have demonstrated such assertive characteristics would probably have been viewed as rebellious and either removed or subdued during their training. The pioneers who pursued registration were themselves Nightingale trainees, but they were also middle class women, used to having power and control over a household. However, they did not reject the Nightingale model of 'docility and purity'; they simply wished in addition to have the entry to nursing practice restricted and the model legitimated through legislation (Montgomery 1998 pp.33–51).

This insistence on self management and self rule, coupled with the Nightingale legacy of femininity and respectability, has been problematic for nursing in terms of its ability to wield real power and influence. It has often created a form of managerial and professional segregation, whereby nursing has become quarantined within the health care system, concerned with nursing matters, but getting little, or at best token, representation on major decision making committees. In this way nursing has tended to become introspective, cordoned off in its own 'state within the state'. Such a situation could be analogous to a form of apartheid or, alternatively, secession. The differences between such a form of segregation and the characteristics of the apartheid regime of the old South Africa include the following factors: until recently, the nursing workforce was not politicised; the segregation was sought, not imposed; and, to a certain extent, nurses colluded in their own oppression.

The quest for autonomy: sameness or difference

By the early 20th century, universal suffrage was becoming a major issue for educated women, many of whom were of a similar class to Nightingale, and concerned to obtain for women the same rights and privileges as men. As Ethel Bedford Fenwick stated, 'the nurse question is the woman question' (in Dock & Stewart 1938 p.254), and many women who were nurses wished to see this (then) all-female career recognised at the same level as medicine, which they viewed as its (mostly) male counterpart. Nurses faced the dilemma of whether to depict themselves as similar to other professions, in particular medicine, or whether to claim to be completely different from other professions, but nevertheless deserving of equal status and power.

This 'sameness/difference' question is a theme which recurs throughout the feminist literature, and has received much attention (MacKinnon 1987, Graycar & Morgan 1990). Catharine MacKinnon describes the dilemma cogently in the following terms:

Two alternate paths to equality for women emerge within this dominant approach, paths that roughly follow the lines of this tension. The leading one is: be the same as men. This path is termed gender neutrality doctrinally and the single standard philosophically. It is testimony to how substance gets itself up as form in law that this rule is considered formal equality. Because this approach mirrors the ideology of the social world, it is considered abstract, meaning transparent of substance; also for this reason it is considered not only to be the standard, but a standard at all. It is so far the leading rule that the words 'equal to' are code for, equivalent to, the words 'the same as'—referent for both unspecified.

To women who want equality yet find that you are different, the doctrine provides an alternate route: be different from men. This equal recognition of difference is termed the special benefit rule or special protection rule legally, the double standard philosophically. (1987 p.33)

MacKinnon (1987 pp.32–33) doubts the legal effectiveness of recognition of sexual equality, whether predicated on sameness or difference. She argues that sex equality is in reality an oxymoron as equality refers to things being the same, whereas sex (in this context) refers to things being different.

Sheehy (1987) outlines four potential equality theories which provide bases for women to argue their case in the development of policies on women's justice issues. The first three are:

1. The 'strict identical treatment' model, which she criticises fiercely, explaining that it 'assumes the continued existence of the current social and political structure and necessarily measures 'equal treatment' by prevailing norms and values';
2. The 'identical treatment with biological exceptions', which she feels hides the pervasiveness of sexism; and
3. The 'treatment according to all differences', in which the differences are focused on and accepted as long-term phenomena. (Sheehy expresses concerns that a theory such as this might entrench differences that have served to disempower women.)

Fourth, Sheehy describes the 'subordination principle', which she favours because it defines women's inequality in terms of subordination to men and sets out to evaluate 'practices, policies, and laws…to assess whether they operate to maintain women in a socially subordinate position'. Thus it avoids a 'legalistic analysis' of whether a particular difference is an unacceptable basis for unfavourable treatment, and seeks to concentrate on what effect a discriminatory piece of law or policy has on the woman and asks the law to 'pronounce on the reasons for gender differences'. In other words, it identifies the problems that the practices, policies and laws reveal so that they can be addressed. This fourth model corresponds most closely with the approach adopted in this book (Graycar & Morgan 1990 pp.40–42).

Early feminists such as the suffragettes focused on the 'sameness' argument—women must have equal suffrage, equal pay and equal educational opportunities with men. Nurse leaders adopted a similar approach to professional autonomy, seeking state registration and self-regulation similar to the medical profession. However, it seems in retrospect that they were naive in their failure to anticipate that nursing work might have been viewed as 'other than professional work' by society in general. Certainly the contemporary nursing literature bears no resemblance to the way in which their work was viewed by the early 20th century courts and tribunals.

The arguments for professional autonomy have been based on a number of propositions which are similar to those outlined by Flexner (1915 pp.576–81). Nursing has adapted its strategies to bid for professional recognition and autonomy in response to its successes and failures.

The elements of the 'autonomous professional' counter story are detailed at the opening to this chapter. Chronologically, these elements are by no means all present at the same time. The development of nursing's quest for autonomy spans the 20th century and for the purposes of analysis can be divided into three sections: regulation and management, knowledge and education, and clinical decision making. This outsider story has sometimes been aggressively resisted by other power groups. However, as the century progressed, nursing achieved greater (albeit still only partial) recognition as a profession in its own right, which could be attributed to their changed strategies.

The quest for clinical autonomy/equality was not evident in the early years of nursing's professional history. A possible reason for this was that in the early 20th century, there was much less medical and surgical intervention, which meant that nurses played a more significant role in patient recovery than is now the case. Patients who recovered frequently did so fortuitously, to some extent sustained by their nursing care, but often irrespective of their medical treatment. This may have given nurses a greater role in clinical decision making than is now the case. Nurses in Australia and internationally have become dissatisfied with the subordinate clinical role which many currently play.

THE NURSING PROFESSION MUST BE SELF-REGULATING

Entry to the nursing profession must be restricted and governed by its own regulatory authority

Early developments in Britain

Nurses were professionally active at the beginning of the 20th century. Developing national and international nursing organisations lobbied governments on the advancement of nursing issues, including education. The demand for legislation to establish a register of nurses was one of the significant developments (Bendall & Raybould 1969 p.3). The nurse registration debate was in the public domain at the same time as Hillyer v Governors of St Bartholomew's Hospital (1909) was being heard and determined. The issues raised about the domestic versus professional status of nurses in the judgments of Farwell and Kennedy LJJ reflect the nurse registration debate.

The support for a register of nurses is thought to have originated from opposition to a proposal by the British Hospitals Association (BHA), an organisation of hospital administrators including those of St Bartholomew's Hospital. The BHA was anxious to organise a register, but believed that only a one-year nurse training programme was needed, as opposed to the three-year programmes developed by most Nightingale schools. This proposal led to a split with the Hospital Matrons Branch of the BHA, which supported a three-year programme. The chief members of this group, led by Mrs Bedford Fenwick, resigned and established the British Nurses Association (BNA), which strongly opposed the type of register proposed by the BHA (Bendall & Raybould 1969 pp.1–2). In the *Nursing Record* of 22 March 1893, Mrs Bedford Fenwick scornfully described the register that the BHA wished to organise as 'a central registry office, similar to that in vogue for domestic servants'. This was not what the BNA envisaged. They wanted a register of the same status as the medical practitioners' register, which was established in 1860. England, unlike many other Commonwealth countries and America, did not achieve this until 1919.

Interestingly, the debate on state registration involved past and current senior members of the staff of St Bartholomew's Hospital. Regarding the opponents of nurse registration, various hospital administrators and medical staff sent a letter to the *Nursing Record* of 30 March 1893 signed by, amongst others, 'representatives of St Bartholomew's Hospital'. This letter disagreed with the registration of nurses on several grounds, including the argument that it would be 'detrimental to the public and injurious to the medical practitioner'. In 1904 a Select Committee on the Registration of Nurses was established as a result of the intensity of the debate.

Miss Stewart, then Matron of St Bartholomew's Hospital, in her submission described its relatively academic training for nurses, and advocated a similar three-year training. Dr Norman Moore, a senior physician at St Bartholomew's Hospital, gave evidence to the Select Committee that having a register of nurses 'would lead to the establishment of an imperfectly educated order of medical practitioners'. He testified that 'to examine 2,000 nurses a year would be a serious business. Serious and expensive' (Bendall & Raybould 1989 p.10).

Despite the nurses' submissions and assurances to the contrary, there was also considerable concern expressed by members of the medical profession about the risk of competition.

[T]he nurses might become serious rivals and undercut the fees ... charged for professional services. Nurses might flourish their certificates in front of the patients and try to make out that 'they knew more than the doctor', while the patients might be tempted to use the nurse as a substitute for the doctor. (BMA Report to Select Committee in Abel-Smith 1960 p.75)

We want to stop nurses thinking themselves anything more than they are, namely, the faithful carriers out of the doctor's orders. The other side are always talking about nursing being a profession and 'graduates' in nursing, just as they do in America. (Sydney Holland in Abel-Smith 1960 p.37)

The remainder of those opposed who testified were all chairmen of Boards of Governors of other major London teaching hospitals (Bendall & Raybould 1969 p.7). There was considerable antipathy amongst Boards of Governors and hospital administrators in general, and those of St Bartholomew's in particular, towards the professionalisation of nursing by means of a standardised curriculum and state registration. The dominant mindset at the time did not support the idea of nurses on a comparable professional footing with doctors. Additionally, Mrs Bedford Fenwick recalled in the *British Journal of Nursing* (22.9.1923) that certain sections of the Press took an active role in 'downing the nurses'.

However, in 1905 the Select Committee published a report that supported the three-year education and registration of nurses, and accepted the need for a system similar to that used to register medical practitioners. Fourteen years and ten Bills to the House of Commons later, the first British nurses registration legislation was passed (Bendall & Raybould 1969 pp.21–22). In England, the practice of midwifery had been regulated separately by the Midwives Act 1902 (UK), and thus medical concerns about infant mortality and morbidity were not so pressing. This meant that in the UK, when nurses sought professional registration, considerations such as competition were brought to the fore in the absence of concerns about safety.

Developments in New South Wales

By 1902 in NSW the Australasian Trained Nurses Association (ATNA) had succeeded in establishing a uniform standard of education, a minimum training of three years, and a process for accrediting hospital schools of nursing (Seymer 1949 pp.268–69). The first legal process for registering nurses, most specifically midwives, was introduced via the Private Hospitals Act 1908 (NSW), and provided for women who were 'lying-in' to be managed by either a legally qualified medical practitioner or a registered nurse. A registered nurse was defined in the Act as one who had been recognised as such by the Board of Health. This was not acceptable to the council of ATNA, who wanted its own health professionals' board, similar to those established for doctors, dentists and pharmacists (Dickenson 1993 pp.24–26). The first Nurses Registration Act was finally passed in New South Wales in 1924, and provided for the registration of general, mid-wifery, mental health and paediatric nurses. Unlike its counterpart in England, this Act received unanimous support from the medical profession, who were particularly concerned about maternal and infant mortality rates and wanted the practice of midwifery regulated. However, doctors still maintained control, as the newly established Nurses Registration Board had four of its seven positions filled by doctors.

The predominance of doctors on the Board was the subject of considerable debate when the Nurses Act was reviewed in 1953. The general consensus was that their presence would enhance the status of nurses, a sentiment shared by the nursing leaders. However, nurses did achieve greater self-regulation by increasing the number of nurses on the Nurses Registration Board to seven out of thirteen (NSW Hansard 2.September 1953 p.482).

The impetus for statutory changes in 1953 came from the nursing profession which was concerned to maintain a monopoly over nursing. After World War II, there was a shortage of qualified nurses—but not of unqualified 'nurses'. The 1953 statute aimed to create tighter controls over the practice of nursing whilst also creating the opportunity for certain overseas nurses to have their qualifications recognised. NSW had for some time demanded a four-year training prior to registration. This was the subject of debate in Parliament, because it prevented nurses who had received only a three-year training in non-British countries from obtaining registration in NSW when there was a registered nurse shortage (NSW Hansard 2.September 1953 p.449).

In order to regulate the practice of nursing by unqualified nurses another grade of nurse, known as an Assistant in Nursing (AIN), was introduced in NSW. These AINs would receive a prescribed period of training and their names would then be entered onto a Roll. Persons who had been working as unrecorded AINs for a period of two or more years would be able to have their names entered on the Roll automatically.

This second level nurse was not welcomed uniformly. In 1947 Georgina McCready, General Secretary of the NSW Nurses' Association (NSWNA), had described AINs as 'a menace to the nursing profession' (Dickenson 1993 p.164). They did not wish for a second level of nurse, as it interfered with any bid for comparable status with medicine. However, the amendment was accepted as a pragmatic solution to maintain some degree of exclusivity and control over the practice of nursing.

Yet this desire for a homogenous, educated, middle class group was unrealistic, given the composition of the nursing workforce. Although the leaders of the profession were probably still predominantly middle class, the registered nursing workforce comprised predominantly working class girls, largely uneducated, and probably in awe of their medical counterparts from both a social and gender perspective. The AINs were scorned by registered nurses and regarded as inferior. In reluctantly implementing these demarcations, the nursing profession created a self-imposed strategy of divide and rule, a hierarchy based on length of training and title of qualification. To some extent they felt ashamed of this second level of nurse, as it undermined the notion of an exclusive area of nursing work. They enshrined their divisions in legislation, and thus effectively managed to 'divide' themselves and so continued to be 'ruled'.

The current situation in New South Wales

The next major legislative change did not occur until the passing of the Nurses Act 1991 (NSW), although there were serial amendments to the 1953 legislation. The 1991 changes were significant, establishing a new disciplinary structure and introducing greater controls to the practice of midwifery. The Bill was introduced by the Liberal Health Minister, Mr Peter Collins, and came about as a result of unrest in the nursing profession about a number of provisions in the previous Act. The proposed new Board did not have any doctors on it, despite considerable lobbying by the medical profession. Dr Refshauge, the (then) Shadow Minister for Health asked the Minister whether he believed that 'the hegemony of the nursing profession is now so complete that it does not need a medical practitioner on its Board?' (NSW Hansard 20.March.1991 p.1445).

By the time of the Second Reading, the NSWNA had brought its considerable industrial influence to bear on both the Government and the Labor Party (Dickenson 1993 p.179). Dr Refshauge expressed his delight 'to see that nurses will now not be controlled by doctors' and congratulated the Minister for 'not giving in to the medical lobby and insisting that a doctor must be on the Nurses Registration Board' (NSW Hansard 9.April.1991 p.1727). Other government initiatives which contributed to nursing's 'hegemony' were the introduction of a Chief Nursing Officer position, the support of basic education at tertiary level for registered nurses, professional rates of pay and clinical career structures, and the introduction of Area Directors of Nursing.

> *Nurses must be able to control standards for the*
> *practice of nursing, which should be recognised*
> *by the courts and tribunals*

Control of scope of practice

Control over who might practise nursing has always really been a matter of expediency, of finding sufficient people to do the job. Despite a desire amongst some nurse leaders to have 'one portal of entry' to the profession, the reality is that there have always been several. Nevertheless, two early midwifery cases provide examples of the courts' acceptance that the purpose of state regulation was to limit at least the practice of midwifery to those people who were certified under the Act.

Both Davies v Central Midwives Board (1918) and Davis v Morris (1923) recognised midwifery as a designated and protected scope of certified practice. However, the first focused far more on the supervision required of a medical practitioner than on the right of certified midwives to practise without supervision, and both cases referred to the requirement for referral to or consultation with a medical practitioner. It is acknowledged that the medical profession had agitated for the registration of midwives in order to safeguard women from dangerous childbirth practices. But the registration also enacted the subordinate relationship of the midwife to the medical practitioner, as there was no converse requirement for a doctor to consult a midwife. This must have gone some way to allaying the fears of competition which were later expressed about nurses in the medical representations to the Select Committee on the Registration of Nurses.

Much of the later case law which addresses nursing's right to control its own professional regulation is concerned with setting standards for practice, and controlling those who remained in the profession, rather than controlling entry to the profession.

Development of standards in nursing

The Nightingale Pledge

The development of standards of practice in nursing has been a priority since Nightingale's time (Nightingale 1952). A twofold approach to maintenance was taken, with practice standards to be maintained through education, and moral standards to be upheld by taking the Nightingale Pledge, which was published in every Australasian Nurses Journal between 1904 and 1954.

The expectation of loyalty and obedience to the doctor was clear in the phrase 'with loyalty will I endeavour to aid the physician in his work'. Over the years, this dual allegiance has created difficulties for nurses (Johnstone 1994 pp.126–35). If the nurse was required only to be loyal to the doctor, in theory there ought never to be any moral dilemmas. But the nurses' concomitant 'devotion to the welfare of those committed to [their] care' has created difficulties for them when they have disagreed with medical management and found their loyalty to the doctor indefensible.

Codes of Conduct and Codes of Ethics: floors or ceilings?

The International Council of Nurses (ICN) published its first International Code of Nursing Ethics in 1953, and amended it in 1965 and 1973 (Sawyer

1989 p.145). In 1973, clause 7 of the ICN Code, which required loyalty and obedience to the doctor, was deleted at the instigation of a group of Canadian nursing students (Johnstone 1994 p.135). In theory, one would imagine that this would have solved the dual dilemma for nurses and any lack of clarity about their obligations. Now their sole duty (to the patient) was clear. However, this shift in allegiance does not seem to have been conveyed to the medical profession, the managers of health care, or to the judiciary.

In 1980 the Canadian Nurses Association and the College of Nurses of Ontario both produced Codes of Ethics. The United Kingdom Central Council (UKCC) developed its Code of Conduct for Nurses, Midwives and Health Visitors in 1983, and several sets of guidelines have been issued to assist in its implementation and comprehension. This UKCC Code was the first to describe itself as a Code of Conduct, rather than of Ethics, although some did not declare themselves as either. Previously it was sometimes difficult to ascertain the intent of a code and its status, whether it was to be used as a 'ceiling' standard, establishing moral aspirations, or a 'floor', setting out the minimum standard for practice (Chiarella 1995 pp.61–74). Pyne stipulated that the UKCC Code was designed not only to provide advice 'on standards of professional conduct', but also to provide 'a backcloth against which allegations of professional misconduct can be judged' (1988 pp.173–75).

Standards and Codes in Australia

Australia was relatively late in developing codes, but was at the forefront of the development and publication of practice standards. In 1983 the ICN initiated a major project in relation to the regulation of nursing (Pratt 1995 p.3). Simultaneously the Royal Australian Nursing Federation (RANF), the national professional and industrial body, published its first set of Standards for Nursing Practice. By 1990 the Australasian Nurse Registering Authorities Conference (ANRAC) had ratified work which commenced in 1986, and had accepted a set of competencies for nursing practice which had been refined and validated. These ANRAC competencies were developed partially using the work of the (now) Australian Nursing Federation (ANF) in its revised standards for nursing practice and partially through research which identified the competencies required to function as a beginning practitioner. ANRAC incorporated in 1993 and is now the Australian Nursing Council Inc. (ANCI). The registration boards have adopted these competencies, now the ANCI competencies, as the entry point for registration and enrolment. The Foreword to the ANCI competencies makes it quite clear that 'it is expected that all nurses registered and enrolled will be able to demonstrate these competency standards' (1999). In addition, ANCI has developed a Code of Ethics and a Code of Professional Conduct.

Some of the major specialist and nursing organisations have undertaken research to identify advanced practice standards. These have included work undertaken by the University of Newcastle (Australian Nursing Federation 1997), the Confederation of Australian Critical Care Nurses (1996), and the Australian Confederation of Operating Room Nurses (ACORN 1996b). In addition, there have been specific practice standards developed by specialist nursing organisations, such as the standards for cleaning operating theatres (ACORN 1996a).

Acceptance of these standards by courts and tribunals

The extent of acceptance of these published standards by the courts and tribunals is a measure of the acceptance of professional control over the standards of practice in the profession. However, the Australian courts have also reserved the right to set their own standards for professions (F v R 1983, Rogers v Whitaker 1992). The extent to which standards developed by nurses have been accepted judicially has depended on: the extent of the code or standard's circulation; the authority of the body publishing the code or standard, and that body's mandate to compel nurses to abide by it; its intent; and whether it was intended to be a 'ceiling' or a 'floor'.

An example of a case where the standards of practice issued by the nurse registering authorities were accepted as being the 'backdrop against which allegations of professional misconduct may be judged' is Morton v Registered Nurses' Association of Nova Scotia (1989). Nathanson J recognised that the existence of standards was 'implicit in the concept of profession' and that standards were 'benchmarks for the practice of the profession. The standards may be written or unwritten. They may or may not be prescribed by the governing statute or regulations' (p.166).

The ANRAC (now ANCI) competencies, upon which undergraduate curricula are based in Australia, have also been accepted as appropriate standards for disciplinary bodies to apply (Cameron 1995 p.214). The competencies are being used by the profession to establish both entry points and exit points. In Versteegh v The Nurses Board of South Australia (1992) Mullighan J dismissed an appeal against the Board. In doing so, he accepted the use of a number of standards, including the ANRAC competencies, to confirm a finding of unprofessional and unethical conduct.

However, the courts and tribunals have been less prepared to accept standards that they considered to be too idealistic or not sufficiently widely circulated. For example, in Heathcote v NRB and Walton (1991) the court rejected the use of the 1983 RANF Standards for Nursing Practice. Ward DCJ criticised the inappropriateness of introducing unrealistically high standards as a means of determining professional misconduct.

In Langley v Glandore Pty Ltd (in Liq) (1997) a more precise set of practical standards, the ACORN standards for the swab and instrument count, were produced in court as expert evidence to establish the requisite standard of care. ACORN is a professional organisation, whose stated objects include the setting of professional standards. They have a regular journal, in which such standards would be published, but membership of ACORN is not compulsory for perioperative nurses. Overall, it seems as though the courts and tribunals are more prepared to accept those standards established as minimum standards by the profession, providing that they are well publicised.

Nursing must be able to control
continuance in the profession

Historical aspects of control over continuance in the profession

A natural sequel to having a registration act which controls entry to the profession is that the registering authority also has the right to control who remains in the profession, and on what terms.

After the success in obtaining registration, there seems to have been little activity in terms of appeals against decisions of the disciplinary bodies of registration boards. This was probably because much of the disciplinary activity which occurred in nursing was not 'overt, but rather covert and subtle' (Cordery 1996 p.195). Matrons were fiercely protective of their sovereignty, and resented any scrutiny in the way they managed nursing affairs. Complaints about working hours, food and local hospital affairs were all emphatically opposed by the Matrons. Maud Kellett, Matron of Sydney Hospital, is reported to have told the NSWNA's first organiser, Natalie Artemieff, that 'Our girls will work twenty-four hours a day if necessary' (Dickenson 1993 p.83). Nurses usually 'left', rather than be dismissed, and the nursing networks were such that it would be difficult for a nurse who had been 'blacklisted' by one Matron to obtain employment with another. Thus the need to deregister nurses did not arise frequently. Without the imprimatur of the employing Matrons, they would have great difficulty in being able to practise.

There seems to have been little incidence of appeals against decisions of disciplinary bodies until the 1980s, although in New South Wales appeal provisions were included in the Nurses Registration Act 1953 (NSW) and in Victoria in the 1956 legislation.

Recent increases in appeals against decisions of disciplinary bodies

The scope and content of disciplinary hearings

Appeals began to be a little more common in the 1970s and 1980s, particularly in Canada. Some of the earlier ones reflected the need to clarify the regulatory legislation. Not all statutes were alike in their regulatory provisions, but all shared similarly protective jurisdictions. The problems encountered when applying the legislation were also similar. For example, there was initial difficulty in determining precisely what constituted 'competence' or 'fitness' to practise (Re Crandell and Manitoba Association of Registered Nurses 1976, Re Mason and Registered Nurses Association of British Columbia 1979). There were also procedural irregularities, possibly due to the relative inexperience of the disciplinary bodies, and the fact that their understanding of the law in practice was rudimentary. (See Gaudrealt v Felstrom et al 1983, Re Reddall and College of Nurses of Ontario 1983, Re Brock-Berry and Registered Nurses Association of British Columbia 1995, R v The Professional Conduct Committee of the United Kingdom Central Council for Nursing, Midwifery and Health Visiting (UKCC) ex parte the UKCC 1985, Murray-Hamilton v Registration Committee of College of Nurses of Ontario 1986.)

A considerable number of cases were concerned with competence to practise (Re Crandell and Manitoba Association of Registered Nurses 1976, Re Mason and Registered Nurses Association of British Columbia 1979, Morton v Registered Nurses' Association of Nova Scotia 1989). Montgomery has argued that nursing professional regulation in the UK (and probably internationally) has been more concerned with professional responsibilities, in contrast to medical professional regulation, which has been more concerned with the professional rights (1998 pp.44–45). Certainly nursing disciplinary committees have treated even minor misdemeanours harshly. However, the conduct with which nursing disciplinary bodies were concerned resembled that of other professions. Questions of mental fitness to practise due to drug dependency (Powell v Nurses Board of South Australia 1986), sexual misconduct (Browne v Percival & Nurses Board of South Australia 1994), and physical abuse and violation of the therapeutic relationship (Re Carruthers and College of Nurses of Ontario 1996), were problems which similarly beset the medical profession (Health Care Complaints Commission (HCCC) Annual Report 1998–9).

The use of doctors to determine nurses' fitness to practise

A recurrent theme has been the way in which doctors are able to give opinions on nursing matters or to substitute their opinions for those of nurses. Nurses' ability to speak for themselves and the acceptance of their evidence over medical evidence in nursing matters are measures of professional autonomy. The validity of doctors as expert witnesses in nursing disciplinary cases is a litmus test for the extent of nurses' self-regulation. It is well nigh impossible to envisage a (court) situation where a nurse might be called to pronounce on the fitness of a doctor to practise medicine.

Solomon J in Re Crandell and Manitoba Association of Registered Nurses made reference to the fact that 'no medical evidence was called' (1976 p.605) and this concern partly founded his disagreement with the Board's decision. However, Anderson J in Re Mason and Registered Nurses Association of British Columbia dismissed the medical evidence, preferring that of the nurses. He spoke favourably of the qualifications and demeanour of the nurse witness, describing her as 'fair and impartial ' (1979 p.232).

The authority of disciplinary bodies

The punitive nature of nursing self-regulation

One of the striking features of a review of nursing disciplinary decisions is their excessively punitive nature. There have even been two recent Canadian cases where the Registration Boards have appealed against the decisions of their own disciplinary Tribunals, on the grounds that they had been too lenient (Holt v Manitoba Registered Psychiatric Nurses' Association et al 1992, Re College of Nurses of Ontario and Quiogue 1993).

There have been a number of cases where the courts have found that the disciplinary bodies were over-zealous in their desire to uphold the standards of the profession (Re Crandell 1976, Re Vialoux and Registered Psychiatric Nurses Association of Manitoba 1983, Re Rioux 1986). One nurse was convicted of professional misconduct for acts which fell outside her scope of responsibility and one of which occurred while she was at coffee break (Pickard v College of Nurses of Ontario 1987). Another was de-registered for administering an incorrect injection, giving an incorrect immunisation and failing to report the matter to the senior nurse or health visitor, despite the fact that she informed the doctor and the mother immediately of her mistake (Hefferon v UKCC 1988). The nurse's unacceptable fault in this situation seems to have been her failure to report the matter via her line management. As Montgomery observed in this case 'the responsibility of conforming to the shared professional role of nurses overrode the freedom of individual action. It is hard to imagine the GMC [General Medical Council] taking such a view' (Hefferon v UKCC 1998 p.48). In another case a nurse was de-registered for incurring numerous traffic offences (Dennis v UKCC p.1993).

In Re Bailey et al and Saskatchewan Registered Nurses' Association (1996) the Director of Nursing Services (DNS), who had reported the conduct of three of her own nursing staff to the disciplinary body, was the President of the Council of the Saskatchewan Nurses Association. Such was her influence on the case that the proceedings were found to be extraordinarily biased. The Investigation Committee did not interview witnesses who might have exonerated the appellants, they disregarded the nurses' concerns about the position of influence the DNS occupied, and they failed to disclose 'literally dozens of documents' (1996 p.236) which were introduced at the hearing. On appeal Hrabinsky J held that the decision of the Discipline Committee was 'null and void', that it would be 'impossible' to have another fair hearing and that the charges against the appellants could not be raised again (1996 p.237). Although this case is extreme, it indicates the zeal with which senior members of the profession have been wont to pursue perceived breaches of standards.

This phenomenon reflects that need for public approbation that was a feature of the ministering angel outsider story. It may also be a component of that outsider story, and resembles a pattern of behaviour, described by Thornton, where women who aspire to domains routinely inhabited by men feel the need to achieve at a higher level merely to be accepted as equal (1996 p.238). Nurses may have wished to prove that they were fit to self-regulate by demonstrating that they would pursue the highest standards of propriety.

Intervention by courts and tribunals

As a general rule, appellate courts in Canada, England and Australia have expressed a reluctance to interfere with the internal regulation of the nursing profession (Powell v Nurses Board of South Australia 1986, Trotter v College of Nurses of Ontario 1991, Re Carruthers and College of Nurses of Ontario 1996). Barry J enunciated this principle in Re Cabrera:

> My impression of the law at the moment is the courts will not interfere with decisions of professional tribunals or administrative tribunals, unless some glaring error is made or the rules of natural justice are not complied with ... This is a case of a professional body exercising its jurisdiction to control its profession, and in the absence of some unfairness in law, the courts do not interfere with such decisions. (1980 p.193)

However, there are numerous examples where the courts have chosen to interfere with the decisions of nursing disciplinary tribunals. Usually this was because the court considered that the penalty imposed was unnecessarily severe and went further than required to protect public safety. On such occasions, the courts have often expressed recognition that interference with nurses' registration threatens their livelihood. There has been a tendency to prefer activities that would assist the nurse to continue with the practice of nursing. This concern for the impact of disciplinary decisions on the lives of practitioners was described by Steele J in Rioux v College of Nurses of Ontario:

> The power to discipline their members, which is conferred upon the self governing professions, is a very great one, involving as it does potential loss of professional standing, pecuniary loss, and, indeed, loss of the very right to pursue practice of the profession. (1986 p.748)

Paradoxically, the imposition of unduly harsh penalties and standards by the nursing profession against its members serves to impede its quest for self-regulation. The excessively punitive nature of some of these decisions has compelled the appellate courts to intervene and substitute their own decisions.

NURSES MUST MANAGE AND CONTROL THE NURSING WORKFORCE AND NURSING WORK ON A DAY-TO-DAY BASIS

Traditional nursing management structures

It was one of the central tenets of Nightingale's management system that nurses should come under the direct control of the nursing superintendent. In order to achieve this goal, she was careful not to challenge medical supremacy in any way. She expressed this view in a letter to Lady Charlotte Canning from the Barrack Hospital, Scutari in 1855.

Bind the Superintendent by every tie of signed agreement & of honor (sic) to strict obedience to her Medical Chief ... But let all his orders to the Nurses go through her. I mean, of course, not with regard to the medical management of the Patients, but with regard to the placing & discipline of the Nurses ... But I would never have undertaken the Superintendency with that condition that the Nurses consider themselves 'under the direction of the Principal Medical Officer.' I am under his direction. They are under mine. (Vicinus & Nergaard 1989 pp.123–24)

This concept of the nurses having exclusive charge of the nursing staff continued from Nightingale's day until relatively recently. In Merritt & Cobar District Hospital (No.3) Kelleher J stated that:

[T]he matron is not a lowly employee of the Board. She is entrusted, subject to direction by the Board, with the complete administration of the nursing functions of the hospital. The Board bears the final responsibility for every act of the hospital's administration, but the matron is the pivot on which the nursing and domestic services are balanced. (1973 p.529)

Earlier in the last century, there was a fairly static nursing hierarchy, with the matron in charge of the nursing staff in the hospital. Traditionally the matron had financial control over the nursing budget, and often also the housekeeping and domestic budgets. The next level below the matron was usually the ward sister, although in larger hospitals the matron would often have a number of assistant matrons to help her with administrative duties. Ward sisters, having achieved their positions, would often remain in them until retirement, so that the only alternatives for career promotion were either to become a sister tutor in the nurse training school or to become an assistant matron (Jenkins 1989).

In the 1970s in the UK, more hierarchical management structures were introduced, which enabled the ward sisters positions to be vacated more quickly and allowed more junior nurses to obtain promotion (Ministry of Health and Scottish Home and Health Department 1966). This was seen as a solution to a twofold problem: that of 'the authoritarian nursing hierarchy' and 'the absence of any career rewards for the nurse who remains clinically active' (Gardner & McCoppin 1989 pp.321–22). In reality, it did little to alleviate either of these problems as it simply made the authoritarian nursing hierarchy bigger and took the most vocal, confident nurses off the ward. Similar structures were introduced in Australia in the early 1980s.

The impact of economic rationalism on nursing management structures in New South Wales

With the introduction of economic rationalism as the driving force in health economics in New South Wales, there has been considerable interest in the nursing budget and in control of nursing staff (Bloom 2000). There has been considerably more academic interest in the UK, however, with organisations such as the Centre for Health Economics at the University of York issuing 11 publications on skill mix and efficiency in nursing between 1985 and 1996. Nurses are both the largest single group in the health care workforce and the majority of the health care workforce (Daniel 1990 p.66). Thus the nursing budget is substantial, and any increases in pay, however modest, have a significant effect on the overall health budget. With the increasing militancy of nurses in the 1970s and 1980s there were some sizeable gains in terms of improved salaries, and nurses felt that they were finally achieving adequate financial recognition (Gardner & McCoppin 1989, Daniel 1990, Dickenson 1993). However, these gains may have served to focus the gaze of an increasingly financially oriented health care system on the net cost of the nursing workforce. The need for 'productivity savings' became the call. Nurses and other health care professionals were asked to 'do more with less', 'work smarter, not harder' and comply with other similar euphemisms. There was much debate about a new pre-payment funding system for health care based on the American concept of Diagnosis Related Groups (DRGs) (Ducket 1992 pp.137–61), but such funding systems required organising hospitals along closer diagnostic lines than was necessarily the current situation.

By September 1990, the proposals for such decentralised management structures were already in the news. Debbie Picone, then President of the NSWNA, described these developments to the delegates at the AGM. However, Picone's concerns were not for the notion of decentralised systems per se, but for nursing's ability to exercise power in those new structures. She identified the pivotal role nurses play in hospital organisation, arguing that 'for 70% of the time a hospital's general services are being directly managed by nurses' (Picone 1990 pp.15–17).

Despite these protests, the 'productivity savings' continued. In 1991–92 one hospital alone was required to achieve $7 million savings, with approximately $3–3.5 million to be achieved through cuts in nursing positions (Staunton 1991b p.20). The seemingly inexorable structural changes led Patricia Staunton, then General Secretary of the NSWNA, to comment that 'the professional integrity of nursing is being seriously challenged as being no longer individually relevant in the senior decision making echelons of our health care services' (1991a p.3). Kokowski complained that 'we are becoming increasingly bitter and angry that it is always nursing positions and our members' conditions that are invariably targeted when budgetary savings are being looked for' (Kokowski 1991 p.3). By 1994, the 'productivity savings' had been so effective there was a declared shortage of specialist nurses. Staunton was caustic, asking 'Is it any wonder that skilled and experienced nurses have looked for work elsewhere, often in other fields?' (1994 p.3).

In March 1995, there was a change of government and the NSWNA was working hard to convince Dr Refshauge, the new Minister for Health, that nurses should be responsible to nurses, both professionally and administratively (Staunton 1995a p.13, 1995b p.9). However, it seems that the hope that Labor would retain nurses' administrative accountability was forlorn. The Refshauge announcement was that Labor had 'kept its promise' to ensure that nurses remained (only) professionally (but not managerially) responsible to nurses, and that nurses would have 'a greater say in decision making' (Refshauge 1995 pp.6–7). Nurses in New South Wales had lost the fight to retain or regain the nursing budgets, and much of their line management control of nursing.

Nurses perceived this as a disappointing loss. The concern of nursing industrial organisations to maintain nursing's control over nursing was motivated by a well-founded mistrust of the economic rationalism driving health care over the previous fifteen years. It had also been motivated by an equally well-founded awareness of medicine's prowess in appropriating health care funds. For example, Duckett (1992) reported that medical expenditure accounts for over 18% of the health care budget, pharmaceutical benefits another 9% and that medical technology costs are also very high, although no exact figure was given. Since doctors comprise a very small percentage of the health care workforce, their level of expenditure is understandably worrisome if viewed in competition with a nursing budget.

However, the Nightingale model of enclosure within a tight fiscal and disciplinary structure was not necessarily to nursing's advantage. Nursing has rarely determined its budget, it has only managed it. In addition, maintaining control over nursing has, by its very scale, been time consuming, and has meant that nurse managers have of necessity been professionally introspective. In the past, nurses who wished to become nurse managers undertook Diplomas in Nursing Administration, taught by nurses and offered by nursing educational institutions (Russell 1990 pp.78–82). These same nurses have been criticised by economists in their approaches to economic issues (Gray 1987).

The preoccupation of nursing with its managerial segregation has meant that nurses remained with their own designated budget, but had no control over its size. Comments from research on nurse productivity undertaken for the NSWNA (Employment Studies Centre of the University of Newcastle 1992) highlighted this problem very clearly.

Bed usage drives costs, but it is not controlled by nurses. Surely allocation should be determined by nurses since they know the appropriate places for patients. Because nurses are kept right out of budgeting [especially in private hospitals] they cannot even see what income they are generating. (1992 p.42)

The largest, most flexible and most constant component of the health care workforce lost over 1000 positions in NSW in six years, without even being fully involved in how the expenditure cuts would be allocated. The impact of economic rationalism has been that nurses are having to make unacceptable decisions about the delivery of nursing care. This can lead to conditions which have been described as inhuman and unsafe, as reported in this harrowing account from a Western Australian nurse.

I stand by the bedside of a patient with cancer, who I know wants my time; she wants to talk to me about her fears and her feelings. She wants to ask me questions, what can I do?

I have someone to pick up from theatre, someone else in pain; I have the 'obs' to do, the 'meds' to do. I am already behind because someone is vomiting. I have to go; maybe if I 'skimp' on other patients (sic) care I can get back to talk to her and the moment will not have passed.

I don't get back to her. Someone's chemotherapy leaks onto them and the bed, that takes a lot of time. A few days later she dies. I go to bed that night (I was late off duty as usual) and now I can't sleep. I hope someone had time to listen to her, because I failed her.

I stand by the bedside of a patient who has just vomited blood, we clean him up and it happens again. We are busy getting 'blood through', taking obs, cleaning him up and trying to get him ready for theatre. The patient in the next bed had his bowels open about half an hour ago. There is no one else to help me, he has to wait and sit in his own excrement, until I have time.

These things go on day after day, week after week. I feel ashamed and guilty, maybe it's me. I'm not up to this, I can't cope, but I look around, very few people are doing any better. I move from that ward because it tears the heart and soul out of me. (Toomer 1998 p.14)

It is difficult to predict whether nurses would have fared better if they had been originally incorporated into a general hospital management structure. The danger would have been that the doctor's handmaiden story would have prevailed, and nurses would have been subsumed within a medical budget, in which they might have fared no better. Until recently, nurses seeking advancement have rarely considered this a possibility, because nursing affairs have been managed within an internal nursing structure, and such affairs have consumed nurses' efforts and energy. Nurses who moved to non-nursing appointments were regarded as having 'left' nursing, as indeed they often had. There was no prevailing philosophy that a move to a non-nursing position would manoeuvre nurses into other key influential positions in health care.

It is unclear therefore just how deleterious this loss of managerial autonomy has been for nursing. Probably not all nurses were sad to say good-bye to the authoritarian management hierarchy which had characterised nursing for so long (NSW Health Department 1996a, 2001). Those nurses now in general management positions have access to much larger budgets than pre-determined nursing budgets, and are able to bring their knowledge of nursing needs to bear on an overall budget allocation, rather than hopefully awaiting the allocated budget and then coping within it. Many nurses are now in senior management and policy positions in NSW and the profession celebrates and owns their success.

The value of nursing will probably be redefined or even re-appreciated by having nurses in general management positions. These (nurse) general managers would still be required to function within the constraints of a health care system dominated by economic rationalism. Yet at least when the ever-decreasing health care 'pie' is divided up, managers who appreciate the value and worth of skilled nursing practice might not be so quick to attenuate the nursing slice.

But the problem will be greater for nurses if these (nurse) general managers do not re-define management practices, but continue to operate within a system which has hardly addressed the subordination of nurses, and which accepts the current role of clinical nurses as the status quo. There would then be a danger that the reality of nurses' oppression would increase because nurse managers would join the 'real' managers and simply implement the pre-existing ruling maxims of management. They might climb up the ladder of success and pull the ladder up after them.

Acceptance of nursing's managerial autonomy by the courts and tribunals

The legal question of whether nurses are clinically controlled by senior nurses, by doctors or by others is a question which this book has already addressed in depth in other chapters, and will not be dwelt upon here. However, there is evidence to suggest that, whatever the courts and tribunals may have thought about the relationship between doctors and nurses in terms of clinical decision making about patient care and treatment, they have accepted that nursing matters such as staffing are directly under the control of nurses.

In Logan v Waitaki Hospital Board (1935), Reed J proposed the following test to determine who controls the nursing staff at any particular time.

Supposing a railway accident to have occurred in proximity to the hospital, and that there were many injured. If the matron had come into the ward and said "Leave one nurse in the ward and the rest of you come and prepare for the reception of the injured." Eliminating any question of being a case of emergency, could any one of those nurses legally justify a refusal to leave the ward on the ground that she was the servant of Dr Bardsley and amenable only to his instructions? (1935 pp.424–45)

When liability for a nursing management matter has been proven, either the hospital or the individual nurse in charge has usually been found to be negligent. Doctors have always been quite anxious to stress that they were not liable for administrative matters in nursing, although they have often complained when they have been excluded from decision making about nursing matters. In Logan, the doctors gave evidence that 'practically all acts of a nurse are professional and the division suggested by the dictum [in Hillyer] is illusory' (1935 p.427).

A further authority of relevance is Laidlaw et al v Lion's Gate Hospital (Hiddleston et al 1969). This was a post anaesthetic recovery (PAR) room case where the management of the nursing staff levels was central to the finding of negligence. Dohm J held that the hospital was meeting the standard of care requirements by providing two registered experienced recovery room nurses, as this was within the acceptable patient–nurse ratio. However, he held that Nurse S was negligent for failing to provide proper observation for Mrs Laidlaw and for leaving her unchecked in the recovery room for a period of time longer than three to four minutes. He also found Nurse S negligent as the nurse in charge in allowing Nurse M to take her coffee break when she was expecting patients from theatre. She was also negligent in failing to obtain relief staff. He found Nurse M negligent for taking her coffee break at a time when she should have known the probability of patients arriving in the recovery room, bearing in mind that she was an experienced recovery room nurse (1969 p.737).

Similarly, in Krujelis et al v Esdale et al (1971), a 10-year-old boy died in the recovery room due to poor staffing management causing inadequate supervision of the child. Dr Esdale, the anaesthetist, five nurses, and the employing hospital were named as defendants. The five allegations of negligence against Dr Esdale were all dismissed. The fourth, that he failed to ensure that the PAR nurses would provide proper care, failed because 'Dr Esdale had no control or jurisdiction over the PAR and no vestige of reasonable anticipation that Ivars would receive anything but the best of care in it' (1971 pp.559–60). The employing hospital was held not to be liable as an entity for poor staffing levels as these were found to be adequate. Five of the six counts of negligence were found to be proven against the nursing staff, three of which related to the management of the PAR.

It would seem that nurses have achieved some degree of recognition of their managerial autonomy. Even with the new decentralised management structures, matters such as deployment of nursing staff within a unit still fall to the nurse in charge. Accordingly, if the 'railway accident test' were applied, the nurse in charge would still probably be held accountable.

CONCLUSION

This chapter has set out to examine the regulatory and managerial autonomy of nurses. In terms of regulation, nursing could be said to be autonomous, although the courts are likely to intervene if it appears that the profession has been over-zealous. In terms of management, nursing has until recently maintained strong line management control over its employees, but has not been able to have significant governance over the overall financial affairs of the health services. Although line management structures have been weakened over the past decade, the potential for nurses to play a greater and more influential role in financial management has increased significantly and nurses have moved into top positions in health care management. The challenge will be to ensure that such gains serve the best interests of the profession in its ability to deliver optimal nursing care.

9

Autonomy in knowledge and education

Elements of the image

- The nursing profession must be self-regulating;

  - Entry to the nursing profession must be restricted and governed by their own regulatory authority;

  - Nurses must be able to control standards for the practice of nursing, which should be recognised by the courts and tribunals;

  - Nursing must be able to control continuance in the profession.

- Nurses must manage and control the nursing workforce and nursing work on a day-to-day basis.

- Nursing has a unique body of specialist knowledge;

  - Nursing education is the formal theorising of women's work (early argument);

  - Nursing is a scientific discipline with the same characteristics of knowledge as medicine, just different content areas (later argument);

  - Although nursing and medicine are separate and distinct disciplines, there is an overlap of workload, due to the fact that the two operate so closely together;

  - Nursing is a caring discipline based on research, which has created a distinct body of nursing knowledge (current argument);

  - The practice of nursing requires specialised training and education;

  - Nursing as a profession requires proper professional remuneration.

- Clinical nursing knowledge and expertise should be given equal weight to that of medicine in clinical decision making.

INTRODUCTION

This chapter sets out to explore nursing's quest for autonomy in knowledge and education, both of which form part of the outsider story of the nurse as autonomous professional. As with the last chapter addressing this outsider story, the chapter is structured to examine the outsider story first and then to consider the extent to which the story has been accepted by the courts and tribunals. This chapter looks chronologically at three arguments about the status of nursing knowledge: the early argument that nursing was the formal theorising of women's work; the later argument that nursing was a scientific discipline with the same characteristics as medicine, just different content areas; and the most contemporary argument, that nursing is a caring discipline based on research, which has created a distinct body of knowledge. These arguments are not mutually exclusive and all still manifest today in the nursing literature. The elements of the outsider story are detailed at the opening to this chapter.

NURSING HAS A UNIQUE BODY OF SPECIALIST KNOWLEDGE

Nursing education is the formal theorising of women's work (early argument)

In the early 20th century nurses considered their work to be important, perceiving that they were transforming the domestic work which women had traditionally performed into paid work (Cott 1977). This was consistent with the changes from pre-industrial to modern industrial work patterns and health care was no exception (Fisher 1993). What nurses probably did not envisage was the lowly status which others would accord to their work. Theoretically, if nurses were able to identify a unique body of nursing knowledge to develop into a curriculum, they imagined the professionalisation of nursing would be relatively straightforward. However, this was to prove problematic.

Nursing as an inclusive discipline

In Chapter 7, Abraham Flexner's criteria were used to identify whether early 20th century nursing met the requirements for professional status. The two most pertinent criteria addressed the need for professions to be:

- learned in nature, and their members are constantly resorting to the laboratory and seminar for a fresh supply of facts; and
- not merely academic and theoretical, however, but definitely practical in their aims (1915 pp.576–81).

The second criterion, the practical aspect of nursing, would be an unlikely topic for dispute. However, the first has created much controversy over the last century. With the introduction of the Nightingale reforms to nursing education and the promotion of professional self-regulation came the need to identify a designated body of knowledge which, when viewed in its totality, comprised professional nursing.

However, Nightingale was of the opinion that the knowledge ought not to be unique knowledge, but should be made available to any woman (sic) who might have charge of the health of another. Nightingale differentiated nursing knowledge—which she considered inclusive, in the sense that it should be available to everyone—from medical knowledge, which she saw as exclusive. She believed that the role of nurses was to teach everyone about health, hygiene, and nursing care, in order to care for themselves more effectively, and that nursing training was about teaching the totality of this knowledge.

Every day sanitary knowledge, or the knowledge of nursing, or in other words, of how to put the constitution in such a state as that it will have no disease or that it can recover from disease, takes a higher place. It is recognized (sic) as the knowledge which every one ought to have, distinct from medical knowledge, which only a physician can have. (Nightingale 1952 Preface)

This makes a significant differentiation between the professional model of nursing and that of medicine or law, for example. These latter disciplines have an exclusive body of knowledge and an exclusive language. Education and training for the discipline is based on learning these. To the extent that nurses work with doctors, they also need to learn this exclusive medical language and knowledge. However, the skills and knowledge specific to the practice of nursing relate to making explicit and understandable those activities designed to progress a patient 'towards health and/or well-being or to a peaceful death' (Henderson 1969).

Problematically for nurses, because much of this knowledge was and is concerned with matters of hygiene and care, society has experienced difficulty in equating it with professional knowledge. This is evident in the stock story of the nurse as a domestic worker. In addition, the aim of nurses is to enable or assist people to perform 'unaided' those activities which progress them 'towards health and/or well-being or to a peaceful death' (Henderson 1969). Thus, nurses have always needed to demystify language and knowledge in order to enable patients and carers to manage for themselves. It is, therefore, not only difficult, but also undesirable, to seek to quarantine an 'inclusive' discipline such as nursing.

The importance of cleaning in the nursing curriculum

In addition to the question of the desirability of a unique body of knowledge, the other troublesome issue transpired to be the content of the nursing curriculum. At the beginning of the 20th century there was strong consensus about such content, which continued to be based on the Nightingale philosophy. From Nightingale's concerns for hygiene arose the obsession with cleaning, which was then one of the cornerstones of nurse training. At this time the work of Ignaz Paul Semmelweiss (1818–1865) on the infectious nature of puerperal sepsis had been given credence by Lord Lister (1827–1912). 'Germ theory' was being recognised as a reality, and the use of antisepsis and later asepsis was becoming more common (Seymer 1949). Nurses then placed even greater emphasis on hygiene and disinfection as a specialised part of their professional role. In 1952 Lucy Ottley, President of RCN UK, wrote that:

Unless we realise the background of the times, this emphasis on 'sanitary nursing', the constant warnings about musty passages and blocked up chimneys, smells from sinks and smells from drains, seem unnecessary. A hundred years ago the lessons had to be driven home with a reformer's zeal. (In Nightingale 1952 p.7)

Those activities revolutionised the manner in which health care and medicine are practised. It seems ironic that such activities, absolutely dependent on nurses' strict and meticulous attention to hygiene, were the same ones which probably engendered nursing's lowly status for the purpose of fixing liability, as described in Chapter 5. By the time of Reidford v Magistrates of Aberdeen (1933), cleaning typified the routine or menial duties alluded to in Hillyer and such duties were specifically discounted as having no relevance to professional nursing.

Prevention of infection included cleaning and disinfection, activities which the nursing profession did not consider to be either menial or domestic. Florence Nightingale wrote that 'it cannot be necessary to tell a nurse that she should be clean, or that she should keep her patient clean, seeing that a greater part of nursing consists of preserving cleanliness' (1952 p.181).

'The supply of proper food and the like'

Another activity specifically identified as being 'routine or ministerial', by Kennedy LJ in Hillyer, was the supply of proper food to the patients. The designation of feeding duties as domestic or routine was further alluded to in later cases (Reidford v Magistrates of Aberdeen 1933, Gold v Essex County Council 1942). Yet activities such as the 'supply of proper food' (Hillyer 1909 p.829) and 'giving a patient his meals' (Gold v Essex County Council p.299) were described in the nursing literature of the time as critical aspects of nursing work. Antibiotics had not yet been discovered, and thus good nutrition and rest were essential for the patients' abilities to withstand or combat infection and promote healing. For this reason, nurses considered that it was essential that they should control and undertake such work.

To give food and stimulants in the way, at the time, of the kind, with the cooking and preparing, that will best enable the poor enfeebled digestion to assimilate it, is one of the greatest nursing arts. (Nightingale 1882)

Thus, many of the activities which nurses would automatically have included in their curricula in fact damaged their bid for professional status.

> *Nursing is a scientific discipline with the same*
> *characteristics as medicine, just different*
> *content areas (later argument)*

Seeking professional recognition

The judicial and societal disregard in the early 20th century for work which nurses believed to be of critical professional importance must have been deeply disappointing. They learnt that they needed other means to attract professional recognition for nursing work. Activities accorded professional status by the courts and tribunals were those activities most closely associated with the work of doctors. This method of achieving professional status has been described previously as extrinsic professionalism. But it is problematic, as it diminishes those aspects of nursing care which might be seen to be unique to nursing and privileges those activities which make nurses more like doctors.

Grosz (1995 p.54) explains why the uniqueness of women (and, in this case, nursing work) is devalued through such a project:

The project of sexual equality takes male achievements, values, and standards as the norms to which women should also aspire. At most, women can achieve an equality with men only within a system whose overall value is unquestioned and whose power remains unrecognized. Women strive, then, to become the same as men, in a sense, 'masculinized', produced within the terms of men's identities and self-representations.

The most common way in which the courts and tribunals originally ascribed professional status to nursing was by relating their work to that of an accepted/established profession, in this case medicine.

The impact of scientific positivism

The early 20th century saw the re-emergence of scientific positivism (O'Connor 1964). There was a drive to 'eliminate metaphysical elements from the sciences and to show that all the sciences, including the human sciences, are reducible to the method of induction' (Emden 1991 p.16). The effect of the ascendancy of scientific positivism in medicine was to devalue further those aspects of work for health which could not be scientifically explained or quantified. As the century progressed, the 1950s and the 1960s in particular were decades where rapid advances in technology changed the way in which people perceived the world, and the forms of knowledge which were valued.

If nursing wished to be seen as an 'equal' profession, the leaders of the profession therefore saw the need to develop a scientific basis, by which they meant grounded in physical science. Here nursing pursued a path of professionalisation similar to that of liberal feminism. In liberal feminism, the claim has been that women have equal rights and equal status, that there is 'a universal standard of humanity, comprising both women and men' (Davies 1993 pp.180–81). In order to achieve this equal status, liberal feminists originally demanded to be treated by the law in the same way as their male counterparts. Davies (1993 p.181) observed that this was intrinsically problematic for women, as the 'abstract non-gendered and non-sexed individual...was culturally seen as male'. Similarly nurses believed that equal power and status would be achieved if they could only manifest the same qualities as a profession such as medicine. They considered that the exclusive, quasi-scientific, professional model espoused by such professions as medicine and law was the 'gold standard' for professionalism (Marriner 1975 pp.134–36).

Undeniably, the success of nurses in obtaining increased remuneration has been significantly enhanced by evidence demonstrating their increasing responsibility for delegated medical tasks. Arguably, this is not a particularly logical method of achieving professional status, as it follows that if medicine is discarding these tasks, it is moving on to something of greater technological or scientific complexity, leaving nurses always a little way behind the medical 'pack'.

The nursing process and nursing diagnosis: 'scientific' approaches to nursing care

In the 1950s and 1960s, nursing education was based on a medical, disease-centred model, usually system-focused, dealing with anatomy, physiology and pathology. Each disease would be taught in terms of signs and symptoms, investigations, treatment and complications. Almost as an afterthought would follow a description of the nursing care for this particular condition (Bloom 1969). Examinations were similarly framed. At this time, there was concern in Australia and the UK about the quality and appropriateness of nurse education programmes, as retention of nursing staff was exceptionally poor. The root of the problem was believed to lie in the education system, and in nursing's lack of research-based education and practice (Briggs 1978, Russell 1990).

Applying scientific method to nursing

Perhaps an early portent of the changes to come was Virginia Henderson's definition of the role of the nurse (1969 p.4). Just as the American Nurses'

Association Code of Ethics transferred the focus of the nurses' loyalty from the doctor to the patient, so Henderson rearranged the focus of nurses' relationships with the doctor and the patient. Henderson's revolutionary definition stated that the nurses' 'unique function' was to 'assist the individual, sick or well, in the performance of those activities contributing to health or its recovery (or to a peaceful death) that he would perform unaided if he had the necessary strength, will or knowledge'. Henderson went further in affirming the nurse's autonomy, and stated that 'this aspect of her work, this part of her function, she initiates and controls; of this she is master'. Henderson addressed the nurse's relationship with the doctor almost as an afterthought, a secondary consideration.

In the 1970s and 1980s, perhaps in a continuation of Henderson's primary focus on the nurse–patient relationship, the methodology of nursing care became more explicitly scientific. Many of these developments originated in America, perhaps because American nursing programmes transferred much earlier into the tertiary sector (Seymer 1949, Mauksch 1984, Russell 1990). An early development was the Nursing Process, hailed as a 'scientific approach to nursing care' (Marriner 1975 p.134–36). This was described as 'the application of scientific problem solving to nursing care' (Marriner 1975 p.1), and was intended to assist nurses to provide patient-centred care which focused on what nurses, rather than doctors, actually did for patients. There was a growing body of opinion in the nursing literature that the admitting medical diagnosis was not the most significant determinant of the required level of nursing care. Factors such as the patients' ability to perform their 'daily living activities', such as elimination and managing their personal hygiene and nutrition, their level of mobility and flexibility and their mental and socioeconomic status were considered more likely to determine nursing practice and staffing requirements (MacFarlane & Castledine 1982, Roper et al 1983).

The publication and dissemination of such opinions was heartening for clinical nurses, many of whom were dissatisfied with the way in which patient care was fragmented (De La Cuesta 1983). Policies and procedures which encouraged assessments of a patient's ability to perform these 'daily living activities' were embraced enthusiastically by nurse teachers and nurse managers alike. New documentation systems were introduced which encouraged nurses to use a systematic (scientific) method of assessment, planning, implementation and evaluation of nursing care. In addition, patient allocation was considered complementary to an holistic approach to care, whereby each patient had a designated nurse or nurses to give them all their nursing care, as opposed to a division of labour based on task allocation. The nursing literature recorded considerable excitement at the thought that at last nurses could document and account for the care they gave in a unique manner (Hart 1986).

Difficulties encountered in the implementation of the 'scientific'
approach

However, the dynamics and power relationships between doctors and
nurses on the ward did not alter. Clinical nurses who wished to implement
the system found themselves in conflict with medical staff resistant to
changes to a system which had always worked perfectly well for them
(Mitchell 1984). Medical staff were annoyed to find that, because of patient-
rather than task-allocation, nurses no longer 'knew' all the patients on the
ward. They also believed that the paperwork consumed too much nursing
time (Re Mason and Registered Nurses Association of British Columbia
1979). There was deep suspicion about the motivation for its introduction,
one doctor describing it as 'a bid for independence from what they [nurses]
regard as medical domination' (Mitchell 1984 p.217). Dingwall et al
(1991 p.216) propose that the nursing process did not succeed overall,
because it did not 'take into account…the real conditions of nursing
work'.

During the 1980s I described nursing as having 'a religion without a
god…Hav[ing] rejected…the medical model as being inappropriate to
[their] needs…suddenly the Word had disappeared, and it seemed as
though there was only a nursing process to replace it' (Chiarella 1988
pp.25–26). There have been a plethora of nursing models over the past two
decades, all of which have attempted to provide theoretical frameworks
for nursing practice to explain the way in which nurses practise nursing
(e.g. Riehl & Roy 1980). One of the reasons for the failure of the Nursing
Process may have been that the development of nursing knowledge continued to be influenced by this 'sameness' ideal of equality, similar to that
espoused by the liberal feminists. The overriding belief persisted that, if
nursing could only look professionally or academically more like medicine,
professional recognition would occur.

The next American-driven innovation was the introduction of the concept of 'nursing diagnosis'. This was a systematic classification of nursing
problems with which a patient might present, and was intended to provide
a standardised nomenclature for the assessment phase of the nursing
process to facilitate nursing care planning. As might be imagined, the medical profession, who have arrogated to themselves the term *diagnosis*,
describing it as the 'sine qua non of the medical profession' in a media
release (AMA 1992), did not react with enthusiasm.

Although some nurses adopted a separatist, radical approach to this
development (Ride 1983), many other nurses made attempts to be concilia-
tory, offering methods of demarcation which they imagined left medicine
intact, but yet identified the nursing domain. Some adopted a health/
illness demarcation, claiming that 'physicians deal with disease whereas
nurses deal with levels of wellness' (Bandman & Bandman 1988 p.123).

Others used a more legalistic demarcation, stating that 'nursing diagnoses are made by professional nurses, which describe actual or potential health problems, and which nurses, by virtue of their education and experience, are capable and licensed to treat' (Gordon 1976 p.1298). Others contended that nursing and medical diagnoses were complementary, and maintained the view that 'the nurse is the authority on the maintenance of daily living activities while the doctor is, for instance, the authority on the diagnosis and treatment of disease' (MacFarlane & Castledine 1982). The preferred models of medical and nursing practice were described as 'overlapping' or 'inclusive', rather than 'exclusive' (Thomas & Coombs in Marriner 1975 p.99, Bandman & Bandman 1988 p.125).

The response of the medical profession was unequivocal. 'The fundamental error is to presuppose that problems of daily living activities can be separated from diagnosis and treatment ... I do not believe that two people can be in charge of one patient' (Mitchell 1984 p.216). There were calls from the medical profession for doctors to be reintroduced to nurse education (Mitchell 1984 p.218), a reduction in specialisation in nursing (Spence 1989) and, following the introduction of nursing into the tertiary sector, a call for a return to hospital-based nurse education (Spence 1989, Yeo 1990). What nurses saw as clinical nursing 'space', previously invisible, was seen by doctors to be already occupied medical territory. They did not consider that nurses had any space which they could legitimately call nursing territory. Cox (1996 p.171) has identified similar difficulties in finding 'space' for women when they aspire to masculine qualities in attempts to obtain employment, and has concluded that 'we have no separate space, no area of culture that we can claim as ours'.

The particular problem of documentation for an oral culture

A further problem for the nursing process was that nurses found recording these new methods of practice complicated. Instead of examining practice change to embrace holistic nursing care, they became fixated with the documentation (Chiarella 1983). When these new reporting systems broke down, either because they were too time-consuming or they had insufficient information on which to base their nursing care, nurses had all their usual work to do and more paperwork (Chiarella, 1985).

The fact that the paperwork was poorly maintained by nurses should have been predictable, if indefensible. One of the characteristics of outsider scholarship is the use of the spoken word in favour of the written as a means of communication (Williams in Delgado 1995 pp.xvii–xix). Lumby (1991 p.473) states that 'nurses have felt limited in their language and power to express what they actually do. Walk into the tea room if you want to find this [what nurses do] out'. Because nursing has an oral tradition, encouraging nurses to describe their practice in writing has been a challenge. In the 1970s and 1980s in Australia and England, only a relatively small number would have been university educated. Lumby explains that 'since Western society values such displays of knowledge and scholarship it has meant that nurses have not been regarded as true academics and ipso facto their work has not been regarded as valuable' (1991 p.474). Street, in her ethnographic study of nursing culture, confirms this dominant oral tradition. 'Clinical nursing has been formed through an emphasis on the development of oral skills. An examination of the conduct of clinical practice readily discloses a basic premise that the expressive capacity of oral communication leads to knowledge development which is passed on and developed orally through a number of nursing structures' (1992 p.20).

> *Although nursing and medicine are separate and distinct disciplines, there is an overlap of workload, due to the fact that the two operate closely together*

Flexible (and not-so-flexible) work boundaries between medicine and nursing

By and large, the leaders of the nursing profession in the 1970s and 1980s took due account of the medical opposition to their attempts for autonomy, but were unrepentant. They wished to have their role and processes of practice recognised and valued, and did not believe that this would make them particularly different. They only felt that it would make them visible.

Because they have been covert they have been undervalued, but many nurses are now accepting that the judgements they have taken-for-granted for so long lie at the heart of nursing and are something of which they should be proud. We can no longer afford to keep these processes hidden. As they become explicit more effective means will be found to help nurses think for themselves. (Bennett, 1986 p.46)

Nurses have always made regular assessments of patients. For example, when patients are admitted to emergency departments, the nurse takes a brief history from the patient and decides whether that patient needs to see the doctor urgently. This form of decision making, known as 'triage', is a well recognised component of the nursing role. When nurses are on duty in the middle of the night, they monitor and assess patients' conditions and determine the necessity to call a doctor. If they were to call for every fluctuation in condition, doctors would never sleep. In clinical settings where doctors are neither present nor available, nurses make decisions and give advice to patients about minor medications and therapies. These activities, which are collectively described as 'nursing management' of patients and are a well recognised component of the nursing role, require the nurse to make a provisional or at least a differential 'diagnosis'. The nurse identifies the possible diagnoses which the particular presenting problem might indicate, and decides which possible diagnoses are most likely, and then determines which are so serious that the doctor should be called to see the patient (Wicks 1999). If nurses did not practise nursing in this way, doctors could not practise medicine. Yet the language of such practice is exclusively the domain of medicine. When nurses adopt this language, they are opposed on the grounds that they are laying claim to medical territory.

At the same time, not all medical territory is so closely guarded. Over the years, there has been considerable uncontested 'slippage' from medicine to nursing. Why this slippage has occurred and why nursing and medicine can often appear to be occupying the same professional 'territory' has been the subject of much discussion in the nurse practitioner debate. But attempts to have nursing's professional status acknowledged through adopting medical characteristics were both unsuccessful and inappropriate. Other strategies were required.

Nursing is a caring discipline based on research,
which has created a distinct body of knowledge
(current argument)

Humanity and caring in nursing: ever present and difficult to deny

Nurses have always attached great significance to the need to assist doctors in their work, and to carry out their delegated medical tasks for the benefit of improved patient care. However, there is evidence to suggest that they derive the greatest personal satisfaction from the nurturing, comfort-giving aspects of their role, which can incidentally include those areas designated as 'domestic' by the courts. Isabel Stewart (1929 p.1) described the 'real essence of nursing' as 'the creative imagination, the sensitive spirit, and the intellectual understanding lying back of [the] techniques and skills'.

That 'real essence of nursing', the nurturing aspect of practice to which Stewart is referring here, has rarely been addressed directly in the case law. It would have been unlikely to have received professional recognition, as it is regarded as 'natural' women's work. But the skill, tact and patience which is required to undertake some of the more exacting aspects of nursing care does not come 'naturally'. Caring for people with horrific wounds and injuries (physical and psychological) is something which most people, regardless of gender, find extremely difficult. To acquire the skill to cope consistently and compassionately with a patient's anxiety, illness, disability and pain, whilst performing for them or assisting them to perform their activities of daily living, requires many years of practice, knowledge and expertise (Wicks 1999).

An early account of a nurse feeding and dressing the wounds of patients who had undergone head and neck surgery, gives an indication of the skill and compassion which was required.

There were many cases of the removal of cancerous growths of the jaw and tongue and these were big and distressing dressings—the nurse had to reassure the patient in a way peculiar to these patients, who were both apprehensive and sensitive about the mutilated experience of the face, and she learnt to approach him with confidence and sympathy, while at the same time getting on with the dressing in a business-like, though unhurried, way. Feedings over the tongue often had to be given at the same time. Such 'unremitting personal care' ... was required of the nurse as to endear the patient to her and perhaps no other case aroused her pity quite so much. (Armstrong 1965 p.107)

The fact that such skilled care was passed off as women's natural work (Abel-Smith 1960) has hindered nurses' quest for professional status, although it has made them admired and revered as archetypal women. Victor Robinson (a doctor), writing the introduction to *White Caps: the story of nursing* argues that 'the nurse is the mirror in which is reflected the position of women through the ages'. Space does not permit the reproduction of his full introduction, but perhaps most strikingly he observes that, ' ... it never occurred to the Aristotles of the past that it would be safer for the public welfare if nurses were educated instead of lawyers. The untrained nurse is as old as the human race; the trained nurse is a recent discovery. The distinction between the two is a sharp commentary on the follies and prejudices of mankind.' (1946 pp.vii–ix)

The development of qualitative research in nursing as a means of identifying a distinct body of nursing knowledge

The emphasis placed on the provision of comfort as an integral part of the professional nursing role is just as critical today. And, as nurses have begun to feel more confident about the value of the caring work they do, they have begun to research such phenomena as the provision of comfort. Recent research on the human nature of nursing identified the facilitation of comfort as being critical to the nursing role (Taylor 1994).

There has also been increased emphasis on nurse–patient relationships (Stein-Parbury 2000). The ways in which nurses are required to touch patients, the intimacy of their activities, requires critical faculty. In writing of the relationship between a nurse and a triplegic patient whose manual evacuation of faeces the nurse has to perform, Taylor describes the depth of the relationship between them. She observes that 'they humoured each other, but they also respected each other. In the everyday world, it takes a lot of understanding between friends before you can joke about something as personal as bowel habits' (1994 p.115).

Although the nursing process and nursing diagnosis did nothing to ameliorate the territorial disputes between doctors and nurses, their introduction revolutionised areas of practice, such as health visiting in the UK, where nurses have traditionally worked in relative isolation. It also provided nurses with a degree of confidence, and changed nursing curricula significantly, so that the invisibility of nursing care and the dominance of the medical model was challenged (Dingwall et al 1991). As the number of tertiary educated nurses increased, so did the confidence to seek other theoretical frameworks which looked at what made nursing different from, rather than the same as, medicine. Instead of looking to medicine to explore nursing, they looked to expert nurses. Significant amongst these new researchers was Patricia Benner, who explored the way in which expert nurses practised (1984) and also examined the phenomenon of caring (Benner & Wrubel 1989).

In addition, feminism has begun to have a significant impact on nursing research and thinking. Speedy observed that the discipline of nursing is developing along a track which 'is incorporating principles within its knowledge base which are surprisingly feminist'. Why 'surprisingly feminist' is unclear, as she continues that 'feminist principles are congruent with principles espoused by nurses today, including the ethic of care, nurturing, the centrality of the patient or client, the dialectical relationship between the carers and cared for, and a healthy questioning of the appropriateness of traditional "scientific" modes of thinking and research.' (1991 p.191).

Research and doctrinal development examining the primacy of care has a strong history in America (Leininger 1984, Chinn 1998). Speedy, whilst embracing these developments in nursing, has issued some caveats.

Whilst caring is vital for nursing practice, research and theory development, it is prudent to consider it from a variety of perspectives, including feminism. Feminists are concerned that to focus on caring as uniquely nursing and 'naturally' feminine will result in further devaluing of women and nurses unless this focus is coupled with an awareness of power relations in the health care system and in the wider society. (1991 p.207)

Over the past decade in particular, some Australian nurses have become internationally acclaimed as phenomenological researchers. The book *Towards a Discipline of Nursing* edited by Gray & Pratt in 1991, has become a standard text for undergraduate and postgraduate nursing courses in certain English, Scottish and American universities. Nurses have turned to the interpretive sciences, such as phenomenology and hermeneutics, to provide accounts of nursing and methods of understanding the lived experiences of nurses and patients (van Manen 1984). They have studied philosophers such as Heidegger, Habermas, Kuhn, and poststructuralists such as Foucault, Derrida and Merleau-Ponty to try to understand the nature of their lives and the lives of their patients. They have rejected scientific positivism as the only way to view the health care world (Gray & Pratt

1991). This has attracted further criticism (Spence 1989), particularly as much of the nursing research which has been undertaken is qualitative in design, and has been accorded lower status as a means of providing evidence about practice (NHMRC 1995). However, such criticism has not deterred nurses, as both qualitative and quantitative research methods are being used to understand the phenomenon of nursing and to inform nursing practice.

Whereas the early research was carried out mainly by nurse managers and nurse educators, probably because they were originally the only possible career paths in nursing, much of the current research is clinically based and driven. The number of clinical Masters and Doctoral students in nursing is growing rapidly. The recommendations of reports such as the Briggs Report in the UK and those made in Australia during the 1960s and 1970s are achieving realisation. Gray and Pratt state that 'the opening up of our possible worlds is dependent upon our willingness to not only deconstruct and understand, but also to reconstruct and transform, our lived-world' (1991 p.486).

The need for contemporary nursing theory further to address questions of power

The power relationships between nurses, doctors, and health managers which create problems for nurses, identified back in 1978 by Briggs and outlined in this book, are as yet unresolved, although they are beginning to be explored (Walker 1993). Holmes observes that 'the complete failure to acknowledge nursing's sociohistorical embeddedness, and to articulate any political position, never mind construct any specific political program, must be considered major weaknesses in contemporary nursing theory.' (1991 p.44).

Holmes is correct, in that the adoption of an equality model of professionalism has maintained nursing in its place of subjugation. If nurses seek to achieve equal professional status using the same markers of status as those used for medicine, then medicine is affirmed in its position of power, not challenged, and nursing is in a position of inferiority to medicine. Thus any subordination is arguably legitimate. Grosz elaborates on the way in which 'sameness' models of equality diminish the 'Other' (in Grosz's argument—women) and privilege those whom they seek to be like.

To achieve an equality between the sexes, women's specific needs and interests—what distinguishes them from men—must be minimized and their commonness or humanity stressed ... In this sense, equality becomes a vacuous, or rather, a formal concept insofar as it reduces all specificities, including those which serve to distinguish the positions of the oppressed from those of the oppressor. One can be equal only insofar as the history of the oppression of a specific group is effaced. (1995 p.52)

The practice of nursing requires specialised
training and education

The link between the judicial recognition of nursing as a profession, the development of a specialist body of nursing knowledge, and tertiary education

There has always been great emphasis placed on the value of 'hands-on' experience in nursing by nurses and doctors alike. Nightingale stated that she 'honestly believes that it is impossible to learn [nursing] from any book, and that it can only be thoroughly learnt in the wards of a hospital' (1952 p.113). Likewise, when the Nurses Registration Bill was being debated in the NSW Parliament, the Honourable Member for Burwood, Dr Parr, emphatically stated that '[n]ursing is learnt not out of textbooks, but at the bedside' (NSW Hansard 2 September 1953 p.447). Walker has proposed that nurses fostered a cult of anti-intellectualism because of their origins of apprenticeship. He argues that over the years nurses were indoctrinated into a 'regime of truth' about what real nurses were. Such a regime, he argues 'embodies truths such as "a good nurse is a busy nurse"; "a good nurse does as she is told"; "a good nurse is a nice nurse"; "a real nurse does hands-on work", and so on' (1997 pp.4–6).

Walker (1997) believes that there is still a strong vein of anti-intellectualism in nursing, particularly in relation to the new sources of nursing knowledge derived from qualitative research. He points out that nurses have been quick to criticise the language used by the philosophers whose work has informed qualitative nursing research. Yet the same nurses uncritically and competently learnt the Latin names for diseases and the medical jargon which has been the trademark of health practice for many years.

This anti-intellectualism has characteristically come from the less aca-demically qualified staff, all of whom would have been educated in the apprenticeship-style system. These staff initially felt threatened by the entrance of the new graduates into the clinical environment, as they feared that more academically qualified staff might be promoted over the heads of the more experienced staff (Bryon & Johnson 1990). However, this has not happened and many of those staff have since undertaken conversion courses to convert their hospital certificates into degrees. But this vein of anti-intellectualism has been used to bolster criticism by medical practi-tioners, who quote these nurses to justify their own opposition (Nelson in Demou 1992).

The achievement of professional status has been linked consistently to the need for better education (Russell 1990). From a legal perspective, as long ago as 1948, Boyd McBride J identified the need for nurses to keep up to date (Bernier v Sisters of Service St John's Hospital, Edson). He referred to the nursing textbooks to determine the standard practice of nurses, and he held that the nurses must take responsibility for keeping themselves up to date, even though they were working in a small hospital (pp.476–78).

McClemens J also addressed the relationship between professionalism and education in the Callan Park Report (1961). In calling for major reforms to the practice of nursing at Callan Park, he stressed the urgent need for greater education, particularly in relation to the more senior members of staff. Dr Bailey, the Superintendent, described his older, more senior nurses as having 'no knowledge of modern psychiatric nursing and little inclination to acquire any'. McClemens J did not entirely rebut this description and proposed education as a possible longer-term solution to the problem (1961 pp.168–69).

It is unclear whether McClemens J considered mental nursing to be a profession. Initially, when describing the difficulties encountered by mental nurses, he described it as 'a vocation' (p.116). When discussing the lack of medical and nursing liaison, he stated that 'the status and prestige of the senior nursing staff needed to be elevated to a professional level by education and other means' (p.13). But clearly his Honour perceived any professional status of mental nurses to be linked to the level of education they possessed.

There were also some Award decisions which demonstrated a link between financial rewards and further education, usually in the form of post-registration certificates (In re Public Hospital Nurses (State) Award 1967, In re Public Hospital Nurses (State) Award 1973). The 1973 NSW decision was the first where diplomas and degrees for nurses were mentioned.

Despite this burgeoning recognition, key Australian professional and industrial nursing organisations noticed that other 'paramedical' professions such as physiotherapy, dietetics, and occupational therapy were receiving better remuneration and recognition as a result of their improved university-based educational programmes. During the early 1980s the RANF, RCNA, the NSWCN, and the Florence Nightingale Committee of Australia combined to identify Goals in Nursing Education. They lobbied, marched and demonstrated until the various State governments across Australia acceded to their demands to move nurse education into the tertiary sector (Russell 1990). The first state to make the transition was NSW, which in 1986 moved nursing education completely into Colleges of Advanced Education where nursing was taught at Diploma level. This transition to tertiary education was the basis of the 1989 Professional Rates Case, which established rates of pay for nurses on the same level as some of the other professional employee groups in hospitals.

This was not sufficient for the nursing organisations, which wanted nurses educated to degree level. After a massive national professional consultation exercise, the same four nursing organisations jointly produced a document *Nursing Education Targets 1989–2000* which identified the directions in which they wished nursing education to proceed. Nursing organisations, both professional and industrial, in each State and at Federal level, lobbied and agitated until they succeeded. All states in Australia now have degree programmes in nursing. These are still undergoing some modification as the service needs for new graduates change rapidly, but there is a growing acceptance of undergraduate programmes and the abilities of the new graduates who have not come through a traditional 'hands-on' programme (Nurses Registration Board of NSW et al 1997).

Nursing as a profession requires proper
professional remuneration

Industrial recognition in the 1970s in New South Wales

If the courts and tribunals are a litmus test for the stock story, the 'way the world is', then the extent to which the courts and tribunals have accepted these developments in nursing practice can provide a measure of nursing's success in converting its outsider story into a stock story. Despite the fact that nurses had relatively little success in their industrial claims in the early and middle parts of the 20th century, the industrial courts and tribunals were arguably the first place where judicial recognition of nursing's intrinsic professional status occurred. The first NSW decisions which acknowledged and rewarded specialist nursing (as opposed to delegated medical skills) were handed down in the mid-1970s. Following the decisions in the National and State Wage Cases of April and May 1975, Dey J determined that almost all groups of nurses had already participated in the 1974 community wage movements and must thus fall into line with wage limitation principles (Public Hospital Nurses (State) Award 1976). Then in May 1976, following decisions regarding nurses pay in Victoria, Queensland, the Australian Public Service, and South Australia, the NSWNA brought a claim before the Industrial Commission which was outside the wage-fixing principles— namely, a claim that there had been changes in the value of nursing work.

In judgment on this claim, Kelleher J identified the source of the changes that had occurred in the role of the nurse as 'identical factors associated with advancements in the medical fields' (1976 p.327) and 'important and responsible tasks which were formerly restricted to medical officers' (1976 p.324). However, he also acknowledged such changes as the move to team or patient allocation, the 'counselling of patients and relatives which is now assuming greater significance' and the formal development of skills in clinical assessment and evaluation, which in turn influenced the nature of nurse education. In addition, for the first time there was a recognition of the stressful nature of nursing work (1976 p.324).

A report was compiled providing a contemporary view of the nature of nursing, which was accepted by Kelleher J and reflected in the award.

The report mirrored the thinking of the nurses in the mid-1970s. There was the 'extrinsic professional' argument—nurses ought to get more pay because they are doing more delegated medical work—but there was also the 'intrinsic professional' argument, albeit generally based on a 'sameness principle'. The influence of the introduction of the nursing process (the scientific approach to nursing care), could be detected in the moves to team or patient allocation and the skills required for clinical assessment and evaluation, the first and final steps identified in the nursing process. There was also recognition of some of the more qualitative aspects of nursing work, such as counselling.

1986 Ministerial Reference Case and clinical career structure

One of the most significant NSW decisions of the 20th century relating to nurses' pay, career structures and conditions, arose from a call to move nurse education out of the tertiary sector and back onto the wards! In 1985, all nurse education in NSW had moved from the hospitals to the tertiary sector. This meant that the ready supply of student nurses as cheap labour for the hospitals had ceased, causing a shortage of nurses to staff the wards (Hart et al 1995). In December of that year, the NSW Premier, Neville Wran responded by unsuccessfully mooting the idea of reinstating hospital-based nursing education programmes. Although the medical profession and some factions of the nursing profession supported this, there was widespread nursing opposition (Dickenson 1993). Patricia Staunton, then Assistant General Secretary of the NSWNA, took the lead in negotiations with the Premier, which led to a ministerial reference to investigate nurses' wages and conditions (Ministerial Reference Case 1986).

Counsel for the NSWNA applied the Work Value Principle, which allowed that substantial increases to wages could be awarded if a case could be made out that there had been significant changes in the value of the work undertaken. The NSWNA argued an overwhelming case 'that there had been changes in the skill and responsibility attached to the work and changes to the conditions under which it has been performed in the last five years to such a significant extent as to warrant substantial increases in salary for all classifications under the Public Hospitals (State) Award' (Ministerial Reference Case 1986 p.4).

Medically delegated 'extrinsically professional' work

The Commissioner accepted that nurses had taken on more medically delegated work. He recognised, when new equipment appeared on the ward, that nurses often had to self-educate via the instruction booklet. He acknowledged they had to develop new skills in cardiopulmonary resuscitation and other areas of patient care 'such as monitoring, interpretation of results and detecting malfunctions, e.g. fetal heart monitors and defibrillators' (p.16). He also acknowledged the development of specialist education programmes and what were described as 'extended role' policies to facilitate the practice of these new skills.

Nurse-initiated 'intrinsically professional' work

Most significant for this chapter was the recognition given to the diversity of the work which nurses undertook, the difficult conditions in which they worked and the complexity and skill which they brought to their practice. Commissioner Wells was sympathetic about the effects of the nursing shortages, necessitating as they did either the closure of beds or, more frequently, the use of agency nurses, or 'specials' as he described them. He commented upon the moral dilemmas with which nurses may be faced, given the heavier workload and higher dependency, and quoted an incident which he must have encountered while on his visits to the hospitals.

I have in mind the situation in the intensive care unit at Liverpool where the Charge Sister, when all beds are full and she is confronted by a new patient requiring immediate treatment, has to decide out of all patients in her care who is the least sick and that person is transferred to another ward. (p.21)

He acknowledged that such transfers meant that patients who were much sicker were being nursed on the wards, and that because of shorter length of stay all patients on the ward were of a higher dependency. He held that 'the extra work, skill, responsibility and stress attending the nursing job today have changed and need to be reassessed in 1986 terms' (p.22). He held that the changes required as a result of the issues raised by the identification of the AIDS (Acquired Immunodeficiency Syndrome) virus included research, education and new protocols. Recognition was also given to the increasing specialisation of community nurses in areas such as palliative care and AIDS.

The public relations functions of nurses were recognised in terms of cultural differences, patient and relative counselling, and liaison between all members of the health care team. The role of the nurse as a resource person and educator for medical and paramedical staff was acknowledged. He later stated 'from the above, I have concluded that registered nurses are now relied on more heavily than in 1981 for expert advice, education and assistance' (p.32). He also acknowledged the increase in 'more sophisticated' documentation, particularly in relation to patient care. He found that this extra documentation in a time of nursing shortage created dilemmas for nurses in terms of their priority setting in patient care.

Before fixing the salaries to meet the circumstances of the case, Commissioner Wells summed up his views thus:

For all the reasons listed above, there is no doubt in my mind that the facts of this case as to change fulfil the obligation in the Principles imposed by the strict test. I find that the changes in the nature of the work under this award constitute such a significant net addition to work requirements as to warrant new rates of pay for all classifications ... In my experience I am not aware of any such degree of change in any industry; in fact, in my opinion, the changes are so great as to border on the revolutionary. (p.42)

The changes made in this award did not only increase salaries. The entire nursing career structure in NSW was changed, leading to similar changes in other States. The existing classifications of charge nurse and supervisor were amalgamated into one classification of nurse unit manager (NUM). Two new clinical classifications were introduced: clinical nurse specialist (CNS), which incorporated the clinical teacher role; and clinical nurse consultant (CNC), which gave recognition to expert nurses (p.46).

The clinical career structure determined under this award is similar to that which exists at the time of writing. This award significantly influenced not only the remuneration for nurses in the future, but also the development of specialist education programmes for nurses. Increasing clinical specialisation in nursing was furthered through the clinical career structure, and education programmes needed to adapt to cater for the needs of specialist nurses. The clinical career structure has also enabled senior nurses who are career oriented to remain in clinical practice and undertake research into clinical nursing issues. The development of a clinical career structure has had a considerable impact on the assertiveness of nurses in their clinical relations over the past decade.

The professional rates case

Late in 1987, less than two years after this momentous decision, the NSWNA made an application to an Anomalies Conference under the Anomalies and Inequities State Wage Principles Act 1987 (NSW) for a finding as to an 'arguable case' in a claim relating to professional rates of pay for registered nurses (Public Hospital Nurses State Award 1987a). The claim was described by counsel for the NSWNA as 'a claim to apply full professional rates to the nursing staff of the NSW public hospitals' (p.559). It was intended to bring the salaries of public hospital nurses into line with those of other 'scientific officers', for example occupational therapists, speech pathologists and medical technologists. The claim was made at this time because the first graduates of the Diploma in Applied Science (Nursing) students were about to come into the hospital system. It was argued that 'the professional standing and responsibility of the graduate nurse is at least as high as that of other health professionals and probably higher due to the range of skills and responsibilities involved in the profession of nursing'. In addition, it was claimed that the introduction of the new programmes 'does no more than equate the graduate with those nurses who were educated by the hospital based training programme'. The Ministerial Reference Case was used to demonstrate the Commission's acceptance of the upgrading of hospital-based training.

Fisher P (Public Hospital Nurses (State) Award 1987a pp.564–5) held that the determination in the Ministerial Reference Case applied to exactly the same claim as the one before him now. He declined to refer the matter of professional rates to the Anomalies Bench, stating that 'the Nurses' Association cannot have cake in 1986 and eat it again in 1987'. However, he agreed to refer the matter of the anomaly between hospital-trained nurses, who had received three years' wages during training, and new graduates, who had not been paid at all during their undergraduate education.

The NSWNA successfully sought leave to appeal the decision. The Commission accepted the findings of the Victorian Commission that 'all registered nurses, whether they are registered as a result of a hospital training course or a College course, are to be regarded as performing the duties and responsibilities of a professional occupation when working as a registered nurse' (Public Hospital Nurses (State) Award 1987b p.4). It also accepted the submission of the Health Administration Corporation (HAC) and the Public Employment Industrial Relations Authority, whose counsel stated that 'nurses could now be regarded as having moved into the professional group'. Further the HAC had conceded that 'there is no longer any justification for excluding them from the professional group in public hospitals in New South Wales' (1987b p.7).

CONCLUSION

In establishing a unique body of knowledge which attracts professional recognition and remuneration, nursing has been only partially successful. Much of its recognition has occurred through an alignment with medicine which has meant that the knowledge, skills and attributes which were most pertinent to nurses were either disregarded as routine or domestic, or remained invisible. However, towards the end of the 20th century, there has been greater recognition of the unique professional contribution which nurses make to health care delivery. This contribution has been made visible through research, education and political action.

10

Autonomy in clinical decision making

Elements of the image

- The nursing profession must be self-regulating;

  - Entry to the nursing profession must be restricted and governed by their own regulatory authority;

  - Nurses must be able to control standards for the practice of nursing, which should be recognised by the courts and tribunals;

  - Nursing must be able to control continuance in the profession.

- Nurses must manage and control the nursing workforce and nursing work on a day-to-day basis.

- Nursing has a unique body of specialist knowledge;

  - Nursing education is the formal theorising of women's work (early argument);

  - Nursing is a scientific discipline with the same characteristics of knowledge as medicine, just different content areas (later argument);

  - Although nursing and medicine are separate and distinct disciplines, there is an overlap of workload, due to the fact that the two operate so closely together;

  - Nursing is a caring discipline based on research, which has created a distinct body of nursing knowledge (current argument);

  - The practice of nursing requires specialised training and education;

  - Nursing as a profession requires proper professional remuneration.

- Clinical nursing knowledge and expertise should be given equal weight to that of medicine in clinical decision making.

INTRODUCTION

This chapter addresses the third element relating to the nurse as an autonomous professional, which continues to be particularly problematic for nurses. It examines some clinical issues and tries to bring some insight into these problems for readers by providing accounts from nurses themselves of the experience of clinical subordination. The chapter describes how nurses have sought greater professional recognition in their clinical practice, and finally examines the extent to which these issues are dealt with (or not) by the courts and tribunals.

CLINICAL NURSING KNOWLEDGE AND EXPERTISE SHOULD BE GIVEN EQUAL WEIGHT TO THAT OF MEDICINE IN CLINICAL DECISION MAKING

Nurse–doctor dynamics in clinical relationships

Nurses have long felt that their clinical opinions and expertise are not given sufficient credence by the medical profession (Briggs Report 1978, Employment Studies Centre Report 1992, NSW Health Department 1996a). Furthermore, judicial attitudes condone this inequality. Doctors are seen as being at least clinically dominant over nurses, and the clinical concerns of nurses, if acknowledged, are acted upon at the discretion of the medical staff. Even when nurses' skilled concerns are heeded, Wicks found that 'the majority of doctors took the information from nurses and passed it on without bothering to attribute any credit to the nurses' skill' (1999 p.138). Nurses' clinical skills and opinions only have legal significance for doctors in their default, when doctors use the defence of reliance on the expertise of nurses as a means of mitigating their liability.

There are those who would argue: 'But there can only be one captain of the ship. Since most people come to hospital for cure, and because doctors control the mechanisms of cure, they must be in charge, and all other members of the health care team must be subordinate to them.' This is the stock story, and it is unquestionably the medical profession's reasoning. Kwong has suggested that most nurses would agree with this argument, that it is only the 'militant nursing educators [wishing] to justify their existence and their claim for glory who might seek ... changes' (1992 p.9).

Nurses do not usually wish to challenge the clinical decisions of doctors, because either they trust their clinical judgment or they agree with it. The nurses' traditional role, as discussed earlier, is to support the patient through the medical treatment towards cure, amelioration, or death. In complex treatment and surgery, the requisite skill and knowledge is such that the nurse would neither wish nor be able to take control. The patient's best interest is served by being cured, and nurses and doctors unite to achieve this. Doctors order sophisticated and sometimes aggressive forms of treatment, which is often administered by nursing staff, who concurrently monitor and optimise the quality of the patient's existence. If the treatment is unsuccessful, all parties agree when enough is enough, and treatment is discontinued and palliation is implemented. At this stage, the patient's existence becomes the critical focus, and nurses often (albeit unofficially) take over patient management at this stage. Here doctors would be advised by nursing staff on the patient's most pressing problems, for which they provide amelioration.

Clinical issues which are particularly problematic for nurses

So, you might ask, where are the problems? There are three main issues for nurses. First, when nurses feel that the patient's existence is being made so intolerable by the medical or surgical treatment that it should stop, but doctors do not agree. Second, where the treatment is not working and does not appear to be likely to work, and nurses believe that the patient would have a better remaining existence if they were palliated, but doctors wish to continue (Wicks 1999). Third, where nurses are concerned that a doctor's practice is at best ill-advised, or at worst dangerous, but the doctor does not heed their concerns.

The first two are particularly complex, as patients and their relatives are understandably seeking treatment and cure. Because nurses have such close proximity to patients and relatives, they become exquisitely intimate with human suffering and can experience it vicariously.

This is both disadvantageous and advantageous. It can be disadvantageous because sometimes nurses feel personally responsible for the patient's suffering despite everyone's best efforts. Because they cannot alleviate the suffering, they do not want the patient to continue to endure it. The patient's suffering can become the nurse's suffering, and it is difficult to bear. Further, sometimes very sick patients cannot clearly indicate their wishes, so everyone is reliant on the wishes of their relatives or other responsible persons.

However, this awareness can also be advantageous because nurses are thus able to bring unique insight into the patient's experience. Nurses have precise first hand knowledge of such critical minutiae as the extent of bruising from repeated injections, the impact of movement or endotracheal aspiration on vital signs, the effectiveness of pain management, the patient's emotional state. Such factors are central to good clinical decision making.

But the effects of proximity can become problematic if the relatives and the doctors still have cure as the priority, and only the nurses have the quality of existence as the priority. In such situations nurses have little ability to influence patient outcomes. Unquestionably, if professional, family and patient views have been considered, nurses may need to concede a difference of priority, rather than a case of right and wrong.

But if nurses believed firmly that the doctor was wrong (undoubtedly the exception, rather than the rule), there should be formal mechanisms for their views to be given equal weight in clinical decision making. More seriously, where nurses are concerned about the manner in which a doctor is practising, or a course of treatment, nurses need a clearly accepted right and an acknowledged positive duty to intervene. There should be no 'protocols' which suggest that nurses do not challenge doctors (Inquest touching the death of TJB 1989), no 'courage' required to make the challenge (Re Anderson and Re Johnson 1967). Nurses should be confident that their primary responsibility is 'to provide safe and appropriate nursing care' (ANCI Code of Professional Conduct 1995). This must suggest that, in any dilemma, their duty would be owed to the patient, not the doctor. But the Code of Professional Conduct, despite its rhetoric, does not alone provide nurses with the authority to challenge medical decision making hierarchies.

The position of outsiders: what it feels like to be subordinated in clinical decision making

This chapter primarily concerns an outsider story, which requires listening to the voices of the 'Other', the voices 'from the bottom' (Matsuda 1987 p.323). Nurses who find themselves in situations such as those mooted above need the authority to intervene and to have their views and clinical contributions legitimated and respected.

To understand why nurses seek this authority and legitimation it is necessary to explain why the alternative—being subordinate to the doctor, whether as handmaiden or subordinate professional—is problematic. It might also help to identify what changes nurses require. Nurses' call for clinical autonomy is not a call to practise medicine; rather it is a call to have some of the more critical aspects of their regular practice legitimated. They seek to have their work and opinions accorded equal weight and respect. They also seek legal authority to undertake tasks which they currently perform clandestinely.

One of the important factors in the call for clinical autonomy is that it is coming from nurse clinicians (Adrian & O'Connell 2000). It is coming from those voices 'from the bottom', but is supported by the managers and leaders of the profession who have driven many of the earlier debates, such as the need for improved education and managerial autonomy. Those more senior nurses experienced the reality of clinical subordination, but escaped it through their career moves. Since education and management were once the only available career paths, which thus attracted the most ambitious nurses, these were the first fields in which autonomy was claimed. Although many highly skilled nurses remained in the clinical areas, the more radical often found the level of subordination unpalatable, and either left or sought promotion.

Thus, until recently the nurses who stayed as clinicians were often either deeply dedicated, or deeply cowed by the system, which was both oppressive and inconsistent. Clinical nurses (in addition to being bullied by senior nurses) have been treated extremely discourteously by senior medical officers. Over the years there have been stories: of a surgeon swearing at nurses and throwing instruments at them in the operating theatres (Anon 1997); of another surgeon demanding that his patients' beds be pushed together during a ward visit to reduce his walking distance (Russell 1996). There is evidence of a doctor demanding that a procedure be carried out late at night, causing considerable inconvenience in preparation, and then cancelling without even an apology (Wicks 1999). Yet another nurse tells of an obstetrician screaming at her when she suggested an alternative form of management in a patient who had been sexually abused (Bonnet 1997). Since nursing has traditionally employed an oral culture, one can only imagine the number of stories which were never published.

A senior surgical manager recalled a surgeon who was so rude to the junior nursing staff that 'either a charge nurse or myself sat in that ENT theatre every week [for three months] until the surgeon learnt to control himself' (Hines 1993 p.24). Pringle reported that operating theatre nurses 'frequently experience male surgeons as being frightening and rude' (1998 p.195). A recent Australian study revealed that two in three nurses have experienced work-based sexual harassment (Weekes 1995).

The UK Briggs Report (1978) listed complaints collected from nurses and midwives about medical activities undertaken without consulting nursing staff. These included admission of patients causing overcrowding; medical research which created significant unrecognised work for nurses; the installation of technical equipment in wards requiring monitoring by nurses; and the planning of new units or other developments. The report concluded, rather lamely, that 'there is obvious scope for improvements'. It hoped to see 'a change of attitude among those doctors to whom one or more of the complaints listed above applies, so that ultimately all live up to the standards of the best' (pp.46–47). And that was it. Out of the 75 recommendations at the end of the report, not one addressed any of the difficulties identified above which were acknowledged to be 'widespread'.

Such findings were not confined to the 1970s or to the UK. The Employment Studies Centre of the University of Newcastle report (1992) described similar behaviour, with added new dimensions. Although beyond the scope of this text in its entirety, the report highlights the frustration which nurses experience in their subordinate roles.

The nurses in this study, as in the later work by Wicks (1999) describe one of the major problems as waiting. They waited for doctors to give permission for patient discharge, usually on the advice of nursing staff. They waited for doctors (who might not even know the patients) to write up discharge prescriptions, summaries and referrals, which concomitantly delayed the patients' discharge. They waited for doctors to write or re-write routine prescriptions with which the nurses were familiar; to review minor cases in Accident & Emergency, which nurses could have dealt with promptly. They waited for doctors to review wounds requiring authorisation of prescriptions for expensive dressings, only to have them ask 'What do you think, Sis?', and for surgeons to attend operating lists, requiring unnecessarily long fasts for patients (University of Newcastle 1992 pp.39–41).

Another recurrent theme, linked to the first, was that of trying to find a doctor ('often any doctor') to sign forms. To authorise pathology and radiology requests for specimens which had already been taken, but which, without a doctor's signature, would not be reimbursed through Medicare. To sign an order for Meals on Wheels; to refer private patients to a social worker, although nurses can refer public ones. To authorise a nurses' decision to remove a drain, because hospital protocols say they cannot be removed without a doctor's written order (University of Newcastle 1992 pp.38–43).

If this lack of authority were not sufficient, the report also identified their added sense of frustration that they spent so much time teaching the junior doctors (often the same ones they would later wait for). This was also acknowledged in the Ministerial Reference Case (1986). Nurses reported having to teach doctors infection control, suturing, basic clinical skills and orientation to the hospital and ward. Organising routine activities such as observations for the convenience of the doctors was also identified as a source of irritation (1992 p.41). The report also called for 'an opportunity to break down rigid, out-dated barriers to such improvements, and to develop a multi-disciplinary approach to health care, where all health professionals are "equal carers" able to perform a wide range of tasks in the most competent and efficient manner' (University of Newcastle 1992 p.52). Ann Daniel has also described the frustration which nurses experience (1990 pp.76–77).

Remarkable folly goes unremarked

Occasionally, a judge has commented on the lack of manifest clinical authority which nurses exercise (Inquest touching the death of TJB 1989); but commonly, even quite extraordinary acts of medical arrogance and/or stupidity pass without any comment on the potential for the nurse to intercede. In the 1994 Inquest into the death of PDP, the extraordinary behaviour of the anaesthetist went unremarked by the Coroner. Yet from the nurses' perspective, his behaviour must have created an intolerable situation.

In this case, reported in Chapter 6, the patient was returned to theatre at the behest of the theatre manager. At some stage towards the end of the second operation the patient's pupils were fixed and dilated and the anaesthetist announced generally that further efforts were useless.

The surgeon and anaesthetist left the nurses in the operating theatre with the patient, who was still attached to an electrocardiograph (ECG) monitor, still intubated, ventilated and with a blood transfusion and drip still running. The nurses were so concerned about the situation that they took the initiative of allowing the patient's wife into the operating theatre to see her husband. One can only imagine the sense of helplessness these nurses must have felt, supporting the anxious wife, unable to state that the patient was dead, but knowing that he was.

The anaesthetist initially testified that he had left the ventilator and the two drips connected in case they might resuscitate the patient again, but later conceded in evidence that there was no chance of improving his condition. The surgeon then arranged transfer to an intensive care unit in another hospital, a proposition which it was left to the deputy director of nursing, the most senior nurse on duty, to challenge. She asked why, 'if resuscitation had ceased and the patient was clinically dead … there was a question of transferring the patient to another hospital?' (1994 p.13).

It is ludicrous that inter-hospital transfer arrangements for a dead patient had to be stopped by such a senior nurse, when his death was so blatantly evident to the 'experienced [clinical] nursing staff' in the operating theatre that they took the unorthodox step of bringing in the patient's wife. Yet this bizarre behaviour and the lack of authority of the clinical nursing staff to put a stop to such a masquerade passed without comment in the judgment.

Similarly, when in the middle of the night a doctor refused twice to attend the cardiac arrest of a 21-month-old child, no specific comment was made about this behaviour. The doctor admitted in evidence that this was a 'silly thing to do', but explained that at the time of the phone calls he had only had three hours' sleep, having left work at 2.00 a.m. (Inquest touching the death of TJB, 1989 p.4).

No comment was made about the nurses' experiences in any of these situations. One might argue that such comment was unnecessary, as their angst was not central to the determination. But Chapter 6 demonstrated that judges often make 'stock story' comments which have no bearing on the facts of the case. Moreover the body of literature concerning error in health care focuses on breakdown of communications and the failure of each and every team member to accept responsibility (Wilson et al 1995, National Expert Advisory Group 1999). Yet unless the stock story becomes that all team members are expected and accorded the authority to take responsibility, and unless such authority becomes an integral part of every clinician's repertoire, challenges to avert such human error will not occur. Solutions to this problem will be discussed in Chapter 11.

Microaggressions and marginality: why these problems are only just coming to a head

These microaggressions, these 'daily incidents of … mere ignorance' are certain to 'wear down the determination of individuals' (Calmore 1997 p.922), and indeed, that is what happens. Nurses become disheartened and dispirited, and they leave. Nurses know the contribution they bring to health care, yet they feel devalued through such experiences. Calmore describes racism as 'reinforced in social relations, institutional relationships and personal behaviour' (1997 p.924). So too is discrimination against nurses, as can be heard from these 'voices from the bottom'. The cases described above are examples where the nurses **were** able to tell their stories, where they gave evidence. Still the anguish of those stories did not seem to be sufficient to alter the status quo.

At the end of the University of Newcastle Employment Studies Centre report was a quote from an article by Ginzberg:

Many of the continuing difficulties lie not with nurses but with physicians. Persons at the top of the totem pole often come to assume that they are there by virtue of right, not as a result of history and tradition. They are loath to cede any part of their authority and privilege and they see no authority why what was should not continue to be. Medicine has long been characterised by a machismo ethic, a milieu within which physicians fail to recognise that a revolution has occurred in the role of women, particularly educated women, in society and in the economy. (Ginzburg 1981 p.32)

In 1996 and again in 2001 further reports highlighted lack of self-esteem, status, recognition of experience and skills, and of a sense of being valued as an important member of the health care team and harassment in the workplace, as reasons why nurses are still leaving nursing and do not wish to return (NSW Health Department, 1996a & 2001). This lack of progress in overcoming the subordination of clinical nurses is a multifaceted problem. However, two possible reasons may be the marginalisation of nurse managers and the previous lack of a clinical career structure.

The marginalisation of nurse managers

In the past, many nurses who moved into management positions, especially those in middle management, have colluded with the medical profession and the administrators to maintain the status quo. Such behaviour has been attributed to the phenomenon of marginality (McCall 1996). The researcher cites Keen's definition of marginality:

Oppressed people who ardently buy into the system become tokens of the system—acquiring power (but never full power) and beginning to act as suboppressors. When you've had the feeling that nurses have more loyalty to medicine or to the hospital administration than they do to nursing, you've probably been right. Rewards provided by an oppressive system are very effective in the creation and maintenance of these suboppressors. (p.285)

However, with the serial restructures which have occurred over the past decade, the middle management layer of nursing has all but disappeared. New, flattened, nursing structures have appeared, with decentralised clinical control of nursing budgets, and with senior nurses by and large having professional accountability, but less hierarchical authority.

The previous lack of a clinical career structure

Another reason for the slow pace of change might be that until the late 1980s in Australia this marginality and collusion by middle managers was accentuated by the absence of a clinical career structure for nurses. Thus the most ambitious nurses were leaving the bedside to further their careers. In this way they were perhaps becoming marginalised themselves. As clinical nursing began to mean less to them, their managerial problems loomed larger and the difficulties they encountered as clinical nurses faded in their memories. The introduction of a clinical career structure has meant that highly qualified, competent and articulate nurses are now remaining at the bedside and challenging the traditional 'machismo ethic' of medicine, not necessarily exercised only by men. Perhaps this is why the debate about clinical autonomy has now taken on a new urgency, and the thrust for legislative change and the introduction of nurse practitioner status is occurring.

Nurses' search for clinical autonomy by entitlement, rather than by benefaction

Nurses do not view the 'space' which they occupy as medical territory which doctors 'allow' nurses to inhabit at and for their convenience. Rather, they see their clinical activities and decisions as necessary for patient wellbeing and ones they are qualified and able to perform. They believe that their time would be better spent doing certain tasks and making certain decisions (which they are clinically competent to do or make) rather than looking or waiting for doctors to do or make them. It is not a desire to replace doctors or to become doctors which leads to the call for clinical autonomy. It is their lack of sovereignty over tasks and decisions, buttressed both by policy and legislation.

Currently nurses do not have clinical autonomy by right. Where they are able to exercise authority in clinical decision making, such status is accorded to them by the medical profession at its discretion. It is a dispensation, and nurses are subject to medical whim as to whether they are able to exercise clinical autonomy. This is not to suggest that all doctor/nurse relationships are unsatisfactory. This is simply not the case. There are many doctors who believe and demonstrate that nurses are their clinical peers, and nurses who work with these excellent men and women are gratified that they have elected to treat them in this manner. The difficulty for nurses is that even these situations are subject to the doctors' choice; but the worth of these doctors is in no way diminished because nurses would prefer to be treated this way by entitlement, rather than by benefaction.

Such arguments, such outsider stories, can be challenging. They are not the stories which we are used to hearing, and thus they tend to sit uncomfortably with our familiar stories, 'the majoritarian narrative' (Delgado 1995 p.194). They can expose what Scheppele calls 'the perceptual fault lines' (1989 p.2082). They can make us irritably aware that the status which certain groups enjoy in society (groups whom we like and admire) is built upon the discomfort of other groups (groups whom we are accustomed to conceiving as 'good' and 'docile') whom we liked to imagine were content with their lot. It does not suit our image of 'the way the world is' to imagine that the 'docile' groups are feeling frustrated and angry, that the peace and calm which they have always embodied is fragile, even illusory. In this way, outsider stories can be seen as troublesome, upsetting or interfering, and the natural tendency is to ignore them or trivialise them, because the established order already works very well for those in power.

Such outsider stories are often described as 'doctor bashing', which is a way of making out that the 'Other' (in this case the nurse) is malicious, unkind or ungrateful, particularly given the way that medicine has so actively involved itself with nursing in the past. But the very response of naming these nurses' stories as 'doctor bashing' demonstrates the difficulty for nurses to make themselves central to the issue. The listener has heard the nurses but still identified the doctors as central. Calmore (1997) identified a similar problem when he offered a Critical Race Theory subject at Loyola Law School in Los Angeles. He received descriptions of this subject such as 'bad-white-people stuff' and 'blame all Whites for everything rhetoric' (p.914). But he explained this was not the aim of his seminars. He simply wished to help his students to understand that 'race is always already insinuated in the most innocent and neutral-seeming concept' (Harris 1994 p.750). And so it is in health care. The stock stories of domestic worker, doctor's handmaiden, and subordinate professional are 'always already' insinuated in any consideration of nurses where doctors are also mentioned.

Medicine's patronage was obtained at considerable cost to the nursing profession: a cost which has been borne by generations of clinical nurses, and which has created the culture of oppression and subordination described in this and previous chapters. The anger with which medicine has attacked any moves on behalf of nurses to assert themselves could also indicate the loss which medicine would suffer were there to be an alteration to the status quo. A system in which one group spends an inordinate amount of its time following up the work of another and acting as the scapegoat should things go wrong is not to be abandoned lightly. In addition, the existing system brings considerable financial rewards to the medical profession due to monopolies on certain practices, such as prescribing, treatments and referrals (Freidson 1970, Fisher 1993). Thus, while medicine has sanctioned the transference of tasks which were not of themselves revenue raising, such as dialysis and venipuncture, with relative equanimity, it has actively resisted the transference of others which were income related, as evidenced by the nurse practitioner debate.

It is hoped that by hearing some accounts 'from the bottom' the reader will have gained some insight into the lives of nurses and the difficulties which they experience. Yet one has the sensation that the stock story of the nurse as doctor's handmaiden or subordinate professional is 'always already' present in the coroners' or the judges' minds. The tacit acceptance of the inability of the nurses to do anything further in the most dreadful situations tells us that the judges rarely feel any compulsion to challenge 'the way the world is', or to examine further the 'agony tales' of the nurses.

The courts' and tribunals' recognition of clinical autonomy

From a clinical perspective, the autonomous professional image is still an outsider story. Cases such as Atcheson v College of Physicians and Surgeons (Alta) (1994) demonstrate the difficulty which nurses can encounter in establishing themselves as autonomous professionals even with the goodwill and support of medical colleagues. There have been a few cases where the courts and tribunals have been prepared to acknowledge the extent of clinical autonomy which some nurses exercise, and to recognise the complexity and skill of their clinical practice. However, the nurses have worked in established domains of practice, such as midwifery; in remote areas where there were insufficient medical staff; or where there was no doctor immediately available, such as in psychiatry or rural women's health.

For example, it has been held that nurses needed to have access to medical records for them to be able to give comprehensive care to their patients when medical staff were unavailable (Callan Park Report 1961, Inquest touching the death of Mrs G 1967[1]). There has been recognition that nurses need to prescribe medications on occasions, and that in emergencies nurses may 'be entitled, as a temporary measure, to substitute [their] own judgment for that of a qualified medical practitioner' (Fitzpatrick & Lockhart v Messiter 1990). There have been dicta recognising the considerable experience of some nurses (Hefferon v UKCC 1988). A midwife's authority to manage

---

[1] No further details of this hearing available; notes obtained from representation file, New South Wales Nurses' Association.

a midwifery case has been accepted unquestioningly. In Gaughan v Bedfordshire HA (1997), the evidence of an obstetrician expert witness was accepted that 'in reality most midwives are more skilled than doctors in delivery, unless more manipulative or invasive procedures become necessary' (p.187). It has also been acknowledged that nurses can and do make medical diagnoses (Inquest touching the death of MAQ 1987/88).

In terms of establishing a standard of care, there has also been a recognition that nurses, just like doctors, can make decisions which do not amount to negligence if there is a responsible body of [nursing] opinion to support them (Gaughan v Bedfordshire HA 1997). There have been a number of recent English cases where the standard of the reasonable professional, known as the Bolam test (1957), has been applied to nurses and midwives (Hill v West Lancashire HA 1997, Corley v NW Hertfordshire HA 1997, Gaughan v Bedfordshire HA 1997).

In Langley & Anor v Glandore Pty Ltd (in Liq) & Anor (1997), the practices of theatre nursing staff came under direct scrutiny. The surgeons, who had been found guilty of negligence, inter alia for a failure to remove a swab from the wound, appealed the finding of the jury 'that the hospital was guilty of no negligence in its care and treatment of the plaintiff' (p.565). They argued that 'the primary duty that a correct count had been made of all instruments, sponges, packs and the like to establish that they had all been removed from the patient's body at the conclusion of the operation, lay with the nurses' (p.564). The Queensland Court of Appeal upheld their appeal, finding that surgeons 'all rely on established counting and checking procedures that the nurses must undertake' because the nurses were the 'primarily responsible accounting parties' (pp.566–68). Similarly, in Elliott v Bickerstaff the Court of Appeal acknowledged that 'important and necessary work preliminary to an operation and upon which the success or failure of the operation may depend must necessarily be left to the hospital sister and her nurses (1999 p.12).

Ison v Northern Rivers Area Health Service (1997) was a dismissal appeal by a women's health nurse who had been working in a senior clinical and autonomous role. The grounds for dismissal were failure to notify women about abnormal Pap smear results and keeping inadequate records. Her defence was that she was overworked and unsupported although she had not advised management of this. Thus it was held that her employer was entitled to rely on 'the expertise and competency of the sole practitioner that the clerical and administrative tasks would be attended to correctly' (p.21). In dismissing the appeal, the judge linked the severity of her penalty to her senior and autonomous position.

The applicant accepted that not only was she responsible for providing a clinical service which was absolutely fundamental to the health and well-being of women who used that service, but she was also responsible for providing such a clinical service at 'an advanced level of nursing practice, [involving] an advanced level of knowledge ... of initiative ... of responsibility ... and therefore of course of accountability (p.24).

A number of recent coronial decisions have found nurses to be potentially guilty of an indictable offence. These indicate higher expectations of nurses, especially when compared to the leniency in relation to events such as Chelmsford. Only two records of NSW coronial inquiries before the 1990s were located where the nurse was referred on a criminal charge (Inquest touching the death of YGJ 1973, Inquest touching the death of RLB 1980). However, between 1993 and 1995 there were three NSW cases involving nurses where the coronial inquest was terminated under s.19 (1) (a) of the Coroner's Act 1980 (NSW). The Coroner was 'of the opinion that the evidence given ... establishes a prima facie case ... for an indictable offence'. In all three of these cases, the Coroner held that the lack of care in relation to the prescription, administration and/or checking of medications was so poor as to amount to reckless or criminal negligence (Inquest touching the death of CS 1993, Inquest touching the death of CRN 1994, Inquest touching the death of NVK 1995).

Such decisions, difficult though they may be for the nurses involved, are the key to legitimate authority for nurses. If nurses are the 'primarily accounting party (sic)', then there can be no question about their authority to demand a recount if they are concerned that a count is incorrect in the operating theatre. If a midwife is to be held to have caused or contributed to the mortality or morbidity of a newborn child, then the midwife's concerns must be heard and addressed if she is managing the case. If a sole women's health practitioner is to be held accountable for her practice in the care of well women, that gives her the right to have concerns and opinions on women's health issues heard and addressed in multidisciplinary forums. Cases such as these give the nurses some opportunity to be recognised as (at least) equal participants in clinical decision making.

The problems with nursing records

Chapter 6 identified occasions when nurses have been disadvantaged because doctors have given evidence about nursing matters. Yet there have been occasions when medical and nursing evidence was in conflict and the courts have accepted both at face value.

Sometimes this has advantaged nurses in regard to both verbal (Savoie v Bouchard 1982, Corley v North West Hertfordshire Health Authority 1997) and written (Briffet v Gander and District Hospital Board et al 1992) evidence. However, on numerous occasions the poor quality of the nursing records has meant that the courts have (understandably) taken them literally and found their depiction of nursing care wanting. Perhaps because nursing has an oral tradition (Lumby 1991, Street 1992), the nursing records have never been the major focus of authenticity for nurses. Greater reliance has traditionally been vested in the oral nursing handover (Parker 1994). Thus, questions such as 'at what time did you take Mr Smith's 6 o'clock observations?', however illogical they may sound to listeners, are a consequence of the fact that fourth-hourly observation charts are often pre-printed with the times 2, 6, 10, 2, 6, 10 (Employment Studies Centre of the University of Newcastle 1992). This results in a number of anomalies. For example, if a nurse has a caseload of eight patients, only one can have their observations recorded exactly on the hour. In addition, the records often take the form of graphs or plans, meaning times are abbreviated or rounded off to save space.

This does not excuse poor recording practices, but it goes some way to explaining them. Clearly this is problematic for nurses who wish their records to be accorded the same authority as those of medical practitioners. Especially when witnesses have poor recollection of events, judges rely on written evidence, meaning that nurses who do not produce accurate records will find it difficult to have their story heard. When nurses' charts and times have been tendered in courts and tribunals, they have been found to be inaccurate, and the nurse witness's credibility has suffered as a consequence. A finding that 'these times were all approximate times, were not accurate times and cannot be relied upon' led to the judge declaring that 'I accept [the anaesthetist's conflicting] evidence in view of the inexactitude of the nurses' times as shown by the contradictions on the charts' (Laidlaw et al v Lion's Gate Hospital (Hiddleston et al 1969)). This (fairly common) inaccuracy elicits considerable irritation in the judgments (Joseph Brant Memorial Hospital et al v Koziol et al 1977, Inquest touching the death of MWF 1993, Farrell v Cant et al 1992, Inquest touching the death of CWCK (T) 1994, Hill v West Lancashire HA 1997). Although medical records have also been the objects of judicial criticism, there is a stronger written culture in medicine and thus a tendency to greater accuracy (Breen v Williams 1996). This has enabled doctors' records, and thus their evidence, to carry more weight than those of nurses.

CONCLUSION

This outsider story is far from simple. It encompasses the sociopathology of oppressed group experiences and behaviour. Yet it is critical for nurses, as the resolution of the legal and policy issues addressed within it are crucial to the recruitment and retention of nurses.

The outsider story of the nurse as an autonomous professional was sought initially through comparable professional standing with medicine. However, as the last century progressed, nurses began to explore different models of professionalism, and developed a greater sense of confidence in their own unique identity. Nursing has pursued its quest for professional autonomy on four fronts: self-regulation, including development of standards; education and research; managerial control; and clinical authority.

In the courts and tribunals, nurses have achieved judicial recognition of self-regulation and development of standards, although there has been a tendency towards excessive disciplinary zeal. Nursing's exclusive control over staffing and administration has also been acknowledged judicially, although the recent restructuring of health services along more general management lines has yet to undergo judicial scrutiny. The acknowledgement of nursing education and research has been more ambiguous, with delegated medical tasks eliciting more veneration than traditional caring or domestic nursing work.

Clinical authority remains the most problematic area for nurses. Previous chapters have examined the interdependence of medicine and nursing. This chapter has attempted to explain what clinical autonomy entails and the consequences for nurses of a lack of clinical autonomy. The current situation is unreasonable for nurses and leads to deep dissatisfaction and resentment.

PART 5

Living in a legal and professional shadow land

PART CONTENTS

11

Bringing the images together

INTRODUCTION

This book set out to identify the status of the accredited nurse. Status was defined as an amalgam of legal and non-legal factors. These are:

- the nature of the nursing role as it is defined by law and as it evolves in practice;
- whether nursing is regarded as a profession, both at law and in society;
- the legal and actual ability of nurses to exercise power in their professional and clinical lives; and
- the legal and actual responsibilities and duties which nurses are expected to shoulder.

The research was undertaken to assist nurses with the difficulties and uncertainties that they experience in their political, professional and clinical lives. These are exacerbated by the incongruity of the law relating to nurses, and its failure to address the reality of nursing practice, particularly when there is a multidisciplinary influence on such practice. Nurses are rarely regarded as central to the delivery of health care—they are regarded as peripheral, even invisible. Their status is frequently determined according to their juxtaposition with other more dominant legal entities, such as doctors or health care institutions, whose status is fixed more firmly.

This chapter explores the personal, professional and clinical problems created by the juxtaposition of the five images of the nurse, the extent to which the law has addressed or compounded those effects, and some possible solutions.

THE JUXTAPOSITION OF THE FIVE IMAGES

The value of the combination of feminist and critical race theory

Feminist and critical race theories have provided the theoretical framework to analyse the contrast between the images of the nurse emerging from the case law and the accounts of nurses themselves. Walker (1993 p.230) states that 'as long as the print media [and in this case, the law] perpetuate images of the nurse which confirm [the stereotypes] then her identity will be imprisoned in those images, and she will be likely to continue to conform with them'. 'For me (says Walker) being a nurse means living on a site of struggle in which the search for validation and recognition always occurs on the social, cultural and ideological territories of others who are not nurses.'

Feminist theory

Nurses are an 'outsider' group in that, despite their majority in the health care workforce, they are significantly less powerful and influential in health care decision making (political, professional and clinical) than are other dominant minority groups such as doctors and administrators. Medical practitioners and administrators were traditionally mostly male. Nurses were (and are) mostly female. Feminist theory has elucidated the exclusion of a mainly female work force from the exercise of power by a predominantly male elite. Feminist jurisprudential analysis of women's work helps to explain why nursing work has been devalued and regarded as traditional women's work (Graycar & Morgan 1990 p.73).

Although more women are now practising medicine and health administration, nurses still struggle to influence administrative, political, and clinical decision making. This is because nursing is still discriminated against as a 'basic' or 'domestic' occupation, even by middle class, professional women. Pringle (1998 p.194) observes that 'there is a recognisable class discourse that now connects doing medicine with being "bright" and doing nursing with being "dumb"'. The implication is that nurses would be doctors if only they were bright enough, and no woman who was 'bright' would consider nursing. Interestingly, she found that nurses 'rarely expressed any desire to be doctors', many considering that a career in medicine would make it difficult for a woman to have 'any kind of civilised life'.

Critical race theory

Thus, nurses experience discrimination from other professional women. Critical race theory, with its conception of intersectionality (Crenshaw 1989 p.167) has helped to examine the nature of nurses' experiences and the stories told about and by nurses. Nurses find themselves in a similar position to black, lesbian, and other 'minority' women who are not considered to conform to educated, middle class, professional standards. Nurses know that they are discriminated against because of gender. In addition they have in the past been subject to many 'microaggressions' from women in other professions, 'daily incidents of...mere ignorance' which 'wear down the determination of individuals' (Calmore 1997 p.922). Nurses have learnt that they are viewed as doubly different (female and not 'bright') and are discriminated against because of this second 'difference' by other women. This is common to many oppressed groups, and Bell submits that 'a good deal of the writing in critical race theory stresses that oppressions are neither neatly divorceable from one another nor amenable to strict categorisation' (1992 p.145).

'Microaggressions' against nurses were found in the very texts which informed this theoretical analysis. Delgado refers to nursing the aged as 'changing bedpans in a nursing home' and goes on to say that '[m]uch of it is so simple, anyone can do it' (1995 p.41). Pringle, who provides a balanced analysis overall, refers to 'basic nursing care' as 'a lot of the menial tasks' and RNs' performance of them as 'a kind of deskilling that sits uneasily with their claims to professionalism' (1998 p.193). Pringle describes caring for the mentally ill and working in long-stay areas as less 'glamorous', an unusual adjective ever to associate with a profession which deals constantly with human waste (1993 p.1895).

The denigration of the skills required to care sensitively for elderly, confused, incontinent patients or the chronic mentally ill is a common experience for nurses. Nurses know how difficult it is to care for such patients skilfully, preserving not only the integrity of their skin but also their dignity and the sensitivities of their families. But they also know how such skills are regarded as 'basic' by non-nurses, how their work can be belittled to simply 'changing bedpans' or 'menial'.

In this way nurses experience what has been described as 'multiple consciousness' (Barnes 1990–91 p.61). They learn that there are multiple ways to view the world, because the world views of other more powerful groups affect their lives. They become sensitised to such views and learn to respond accordingly. Developing multiple consciousness is seen as a valuable survival technique for outsider groups. Delgado observes that it provides 'a better grasp of reality. It's kind of like looking through a pair of binoculars. Binocular vision is always better than the kind you get by looking at something just through one lens'. He also notes that it is a valuable analytical tool for outsider scholars. 'Multiple consciousness enables the outsider to see defects in the prevailing order before one immersed in that system could...in scholarship, this confer[s] an advantage, particularly with respect to grasping and deploying postmodern theory' (1995 p.122).

The multiple consciousness of nurses: for better or worse

By identifying and examining the five images of nurses from the case law and the nursing literature, this book has tried to construct the multiple consciousness of nurses. However, care must be taken not 'to get so engrossed in critical race theory ideology that we [lose] contact with real world problems' (Bell 1992 p.145). The aim is to address problems in practice, to confront the professional, political, and clinical difficulties which nurses experience. These difficulties are inherent in the inconsistency of the law relating to nurses, and the failure of the law to address the reality of multidisciplinary nursing practice. This means that nurses are uncertain of their duties and/or obligations to the patient, and of their ability or prerogative to intervene when they consider that the patients' best interests are not being served.

Such uncertainty is further exacerbated by the fact that the stock stories support the view that health care is legally and socially constructed as a medical act. As Delgado points out, 'it has to do with one's perspective, one's baseline. If you start out from a certain position, a given practice will look neutral. From a different perspective, the same practice will look one-sided, biased, unfair' (1995 p.71). Thus nurses, made invisible within medicine, and represented by it in key decision-making activities, rarely have the opportunity to challenge the 'neutral' construct or voice their uncertainties. When they obtain such opportunities, their voices are interpreted through the ears of those who have already accepted the stock stories, and their views often tend to be seen as 'socially disruptive' (Bell 1992 p.143).

The juxtaposition of the five images, those 'stock' and 'outsider' stories, in the daily lives of nurses has created professional and clinical difficulties for them. But this is not to depict nurses simply as victims. Many nurses love their work and take great pride and pleasure in their professional interactions with patients (Wicks 1999 p.73). But there are also real difficulties which nurses have to resolve in a culture that accepts the 'stock stories' of nurses as domestic workers, doctors' handmaidens, or subordinate professionals. Nurse leaders have actively promoted the 'outsider' stories with varying degrees of success and have also (possibly ill-advisedly) attempted to use the 'stock' stories to their advantage.

The five images which have emerged from the case law (domestic worker, ministering angel, doctor's handmaiden, subordinate professional, and autonomous professional) are not separate or distinct in the daily lives of nurses. To some degree these images are all 'always already' present (Lather 1991). Each of these images carries with it certain expectations of behaviour and relationships with others. These expectations differ quite considerably according to which image is being portrayed. For example, nurses may be expected to behave:

- as autonomous professionals by themselves, the patients, and the nursing hierarchy;
- as ministering angels by the patients and themselves;
- as doctors' handmaidens or subordinate professionals by the hospital administration and the medical staff.

Each of these groups occasionally transfer their expectations to other images, without necessarily informing the nurses involved. Thus the stock stories (with their concomitant expectations), which the courts and tribunals have accepted and which doctors and administrators have promoted, coexist with the outsider stories which nurses themselves promote and believe. Additionally nurses have, to some extent, internalised and accepted the authenticity of the stock stories in terms of their subordination, and this has affected their relationships with doctors and administrators.

It is significant that many of the 'stock story' descriptions of nurses as both doctors' handmaidens and subordinate professionals are found in the obiter dicta, the discussion part of a judgment. Rarely do they form part of the ratio decidendi, the actual decision, of the case. For example, in several cases judges expressed the opinion that doctors had 'absolute' or 'supreme' control over nurses. However, in these same cases, they gave judgments which in one way or another absolved the doctor from any form of liability for the nurses' acts (Van Wyk v Lewis 1924, Ingram v Fitzgerald 1936, Paton v Parker 1941, Cassidy v Ministry of Health 1951). It seemed almost as though the judge, having in some way distanced the doctors from their relationships of authority with the nurses through the non-liability decisions, felt moved to re-establish it through the obiter dicta. This even occurred in cases where the nurses were not under scrutiny (Pillai v Messiter [No.2] 1989). Such unwarranted comments are important as they feature in stark contrast to the times when the judges have been silent on the moral plights of nurses, which have been discussed in previous chapters.

Simultaneously, doctors and administrators have become cognisant of the nurses' 'outsider' stories and as individuals have rejected them, partly internalised them, or even supported them. The juxtaposition of these stories has created political, professional and clinical anomalies and inconsistencies for nurses. It had caused dissonance for nurses in their professional identity, their relationships, and their patient care. They could feel and/or act, be perceived and/or be treated, as autonomous or subordinate professionals, ministering angels, doctors' handmaidens, and domestics—all in one shift. Because there are so many different expectations of them, nurses cannot anticipate either their treatment or expectations in their 'professional' roles. A great deal of regulatory documentation is silent on the nurses' role. Some do not address the reality of nurses' practice, but only the reality of the exercise of medical power. This means that nurses have little or no guidance in difficult professional or clinical decisions.

The 'tyranny of niceness'

In the midst of such uncertainty, a nurse's behaviour is far more likely to be determined by personality than by law or policy. Moreover, because nursing has been governed by what Kim Walker (1993 p.145) has described as 'the tyranny of niceness', it has been unlikely that their personalities have been particularly well groomed to take on assertive roles. Walker, who believes, like Ethel Bedford Fenwick, that 'the nurse problem is the woman problem' (In Dock & Stewart 1938 p.254), describes 'being nice' as follows:

> The pre-eminent value inherent in the technique of sensibility I call 'being nice' is one that insists that overt conflict must be avoided wherever and whenever possible. This sensibility is sanctified in our culture in the notion that a good woman does not contradict. A nice woman does what she is told ... By extension then, a good nurse takes what she finds (or is given) and does not question. A nice nurse therefore must be a good nurse.
>
> The behaviour this technique initiates is one of backing off, assuming a passive posture, or silencing oneself. It is a technique of sensibility which shapes (us) in pervasive and powerful ways. The reciprocal behaviour such a technique of sensibility elicits is one that is generally tacit, it does not usually ever come to expression. The combination of value, behaviour and response leads to a form of silent but mutual agreement between the individuals engaged in the conflict situation...it gently insists that no further dialogue is needed to resolve the situation. (Walker 1993 p.145)

THE SPECIFIC CONSEQUENCES OF THE JUXTAPOSITION OF THE FIVE IMAGES OF THE NURSE

This juxtaposition has been problematic for nurses in the following ways:

- Acceptance of the proposition that doctors can represent and/or substitute for nurses.
- Acceptance of medical control over patient care.
- Fragmentation of the nursing role:
  - The devaluation of nursing care;
  - The privileging of delegated medical work.
- Poor remuneration and living and working conditions.
- Reciprocal use of the defence of reliance.
- Lack of support for independent moral agency in nursing.
- Invisibility of nurses when the courts and tribunals are dazzled by doctors: the 'myth of meritocracy'.

Acceptance of the proposition that doctors can represent and/or substitute for nurses

Doctors have represented and substituted for nurses in giving expert evidence in court and also in providing exclusive or majoritarian opinions to key decision making and funding allocation committees about issues which involve both medicine and nursing. This likewise applies when it is accepted that a reference to a doctor in a statute or policy document also tacitly implies the presence of a nurse. These representations and substitutions are commonplace in the political and professional lives of nurses. However, in their clinical lives, substitution of doctors for nurses is not so common, although beginning medical practitioners often learn aseptic techniques and other clinical skills from nurses. The decisions relating to the doctor's handmaiden image provide evidence for the argument that the courts and tribunals consider that nursing is a subset of medicine, and that nurses exist to support the 'real' work of medicine. Since nursing is contained within medicine, having a doctor present is the same as having a doctor and a nurse. Decisions relating to the subordinate professional image provide evidence for the assertion that nurses are a professionally separate but subordinate part of a medical team. In either situation the impression of medical superiority and dominance is conspicuous. It presents a persuasive image of medicine's awareness and containment of nursing, and bolsters the legitimacy of its ability to represent nursing.

The 'containment' of nursing within medicine

Containment as a doctor's handmaiden In the doctor's handmaiden chapter this containment can be observed in a number of ways. Nurses are described obiter as physical body parts of doctors: as their eyes and ears (The Callan Park Report 1961, Inquest touching the death of MAQ 1987/88), as hands under the control of the doctor's brain (Davis v Morris 1923, Logan v Waitaki Hospital Board 1935); and doctors are described as 'working through the nurse' (The Callan Park Report 1961). Thus, when a nurse performs work as requested or instructed by a doctor, it is as though the work were performed by a doctor, thereby alleviating any requirement to recognise the presence of a nurse in statute (RCN v DHSS 1980). Particularly in the industrial decisions, work identified as deserving increased remuneration was that which was delegated to nurses by doctors (In re Public Hospital Nurses (State) Award 1967), a perception which nurses have exploited in their award applications (In re Public Hospital Nurses (State) Award 1976, In re Public Hospital Nurses (State) Award 1986).

These perceptions, emanating from the judgments, reinforce the image of nursing as subsumed within medical knowledge. They suggest that nursing is really only an abbreviated, but inferior, course in medicine. Dr Brendan Nelson, then AMA president, argued in opposition to nurse practitioners that 'while nurses received good training and had a good understanding of most medical problems, their depth of that understanding was more superficial than a doctor' (In Demou 1992 p.2). Dr Peter Arnold, also on the topic of nurse practitioners, observed that 'nurses have not had the doctors' level of training in the clinical and pre-clinical sciences' (Arnold 1992 p.5). These statements imply that if nurses wished to practise medicine they would need only to study more of the same, but in greater depth. Such opinions, expressed both in and out of court, foster the myth that doctors know everything about nursing as well as everything about medicine. Accordingly, having a doctor on a committee is equivalent to having a doctor and a nurse.

Containment as a subordinate professional There are also numerous dicta which identify the nurse as under the control of a doctor, even though performing duties classified as professional. Such dicta were often inconsistent with the allocation of liability for negligence in the respective cases, but are nevertheless sufficiently commonplace to highlight the 'stock story'. In contrast to the doctor's handmaiden image, where medical control is undisputed, here nurses are expected to be answerable for their actions, but are unable to control the environment in which those actions take place.

Substitution in courts and tribunals and on committees

As a result of such 'background assumptions, interpretations and implied exceptions' (Delgado 1995 p.71) about the nature of medical control over nursing, courts and tribunals have regularly and unquestioningly accepted medical evidence about nursing matters. Such evidence includes damning factual evidence (Le Page v Kingston & Richmond Health Authority 1997), expert evidence about the requirement for professional nursing care (Lee v McLennnan 1995), and expert evidence about standards of nursing practice in an appeal against a professional misconduct decision (Heathcote v NRB & Walton 1991). Examples have been provided of the omission of nurses from policy documents and legislation relating to nursing care, and from committees discussing issues significant for nursing care.

Such substitution creates obvious problems for nurses, in that their opinions about particular practice or policy difficulties are not afforded the same degree of significance as medical opinions, if they are heard at all. How frustrating and difficult medical subordination can be for nurses, and how the perspectives of nurses and doctors can differ about clinical activities has already been discussed. The amount of time which nurses spend waiting for doctors to arrive to perform administrative or clinical tasks which they could have performed themselves with the appropriate authority provides a perfect example of a problem which affects nurses, but not doctors (University of Newcastle Employment Studies Centre 1992, Wicks 1999). Doctors, in all good faith, are bound to view the world from a medical perspective. Indeed, some do not perceive that there is, or ought to be, any difference between a medical and nursing perspective. Any perception of difference, it is suggested, is only seen by a few ambitious nurse leaders (Buhagiar 1992b).

The invisibility of nurse-initiated work

Unless nurses are able to articulate publicly their own concerns about nurse-initiated work, they many not even be evident to medical staff. Doctors are aware of those activities which nurses perform on their instructions, but tend not (nor do they need) to concern themselves with nurse-initiated work. Nor would they necessarily be aware of such aspects of nursing work. Modern nursing educational curricula do not look like medical curricula, because nurses do more than just delegated medical work. The occasions when nurses would involve doctors in nurse-initiated work would be if they believed that it would impact on the medical management of the patient. But doctors cannot know the experience of being a nurse, and cannot (by definition) be there when the nurse is alone on duty with the patient.

This lack of understanding can and does lead to problems for nurses in practice, because the health care world is legally and socially constructed as a medical world, and nurses are expected to fit into it. The considerable influence of doctors means that they are still more able to dictate the way in which health care is organised and delivered, which in turn impacts on the way in which nurses carry out their care. As English and Australian reports have identified, this leads to a practice environment which is often bureaucratically onerous for nurses (The Briggs Report 1978, NSW Health Department 1995, Wilmore 1997). Nurses also clandestinely perform activities well within their capabilities, but on which the legislation is silent regarding the authority of a nurse, because it is assumed that such activities will be carried out be a doctor. Cases such as RCN v DHSS (1980) promote the sham that treatment given by a nurse acting on the orders of a doctor is in fact treatment given by a doctor. In such situations, the nurse becomes the invisible interface between the doctor and the patient. Yet at that interface there is the need for a range of skills, knowledge and attitudes which are critical to the patient's safety and well-being.

Paradoxically, because nurses are viewed only as an extension of medicine, clinical difficulties which relate specifically to doctors are rarely addressed because the committees which could address them are invariably dominated by doctors.

Acceptance of medical control over patient care

Control over hospital patient care

One of the most significant problems for nurses is the acceptance throughout society, health care and government that in-patient care is medically controlled. Patients in hospital have the name of the admitting medical officer (AMO) on their wrist band, despite the fact that some (particularly public) patients might only see the AMO perhaps once or twice during their stay. To problematise such a system may be seen as heretical. After all, the right and authority of doctors to head the health care team is accepted as a 'given' (Pringle 1998), not viewed as a privilege or even as controversial. It is a neutral observation, a statement of fact. As Delgado (1995 p.7) observes, '[n]eutrality works best when it is able to call up and rely on as many of these culturally inscribed routines and understandings as possible. These understandings, read into the culture long ago, now seem objective, unchallengeable and true'.

But although sick people attend doctors for cure or palliation, they stay in hospitals because their treatment or illness means that neither they nor their relatives are able to care for them and professional nursing care is required. Doctors acknowledge that 'we depend absolutely on our nursing colleagues in order that our (sic) patients be looked after properly' (Buhagiar 1992c p.6). Once (often before) people no longer need to be 'looked after properly' by nurses, they are discharged. The nurse manager or senior nurse clinician into whose unit they are admitted may have greater knowledge of the patient, yet their ability to influence the care and treatment will be informal. This can be particularly galling for expert clinical nurses who may be dealing with junior and inexperienced medical officers (Pringle 1998).

Yet the stock stories ignore the fact that the provision of nursing care underpins the patient's hospitalisation. Rather, they confirm that the doctor admits the patient and the doctor's role is central, with the nursing role seen as either part of the medical treatment (doctor's handmaiden) or subordinate to the medical treatment (subordinate professional). In reality, both medical and nursing roles have very distinct foci, and both are critical to the patient's eventual recovery. Both doctors and nurses acknowledge that there can be some overlap of tasks, depending on the setting in which the patient is being cared for.

Nursing and medical tasks have adjusted over the years. With the progress in medical technology and treatment, acts which were once the domain of medical practitioners often fall into nursing usage because it is more convenient to have the task performed by a nurse. Nurses have taken on these tasks, probably because it saved them the bureaucratic burden of having to find a doctor but also because they recognise that junior doctors are very busy and work long hours (Pringle 1998).

Control over nurses working in isolation

When nurses work in clinical settings where there are no doctors available (e.g. remote nursing outposts) they often feel compelled in the interests of patient care to perform tasks which might traditionally be the domain of a doctor. For the nurses who are currently performing them, many of those tasks are outside their scope of practice as circumscribed by legislation (Chulov 1998). However, doctors have been content to allow these activities to continue clandestinely, and have supported them by post-hoc authorisation of prescriptions and ordering of investigations (NSW Health Department 1992). Yet as nurses have sought to have these practices legitimised, the medical profession has invoked the subordinate professional image. They have claimed, both in court (Atcheson v College of Physicians and Surgeons (Alta) 1994) and out of court (Buhagiar 1992b, Nicholson 1993, Napier 1998a & b), that such tasks may only be performed by nurses under the instruction of a medical practitioner. The doctors have publicly argued that nurses might not be safe to perform such tasks, despite the fact that privately they had condoned such practices for years.

In Alberta, Canada, the medical registering authority took their objections to nurse pratitioners to court, and the court acknowledged its right to do so (Atcheson v College of Physicians and Surgeons (Alta) 1994). This decision was reached despite acknowledgement that the nurses' services were reported to improve patient care and that nurses in remote areas, where no doctors were available, offered similar services. The medical registering authority did not therefore litigate because there was a threat to its protective jurisdiction. It did so because it had the legislative authority to do so. This fact in itself, and the court's recognition of this right, is central to the argument about gratuitous medical interference in nursing matters. This was an action, to quote Charles R. Lawrence III 'in defense of privilege disguised as merit' (1997 p.759). The conundrum is that the nurse practises as an autonomous practitioner, but attempts at legitimisation invoke the subordinate professional response from some vocal aspects of the medical profession.

Medical ownership of health care procedures

Although nurses might take on tasks previously performed by doctors in the interests of improved patient care, and many tasks might ultimately fall into accepted nursing usage, nurses have no legitimate or even cultural mandate to do so. Nurses may only perform many clinical procedures with the authorisation of the medical profession. The exception would be basic nursing care, for which there are no challenges from doctors or other health care professionals, although there may be some from unskilled workers. They cannot simply assume the task in the best interests of patient care. Medical sanction is required for them to perform these aspects of their work. While this sanction is not usually withheld, it is the ownership of the tasks which is so vexatious, because it begs the recognition of a partnership in care. Health practices are usually viewed as medical care unless the medical profession allows it to be otherwise.

This is not to suggest that nurses do not undertake innovative projects. There are numerous examples of this in the literature. The difficulty is that the projects they choose to undertake must either be medically sanctioned or must fall outside of medicine's bailiwick. Then if they fall outside the traditional scope of medical practice, health funding is not usually provided for them. An example of this is the way in which many nurses have embraced complementary therapies, such as hydrotherapy, aromatherapy and therapeutic massage, into their patient care (Venamore 1997). Although some hospitals and nursing homes have supported nurses in these endeavours, the AMA (1997) has insisted that any compulsory insurance scheme should be limited to registered medical practitioners, and opposes benefits for non-medical services or 'services provided by the practitioners of exclusive dogmas'.

Fragmentation of the nursing role

The devaluation of nursing care

The courts and tribunals have found it difficult to accord professional status for much of the 'basic' work which nurses considered so essential earlier in the last century. This includes activities such as cleaning (Re Hedley Gordon Rowe and Capital Territory Health Commission, Re Judith Adella Cooney and Capital Territory Health Commission 1982), feeding patients (Gold v Essex County Council 1942), and providing physical and emotional care involving cleansing, comforting and the management of elimination (The Callan Park Report 1961). Such work has been described in this book as 'intrinsically professional' work, as it is nurse-generated and nurse-driven. However, before a hospital's vicarious liability for its professional staff was decided, there were a series of decisions in which these aspects of nursing care were designated to be domestic, menial, or routine (Hillyer v Governors of St Bartholomew's Hospital 1909, Lavere v Smith's Falls Public Hospital 1915b, Logan v Waitaki Hospital Board 1935, Vuchar v Trustees of Toronto General Hospital 1937). Eventually, nurses internalised such views and tried to rid themselves of some of this basic work through the industrial courts and tribunals (In re Hospital Nurses' (State) Award 1936b) because they thought that it was impeding their quest for better pay and conditions. This phenomenon of people feeling ashamed of those things that are in fact important to them has been described as 'false consciousness'.

The skill and discretion required to undertake 'basic' nursing care The reality is that, although nurses might now only rarely perform cleaning for disinfection purposes, they still have to undertake such work, because it can be central to nursing practice (Anon 1998b). 'Basic nursing care' is, in reality, far from basic and skilled nurses are required to perform it well. Taylor (1994 pp.107–15) describes in detail a scene between Jane, the nurse, and Max, a triplegic patient, where she is assisting him to evacuate his bowels. Taylor's research focuses on nurses undertaking 'basic' nursing care and identifies how delicate and complex it really is. When they perform such work, its value and necessity transcends its physical messiness. Despite what those who do not undertake this work might think, it is not basic—it is extremely psychologically complex. Cleaning patients who are soiled with excreta, blood, or vomitus, who feel ashamed of themselves for being 'dirty' or for 'losing control', and restoring both their hygiene and their sense of self worth in the process, requires the highest order of skill. The 'privilege of intimacy' (Chiarella 1990) this work confers and the 'environments of permission' (Lawler 1991) required for the work to be performed, mean that the nursing staff know its worth, whilst understanding society's abhorrence of its reality.

But the paradox is to recognise that other people, those who do not know or understand the world of nursing, by and large do not want to know or understand it. Even today the public have a fairly sanitised view of nursing work (Hallam 2000). In addition, it is central to the professional nature of nursing practice that nurses do not discuss the intimate nature of their work. Nurses do things to other human beings which have the potential to strip them of their dignity. One of the reasons why, most of the time, nurses do not strip patients of their dignity is that it is understood that what transpires between nurses and patients will never be discussed in public. Good nursing care is able to make even the strangest experiences seem comfortable. Nurses manage, according to Lawler, to be almost 'invisible' as they perform the most private of functions for the patient (1991 p.179). Taylor describes the scene behind the screens as a nurse washes her patient's genitalia.

Jane is looking intently at the scrotum, lifting carefully the folds to ensure a thorough wash, and painting lotion gently on the grazed area. The penis is washed with equal care and their conversation continues throughout. They could have been having this conversation in a sitting room, it is so unselfconscious. (Taylor 1994 p.111)

Work that 'anybody can do'?   Perhaps the extraordinary intimacy of this work tends to inhibit nurses from going out onto the streets and describing the level of expertise that is required to deliver such care with extreme sensitivity and skill. Delgado is wrong (1995 p.41). 'Anybody' could not do this work. But nurses, for entirely professional reasons, do not discuss these aspects of their work. If we did, how could the next patient feel comfortable? In all the industrial decisions described in this book, the intimate nature of nursing work has never been discussed. Even where changes other than medical changes have been acknowledged in these decisions, they have been in such areas as health law, health economics, and health management (The Ministerial Reference Case 1986).

Perhaps this is partly because nurses have always done this intimate work, and usually only changes to practice are considered to deserve increased pay. But this provides an unsatisfactory model for re-assessing work value when such work was never valued originally. The view that any 'nice' person can deliver this kind of care diminishes the sensitivity and skill required to manage such situations.

In contrast, note the way in which psychiatrists and psychologists have managed to imbue handling sensitive issues of the mind with the requirement for highly specialised skills and knowledge. Yet the management of equally sensitive issues of the body is not granted the same status. Because it involves manual work, 'getting one's hands dirty', it is considered to be menial or domestic. Yet to practise such work without intellectual engagement would be crass, and could of itself lead to psychological damage. If the courts and tribunals were to value this work similarly, the entire award system would need to be revisited.

The domestic designation of this type of nursing care continues to affect decisions about nursing care. When workers' compensation cases are heard, much physical nursing care is compensated on the basis that it will be provided by an unskilled carer (Burford v Allan 1997). The courts regularly accept the argument of counsel for an insurance company that tending to an incontinent patient could just as easily be performed by a domestic worker. Such decisions are further influenced by the fact that the evidence on such matters is often given by a doctor (Lee v McLennan 1995) or, even when a nurse also gives evidence, the doctor's 'expert' opinion on nursing is preferred (Burford v Allan 1997).

The privileging of delegated medical work

Allocation of 'extrinsic professional' status In the early liability cases, at the same time as the courts were holding this 'domestic work' to be unprofessional, they were also designating as professional those aspects of nursing work which were either delegated from doctors or consequent on medical treatment. I have described such work as extrinsically professional, as it derives its status from its association with another profession, namely medicine.

Assistance in the operating room provides a good example. Although nurses assisting a surgeon were referred to as professional, there were always dicta to make sure that the surgeon's control over the nurse was not eroded in any way (e.g. Hillyer v Governors of St Bartholomew's Hospital 1909). Other nursing work which was ascribed extrinsic professional status included the administration of medicines (Strangeways-Lesmere v Clayton 1936), dressings, and the application of heat (Dryden v Surrey County Council 1936, Morris v Winsbury-White 1937). With the latter, the status was further differentiated dependent on whether the heat was ordered as a medical treatment, when it was professional (Vuchar v Trustees of Toronto General Hospital 1937), or as a measure for comfort, when it was not (Fleming v Sisters of St Joseph 1937).

As regards treatments and medications ordered by doctors but delegated to nurses, the courts have usually found that these were professional nursing activities for which the doctor has no responsibility (Logan v Waitaki Hospital Board 1935, Strangeways-Lesmere v Clayton 1936, Vuchar v Trustees of Toronto General Hospital 1937). However, these activities still have their genesis in the orders of the doctor, and are thus professional because of their association with medicine, rather than because nurses performed them. Other routine nursing activities such as removal of packs and swabs (Morris v Winsbury-White 1937) have also been considered to be skilled work over which doctors have no control. These fall into a similar category as treatments because they had their genesis in surgery.

The paradox is that the stock stories of domestic worker, doctor's handmaiden, and subordinate professional all demonstrate that medically derived (extrinsically professional) work is privileged. In contrast, the outsider story of nurses as autonomous professionals seeks to have the other, nurse-generated, caring (intrinsically professional) aspects of their work privileged.

The reliance on this 'extrinsic professional' designation in the industrial courts and tribunals However, nurses still wish to survive and prosper in this climate. Somewhat understandably, they have capitalised on this 'extrinsic professional' designation in the industrial courts and tribunals to demonstrate how much their scope of practice has advanced. This is hardly surprising. Nurses have had to survive. They learnt in NSW from the first excessively harsh award decision that being described as hard workers did not enhance their remuneration (In re Hospital Nurses (State) Award 1936). The NSWNA argued that student nurses worked long arduous hours as hospital workers, and for that reason required adequate recompense at its commercial value. The Full Bench disagreed with their argument, holding that 'trainees in this calling should be regarded as pupils in a profession rather than employees in an industry' (In re Hospital Nurses (State) Award 1936b p.252).

It was therefore hardly surprising that nurses quickly (and with some success) began to emphasise medically derived activities as a means of achieving improved professional status and remuneration. For example, they successfully made claims in New South Wales in 1953, 1967, 1976 and 1986.

This is not to suggest that nurses ought not to be remunerated for such changes. Nursing care has become more specialised in line with increasing medical specialisation, requiring a concomitant increase in knowledge and skills. Recent research amongst operating room nurses demonstrated a statistically significant relationship between technology-related work overload, and increased stress (Johnstone 1997).

The predicament that has emerged is that this strategy for seeking remuneration has created the problem that basic nursing care itself is rarely seen as worthy of significant reward. It also implies that medicine is where all major changes in health practice are generated. The 'stock story' is that 'members of the medical profession are in charge of the patients treatment and the nurses provide nursing in accordance with the doctors directions' (In re Public Hospital Nurses (State) Award 1967 p.338). Accordingly, Kelleher J (Public Hospital Nurses (State) Award 1976 p.324) prefaced his acknowledgement of nursing role changes by saying that 'the increase in complexity in...nursing care...has resulted from advances in medical science and technology in medical, surgical and obstetric fields'.

The impact (or lack of impact) of nursing innovations and research on the 'stock story' In fact, there have been many significant improvements in health care which have been nurse-generated, but if they have related to 'basic' nursing care, for example pressure sore management (Joanna Briggs Institute for Evidence Based Nursing Practice 1997), they have not received significant publicity. Quite a number of nurse-generated innovations have related to safety issues (Strzlecki & Nelson 1989; Pereira, Lee & Wade 1990, Clulow 1994). Because of this they have sometimes had the effect of reducing the nursing workload (Redfern 1997), leaving nurses free to undertake more delegated medical tasks. Other research and investigation has been undertaken by commercial firms, using nurses as advisers. There has also been the added problem that nursing innovations have not attracted acknowledgement in documents such as hospital reports, because nurses have tended 'to generate and disseminate knowledge by means other than...traditional forms of publications [such as published journal articles, authorship of books etc.]. Nursing publications are more likely to be in the form of patient teaching brochures, nursing practice and policy statements etc' (Lane & Sivaram 1999).

On some occasions, nursing innovations have worked against nurses in the award decisions. For example, the introduction of intensive care units, an initiative driven by nurse managers, led Richards J to accept the evidence of the Hospitals Commission of NSW that this would take the strain off ward nurses (In re Public Hospital Nurses (State) Award 1967). There is also the difficulty that some nursing research has been concerned with reducing the need for clinical interventions, rather than promoting them. For example, nursing research has demonstrated that the provision of pre-operative information reduces the need for post-operative analgesia (Hayward 1981). Such findings are unlikely to attract major sponsorship from the drug firms. As Neyle and West observe: 'the argument that research dollars should be directed towards doing the most good to the greatest number of people with the least possibility of dire consequences, although attractive, does not yet appear to hold much sway amongst funding bodies' (1991 p.282).

Since the Briggs Report (1978) it has been argued that for nursing to enhance its professional status it must become a 'research-based profession'. A related and significant problem has been that the National Health and Medical Research Council (NHMRC) has a longstanding policy of giving large research grants only to researchers with a proven track record (Sax 1989). The rationale for this has been that public funds must be distributed judiciously to those who are most likely to use them successfully. This differs from the philosophy of affirmative action, which seeks to give those traditionally excluded the opportunity to achieve in fields which have commonly been the domain of a single dominant power group (Hall 1997). For nurses, this has meant that, in order to succeed both in obtaining a significant grant and developing research expertise, they have needed an experienced researcher to apply for the grant with them, and the most obvious person has usually been a doctor. Many nurses obtained their research expertise working as research assistants on medical research grants. Even if the research were nursing-related, the most successful means of giving the application credibility would be for nurses to team up with medical practitioners and have the doctors' names as first researchers.

In 1994 only 0.4% of all research applications to the Medical Research Council of the NHMRC were nursing-related (Whitworth 1994). The introduction of professorial positions in nursing has begun to address this problem; but there have been instances where research ideas which were nurse-generated have become research projects which were doctor-led, for the very reason that the research grant would not have been made if they had not. This has compounded the problem that advances in health care have been viewed in the past as solely doctor-generated, and therefore doctor-owned, whereas in fact some of these advances were nurse-generated. Thus for nurses to further their autonomous professional status, they have needed to take on subordinate professional roles.

Poor remuneration and living and working conditions

Nurses treated like domestics and handmaidens

Several images have combined to downgrade the remuneration, and the living and working conditions of nurses. The domestic worker and doctor's handmaiden images have meant that nurses have not been regarded as professionals, and thus not deserving of professional remuneration, unless they were performing delegated medical tasks. Their working hours were also more akin to those of domestic workers than professional staff. In NSW in the 1936 Award, the appalling living conditions were acknowledged, but no provision was made for improvement because such improvements as were necessary would require a large expenditure. In the 1953 NSW Award no conditions were set for accommodation because the judge felt that there was no point in attempting the impossible. This led to significant deterioration in the existing occupation standards (Russell 1990 pp.60–61).

In the 1930s and 1940s even the Matrons were 'over-worked and underpaid. When the domestic staff, cooks and laundresses, failed to appear they filled the gap' (Russell 1996 p.34). Despite their being described as 'the pivot on which the nursing and domestic services are balanced' (In re Merritt & Cobar District Hospital (No.3) 1973 p.529), they were treated more like domestics than professionals. For example, in re Public Hospital

Nurses (State) Award (1967) it was held that the matron did not need a laundry because she could do her handwashing in her small kitchen sink.

Nursing's devotion leading to poor pay and conditions

The ministering angel image has meant that there has been a tendency in the industrial courts and tribunals to view goodness as its own reward. The desire to protect the quasi-charitable status of hospitals, evident in the early nursing negligence decisions and referred to in Cassidy v Ministry of Health (1951) by Denning LJ and in Ellis v Wallsend District Hospital (1989) by Kirby P, initially created a concomitant reluctance to reward nurses financially. Nursing, subsumed within the nature of the work carried out by hospitals, was not able to attract the remuneration of other professions. The work of hospitals was described as 'providing medical and surgical services for the sick, and providing them with accommodation and expert care and attention during illness, and in some cases also services designed to prevent illness or ward off future suffering' (In re Hospital Nurses (State) Award, 1936b p.251). Nurses were described in this award as 'devoted' women 'willing to make sacrifices in the work which they have undertaken'. These sacrifices included an expectation that the nurses would work excessively long hours in highly questionable conditions.

Many nurses have also actively opposed the idea of industrial militancy because it did not sit well with the ministering angel image (Russell 1996, Hallam 2000). Even today, when nurses are reported to be far more prepared to take industrial action, their decision to do so would still be influenced strongly by the specific issue generating the industrial action (Burns & Goodnow 1995). In the last fifteen years, as a result of the move to the tertiary sector, nurses in New South Wales have achieved professional rates of pay commensurate with other health care professionals (In re Public Hospital Nurses (State) Award 1987a & b). This achievement reflects the way in which nurses have successfully promoted their autonomous professional image. But there is still much to be done. This book has demonstrated that the interpersonal, physical aspects of nursing care are not automatically financially rewarded, despite the fact that the nurses themselves are very highly regarded for their ethics and honesty (Anon 1998a).

Reciprocal use of the defence of reliance

One of the most contradictory elements in the judicial treatments of nurses and doctors is the use by doctors and nurses of specific stories in courts and tribunals to exonerate themselves. It borders on the schizophrenic because the stories they use are those which they usually promote. For example, nurses have taken on the 'stock story' of the doctor's handmaiden (i.e. not responsible because the doctor is in control) and doctors have told the 'outsider story' of the autonomous professional (i.e. not responsible because the nurse is in control). This is inconsistent with the stories which nurses and doctors tell out of court, as inferred from the relevant medical and nursing literature.

The courts and tribunals have also been inconsistent on numerous occasions, particularly in the case of doctors. When considering the question of a doctor's liability for the act or omission of a nurse, they have stated in dicta that doctors had supreme control over nurses—whilst simultaneously holding in the ratio that the doctor in question was not liable for the actions of the particular nurse. Conversely, when examining a doctor's liability for an act or omission which appeared to be both a medical and nursing responsibility, the courts have held in the ratio that nurses were in supreme control of nurses—so again the doctor was not liable. The courts have tended to accept the reliance defence more readily from doctors than they do from nurses, probably because of the authority of medical evidence.

Nurses telling stock stories

When nurses come under scrutiny before the courts and tribunals, and a doctor is also involved, they have successfully pleaded the doctor's handmaiden image as a defence, and argued that they were only following orders (The Chelmsford Report 1990). Although this is not as common as its medical counterpart, resort to such a defence is remarkable in light of the efforts which nurses have made over the past century to be acknowledged as professionals.

Yet, it is not difficult to see how it might occur. The Chelmsford Report (1990) provides evidence of the shocking fact that a succession of highly trained matrons had allowed one man effectively to cause the deaths of at least 24 people as a direct result of the deep sleep therapy over a period of 16 years (Vol 1 p.50). Counsel for the nurses, one might imagine, had a massive task to perform. Somehow they had to make it appear that these nurses were blameless victims, rather than collaborators, in these dreadful events. Although there was evidence of some attempts by nurses to challenge the doctors, these were ineffective and the usual response was to leave Chelmsford. To quote Sarmas (1994 p.721) 'it was necessary to construct powerful images'. And construct them they did. In the hearing, the matrons gave evidence of the unequal power relationships between the nurses and the doctors, which was corroborated by expert nurse witnesses (Vol 5 pp.105 & 113). Examples were provided of the 'era where nurses walked with their hands behind their back behind the doctor, never spoke unless spoken to', not 'allowed to think' (Vol 1 p.148), a time when 'the doctors reigned supreme in the system' (Vol 1 p.126).

Given the acceptance of the stock story of the doctor's handmaiden and the very successful outsider story of the ministering angel, it is unsurprising that

Commissioner Slattery accepted these stories. Fisher (1987), who conceptualises humans as *homo narrans* (the story-telling animal) says that stories need to have 'good reasons', to be rational, and that rationality is affected by the fact that humans are narrative beings. So for the matrons' story to be accepted by the Commissioner it needed to 'ring true with the stories [he knew] to be true in [his life]' (Dowling 1993). The Commissioner made sympathetic references to 'the traditions of the nursing profession' which he found that the nurses 'tried to uphold'. Yet these nurses, dominated or intimidated or not, allowed Dr Harry Bayley to continue to practise and cause patients to die for 16 years. So powerfully did the doctor's handmaiden image 'ring true', that the Commissioner made the comment only that it was 'a little surprising that only two nurses during the period 1963 to 1979 were known to have complained to Health about events at Chelmsford' (Vol 1 pp.163–64).

The difficulty for nurses in the acceptance of this stock story is that 'it served to reinforce rather than challenge the stock stories which rendered [their] experience[s] and [their] reality invisible' (Sarmas 1994 p.724). The implications of the Commissioner's findings are discussed in the section entitled 'dazzled by doctors'.

When courts and tribunals spontaneously adopt the 'stock story'   In the appeal against the decision of the Nurses Tribunal in Heathcote v NRB and Walton (1991), the judge seemed to adopt the doctor's handmaiden defence, even though it had not been introduced by counsel. Appellant counsel's argument appears to be based on the definition of professional misconduct in Qidwai v Brown (1984), namely 'whether the practitioner was in such breach of the written or unwritten rules of the profession as would reasonably incur a strong reprobation of professional brethren of good repute and competence'. Heathcote's 'professional brethren' averred that her conduct did not incur their strong reprobation, regardless of whether they thought her actions were appropriate.

Yet, none of the expert witnesses suggested that Heathcote was 'only following orders'. The evidence centred on the contextual issues of nursing in remote areas and the difficulties created by the practice environment. Ward DCJ accepted the 'exigencies existing which so often include aberrant human behaviour, insufficient facilities and misunderstandings due to language use' (1991 p.21). But he then went on to describe Heathcote's behaviour as 'the wisest and proper course of getting in touch with the doctor' because she 'was not allowed in nursing procedure, even at that stage of difficulty in management, to prescribe or administer even sedative medication to settle the patient' (1991 p.13).

Doctors telling outsider stories

When doctors come under judicial scrutiny, and a nurse is also involved, their counsel have often invoked the autonomous professional image as a defence. It has been argued that nurses are professionals too, and doctors are entitled to rely on nursing skills to support medical practice. This defence has been highly successful for doctors, whose counsel have argued that nursing care was not the business of doctors (Laidlaw et al v Lion's Gate Hospital, Hiddleston et al 1969), or that they had little control over the way in which nurses practise (Krujelis et al v Esdale et al 1971). The language in such judgments has been particularly telling. Medical experts have testified that a defendant anaesthetist was 'entitled to rely on' the nurse (Laidlaw et al v Lion's Gate Hospital, Hiddleston et al 1969 p.739). A defendant anaesthetist averred that he had 'no control or jurisdiction over the PAR' (post-anaesthetic room) and that the PAR staff had 'complete jurisdiction, without consulting with anyone' (Krujelis et al v Esdale et al 1971 p.560). Surgeons have testified that the nurse's sponge count was 'relied upon by the surgeon' (Karderas et al v Clow et al 1972 p.311) and that they 'all rely on established counting and checking procedures that the nurses must undertake' (Langley & Anor v Glandore Pty. Ltd (In liq) 1997 p.64:566 & p.64:568). Paediatricians have argued that they were entitled to leave fluid requirements for children to the discretion of the nursing staff (Inquest touching the death of TJB 1989).

Experienced doctors have argued that they are entitled to rely on the expertise of nursing staff, even if the nurses are inexperienced (Gleason (Guardian ad litem of) v Bulkley Valley District Hospital 1996, Granger (litigation guardian of) v Ottawa General Hospital 1996). Yet when a junior house officer, herself inexperienced, made a serious omission in examining a patient, she was exonerated because the more experienced nurse failed to alert her to the specific problem for which she should have examined the patient (Inquest touching the death of HAB 1992). One physician received little criticism despite the fact that he refused to attend the cardiac arrest of a two-year-old child (Inquest touching the death of TJB, 1989). He was able to argue that the nursing staff ought to have told him earlier and more than once of their concerns for the child. Even areas of medicine which have been absolutely sacrosanct, such as diagnosis (AMA 1992), have been argued to be legitimately within the nursing domain when doctors have found themselves under pressure (Inquest touching the death of MAQ 1989).

At first glance the use of this defence seems remarkable. Dominant medical groups and individual doctors have published their views on the relative positions of nurses and doctors too often for it to be imagined that they perceive nurses as anything other than subordinate. One of the successes which the AMA representative claimed (erroneously) in the Stage Two Nurse Practitioner Project negotiations was 'the dropping of any reference to "independent"' (Nicholson 1993). Nurses wishing to advance nursing practice have been described as part of a 'militant tendency within nursing' (Currie 1984), as 'militant nurses' making 'claims for glory' (Kwong 1992), as having a 'grossly inflated opinion of their abilities' (Buhagiar 1992a), as being 'semi-qualified people' (Napier 1998a), and as 'wingers in the forward pack' (Phelps in AMA et al 2000).

Nursing's 'sword' becomes medicine's 'shield'

Why would the courts and tribunals do this? Why would they so readily accept this 'outsider story'—that nurses control and manage their own clinical practice—when the rest of this book has demonstrated that an authoritative 'stock story' is that nurses are controlled and dominated by doctors? Does this mean that times are changing? Are courts and tribunals gradually recognising nurses as autonomous professionals over whom doctors exercise no control? This is possible, as nurses are currently enjoying a higher profile on NSW and UK key decision-making bodies (NSW Health Department 2000). Perhaps doctors have decided to abdicate their control of health care and have somehow communicated this to the judiciary? This is an unlikely explanation, given the recent opposition to nurse practitioners in New South Wales (Napier in Anastasopoulos & Vale 1997, AMA 1998). Moreover, why would the courts and tribunals accept such outsider stories, these 'stories from the bottom', as authentic? And why would this be when there is strong evidence provided in this book, from all the dicta, of a judicial cultural mindset of medical supremacy in doctor–nurse relations.

The answer is twofold. First, stories told by outsider groups can become authoritative when used by dominant power groups. Second, there is a difference between the exercise of power and the shouldering of responsibility. These issues will be explored below.

When stories 'from the bottom' are told by people 'at the top' Critical race theory demonstrates how a dominant group can take the arguments of a subordinate group and use them to their advantage. For example, Powell (1997) points out that black people have argued for many years that race is an illusion, rather than a scientific fact. The 'permanence of racism' would suggest that this argument has not been widely accepted by the American community at large (Bell 1992). However, Powell goes on to explain that this argument has now been adopted by conservative white elements in American society to the disadvantage of blacks. He explains that in America, this line of argument from the new right has led to the (US) Supreme Court using the reasoning 'to attack the validity of race-conscious programs such as affirmative action, set-asides, and redistribution in voting' (1997 p.790). Recently in the US Supreme Court, Justice Antonio Scalia turned the affirmative action argument on its head and gave dire warnings of what would happen if the law did not become completely 'colourblind'. He held, 'To pursue the concept of racial entitlement—even for the most admirable and benign of purposes—is to reinforce and preserve for future mischief the way of thinking that produced race slavery, race privilege and race hatred' (Adarand Constructors Inc. v Pena 1997).

This provides insight into why the 'nurse as an autonomous professional' argument has been so easily accepted as a medical defence. Medical opinion has long held a privileged place in court (Bolam v Friern Hospital Management Committee 1957, Kennedy & Grubb 1994). In the past judges have accepted the authority of medical opinion, although landmark Australian cases such as F v R (1983) and Rogers v Whitaker (1992) indicate something of a shift in attitude. But as Daniel (1990 p.1) points out, 'the medical profession assumed sovereignty in the domain of health services ... [basing] its authority on the esoteric, scientific knowledge which it commanded and on its exclusive mandate to apply this knowledge to the care and treatment of the sick'.

This book has demonstrated on numerous occasions that judges acknowledge the authority of doctors to speak on all health matters. Whitty (1998 p.150) observes that 'there is a long history of judicial deference to doctors as members of an eminent profession, exercising their expertise for the best interests of the public'. Even overtly self-interested activities of medical groups such as the AMA, the 'strongest, most powerful trade union in Australia' (MacKay 1995 p.344), are respectably cloaked within the objective of 'the promotion and protection of the honour and interests of the medical profession as well as the furtherance of medical science' (MacKay 1995 p.348). Such entrenched authority means that even a defence which runs contrary to the established mores of the defending group is accepted without question.

Accordingly, at the behest of the medical profession, judges seem to accept without comment an outsider story that is contrary to the stock story of medical domination that they have been affirming in dicta for many years. If the 'stories from the bottom' are told by the 'people at the top', they are able to take on an authority which they do not possess when told by outsiders.

Autonomous professional story: a story about the shouldering of responsibility, not the exercise of power   The second part of the twofold explanation of the court's acceptance of this outsider story is that the acceptance is usually only partial. This supremacy, this autonomy, is not about the exercise of power. It is about the shouldering of responsibility. For nurses, the two are apparently not the same. After the courts and tribunals have accepted that the nurses are at fault, that the doctors can rely on them to bring problems to their attention, that the doctors have no responsibility for what nurses do—the nurses still have no power to influence clinical outcomes.

There are several cases that demonstrate that the only strategy nurses possess is to bring a problem to the attention of the doctors. They cannot force them to act. Cases such as MacDonald v York County Hospital and Dr Vail (1973) and Bolitho v City & Hackney HA (1998), decided as they were on the question of causation, serve to highlight the nurses' dilemmas.

The patient in the first case lost his leg, the child in the second case suffered catastrophic brain damage. In both cases the nurses had expressed their concerns about the patient on a number of occasions. In both cases the doctors did not respond to the nurses' concerns, originally in MacDonald and repeatedly in Bolitho. In MacDonald the nurses were found not to be negligent on grounds of causation. In Bolitho, although the doctors' failure to attend was found to be a breach of duty, they were found not to be negligent. In both cases the finding of no negligence was because the doctors gave evidence that they would not have altered their treatment even if they had seen the patients. In both cases the doctors did not see the patients until it was too late even to attempt to prevent the damage occurring. Both cases were determined by the judges without comment as to the difficulties the nurses might have experienced.

In Re Anderson and Re Johnson (1967) and the Inquest touching the death of PDP (1994), the fact that doctors failed to take action on the expressed concerns of the nursing staff similarly elicited no comment. Both these patients also died.

In all of these four cases the nurses expressed their professional, clinical opinions to the doctor on the patients' conditions. In the first two cases, the doctors gave sworn evidence to the fact that, regardless of the outcomes, they would not have heeded the nurses' concerns and changed the treatment. In the latter two cases, the facts emerged that the doctors manifestly did ignore the nurses' concerns and continued on their clinically determined route to the detriment of the patient.

The fact that no judicial comment was made on any of these issues suggests that the judges did not consider this to be remarkable. Plainly the doctors were exercising their clinical judgment and autonomy, which cannot be interfered with. Perhaps the judges held similar views to those of the AMA that 'only medical practitioners have the knowledge and skills to provide comprehensive patient care', and that nurses should 'only work within strict protocols and guidelines as determined by the medical profession' (1996). Yet such views deny the possibility that the nurses might have been right; that the nurses on these occasions might have known more than the doctor, as elsewhere doctors have testified (Gaughan v Bedfordshire HA 1997) and judges acknowledged (Cassidy v Ministry of Health 1951). In the above cases where the patients died or were seriously injured, it seems that the nurses' concerns were valid, and were worthy of concession and investigation. But this possibility draws no comment from the judges. Arguably in Re Anderson and Re Johnson (1967) the nurses were not under scrutiny, thus perhaps the judges did not comment because the nurses would have had no right of reply. But in the other cases the nurses were under scrutiny. In addition, as this book has demonstrated, on the matter of medical dominance, the courts and tribunals have not demonstrated any hesitancy to comment.

So even with the assistance of the defence of reliance, nurses still do not attract autonomous or even equal status. They are still only subordinate professionals. Thus, the professional 'arithmetic' looks something like this: 'Autonomous' nurse with responsibility + autonomous doctor with power = subordinate professional nurse.

Outside the courts and tribunals, nurse leaders have sought recognition as professionals in their own right, with their own responsibilities and duties to the patient, but as yet have had limited gains in practice. Ironically, the most significant clinical manifestation of this recognition inside the courts and tribunals has operated as a shield for doctors, rather than as a sword for nurses (with apologies to the maxims of equity).

Making new harmonies

I was unable to find any cases where the autonomous professional defence was invoked but did not succeed. The fact that it is often so successful for doctors is an important issue for this book because this defence much more closely approximates the nurses' responsibilities in everyday clinical practice. Doctors also have to survive, and in practice they do rely on nurses significantly. Doctors have to rely on nurses, because they simply cannot be present for all the patients allocated to their management twenty-four hours a day. Even some of those doctors most critical of nursing's push for autonomy describe their collaborative relationship with 'the majority of nurses' (but not the militant ones with over-inflated opinions of their abilities?) as one of 'mutual trust and cooperation'. They have stated that doctors 'depend absolutely on their nursing colleagues' (Buhagiar 1992b). They have written that 'all doctors acknowledge the special skills and expertise of various nurses in specialty roles—indeed, junior doctors learn much from them' (Arnold 1992 p.5), and that nurses and doctors ought not to become 'competitors after such a long, harmonious relationship' (Miller 1992 p.8).

But the Macquarie Dictionary defines a 'harmony' as a 'consistent, orderly or pleasing arrangement of parts'. The stories that this book has illuminated suggest that the existing 'arrangement of parts' between doctors and nurses is significantly more pleasing to doctors than it is to nurses. This 'arrangement' is also inconsistent, since the medical testimonies of nurses' autonomy correspond neither to medical behaviours in practice nor to medical responses when under challenge. There is an underlying 'refrain' of medical domination which has not always been evident when doctors have come under scrutiny in the courts and tribunals, but which regularly surfaces when nurses try to exercise equal clinical or political decision-making power. This inconsistency provides doctors with the advantage of claiming reliance on nurses. Simultaneously, their monopoly on the clinical and political control of health care delivery has determined that they have not had to share the exercise of power, unless they have wished to do so.

Even when nurses have succeeded in obtaining some recognition of their clinical consequence and expertise, the battles have been bitterly fought and hard won. The announcement of the NSW Government's decision to implement nurse practitioner services drew scathing censure from the AMA (NSW Branch). The Branch President described the decision as a: 'retrograde step used only in countries where health care is inadequate'. The Press Release continued to state that it was a 'black day for rural health', claiming that the Government had 'cave[d] in to nurses' because they had 'threaten[ed] the Health Minister with industrial action and [held] him to ransom' (AMA, 1998).

It should be added, however, that some of the protracted negotiations and discussions which nursing organisations have undertaken with other professional medical colleges have obviously been worthwhile. The Royal Australian College of General Practitioners has been far more moderate in its response to date, stating that the decision of the State government only 'formalises a process already in place and established by need' (Humphries 1998 p.3).

But recognition of the vital, significant and responsible role which nurses play in the delivery of health care should not occur only as a by-product of medical exoneration. Recognition by happenstance does nothing to establish any positions of authority for nurses, unless it is required by doctors that they hold them. More developments like the decision to implement nurse practitioner services are required: developments which legitimate existing situations for nurses, and which are not contingent on the whims of doctors.

Lack of support for independent moral agency in nursing

The 'refrain' of medical domination referred to above is apparent in the difficulty which nurses have repeatedly experienced in exercising independent moral agency. The exercise of moral agency is typical of a full professional, and is clearly what the Codes of Ethics and Conduct and the professional tribunals expect from nurses.

There are two sorts of clinical situations which are problematic for nurses and about which the courts and tribunals are uncharacteristically silent. There is a lack of comment when either doctors disregard the expressed clinical concerns of nurses, or nurses make little or no attempt to intervene to prevent doctors from behaving dangerously. Such lack of comment becomes almost a tacit acceptance of their moral barrenness.

The subordinate professional stock story demonstrates that nurses are expected to inform the doctor of their concerns, but then the responsibility to act rests with the doctor. Both the doctor's handmaiden and the subordinate professional stock stories suggest that there is no judicial expectation that nurses will intervene proactively on behalf of the patient if the doctor is behaving inappropriately or dangerously. They are neither expected nor able to insist, and the doctor is under no obligation to act on their concerns. Nurses frequently describe such situations as intolerable (Johnstone 1994, Bonnet 1997, Zwickler 1997). The difficulty for nursing recruitment and retention is that when nurses are repeatedly faced with this problem, they often become deeply disheartened and demoralised, and may leave nursing (Toomey 1998).

Doctors are not required to heed nurses' clinical concerns

In situations where nurses are concerned about the medical management of a patient, they have no authority to intervene if doctors will not listen to their concerns. The options would be either to seek support from other, more senior nurses, or to go over a junior doctor's head and speak to a more senior medical officer. Both actions would require the nurse to be very concerned indeed, as the possibility of such behaviour ever being necessary is not canvassed in any health care policy or legislation. In addition, in the current health care climate such an action as this may still not achieve anything.

In the Inquest touching the death of TJB (1989) the nursing staff wanted the admitting medical officer (AMO) to insert an intravenous line in a dehydrated child. After one of the nursing staff had unsuccessfully expressed her concerns to him, the nurses (remarkably) approached the Director of Nursing who referred the matter to the Chief Medical Officer. Either the AMO ignored the concerns of senior nursing and medical management, or they did not speak to him, as he did not insert an intravenous line into the child, an action which it was accepted would probably have saved the child's life. The Coroner acknowledged that nurses making a direct approach to the AMO might be contrary to 'protocol' and conceded that some doctors might 'resent' it.

This case can be compared with Bolitho (1998), in which the 'highly experienced nurse' was more proactive. Her concern was such that she went immediately over the house officer's head and rang the registrar. Over a four-hour period before the child's ultimate arrest and catastrophic brain damage, the nurse continued to call both the doctors, but neither came to review the treatment.

How would the nurses have felt in such situations? They knew that whatever treatment had been prescribed and administered was not working, and in both histories the nurses were concerned that the children were deteriorating. It is true that the children might not have improved even if the doctors had appeared and examined them, but the fact remains that they did not. In both cases the nurses' concerns were such that they had gone over the heads of the usual immediate medical contacts, but after that there was nothing more that they were able to do. There is thus a lack of reciprocity, in that the nurses have discharged their duty to protect the patient, but this does not impose a reciprocal duty on the doctors to act on the nurses' concerns.

Nurses are not expected to intervene to prevent imminent harm to the patient

The second scenario, where the nurse is of the opinion that the doctor is about to do imminent harm to the patient, is particularly compelling. Imagine the patient bleeding to death from the ruptured aorta, while the scrub nurse politely asked the refractory surgeon if he wanted a drain (Inquest touching the death of PDP 1994). Recall the highly experienced midwife watching silently while the 'angry' obstetrician pulled too long and too hard on the baby's back (Strelic v Nelson & Ors 1996). Remember the nurse standing by while the resident amputated the head of Smithy's femur in the ward (Zwickler 1997); and the sister at Chelmsford expressing her concerns about the administration of ECT to Mr Peter Clarke, who died about 10 minutes after its administration (The Chelmsford Report 1990). Such images cannot be ignored for want of the courage to address them. As recently as 1996 a NSW judge expressed a belief that the midwife was: 'torn between the allegiance which she believed she owed as a nursing sister towards the medical profession and telling what had happened' (Strelic v Nelson & Ors 1996 p.20).

There should be no doubt in any nurse's mind where allegiance lies. It should lie in exactly the same direction as the doctor's allegiance: towards the patient. The difficulty is that, because of the extent of medical ownership of health care, it has been possible for nurses (and judges, and legislators, and policy makers) to imagine that such allegiance could be owed vicariously via the doctor. Such a route for allegiance might work while the doctor is right. It does not work if the nurse is right and the doctor is wrong.

These situations and judicial responses are unacceptable. There should be mechanisms for situations such as these where the nurse would be able to invoke either a second opinion or some form of clinical review, as a matter of policy or law. It is unlikely that such situations would arise on a regular basis. They would be the exception, rather than the rule. But it is common knowledge that they do arise, and if mechanisms for second opinions or clinical review might protect the lives of any future children in situations similar to those above, they would surely be worth the debunking of a few medical domination myths.

This is not to suggest that there are no legal mechanisms for dealing with doctors who make clinical mistakes: medicolegal textbooks are full of them. This is about possibly being able to prevent such mistakes ever being made, by judicial recognition of the fact that an experienced clinical nurse with adequate clinical authority might have made a difference to the outcome. The possibility that an experienced nurse might be right about the clinical management of a patient must be identified and validated in policy and law, not left as an unspoken secret. Otherwise the ability of a nurse to influence the quality of patient care will continue to be a question of the strength of the nurse's personality, not of legal or policy entitlement.

Human beings make mistakes (Reason 1990) and health care professionals are no exception (Brennan & Leape et al 1991, Wilson et al 1995). The aviation industry has already undertaken a considerable amount of work and has developed the concept of crew resource management. This creates the imperative for each member of the aviation team to speak out forcefully if they believe that there is any problem (Flight Safety Foundation 2000). Such an expectation is an imperative for health care practice if cases such as the ones discussed above are to be avoided. There needs to be provision made for some form of intervention which is instantly recognisable to both doctors and nurses as a 'major clinical dispute procedure'. It could only be invoked if the nurse believed on reasonable grounds that the patient's life or well-being was in serious danger. A refusal to acknowledge and act upon the nurse's concerns in such a situation should carry significant sanctions for medical personnel. This would provide the nurses with some framework within which to operate, and would provide some legitimate recognition of their moral agency. But such an expectation would require a significant change to the existing stock stories and would require a far more egalitarian relationship between the medical and nursing staff.

Invisibility of nurses when courts and tribunals are dazzled by doctors: the myth of the meritocracy

The fact that the courts and tribunals have never formally addressed the dilemmas of nurses in such situations is regrettable. It cannot be argued that courts and tribunals are reluctant to get involved in policy debates generally. Consider a case such as CES v Superclinics (Australia) Pty Ltd (1995). Justice Margaret Beazley (1998), making reference to this case and others, has made the point extra-curially that 'the outcome of cases can be due, not to the hard analysis of medical and other evidence, but to the life experiences and philosophies of judges'. Yet the possibility of any change to the 'stock story' relationship between doctors and nurses was not canvassed in any of the judgments found in this research, other than the tentative suggestion of Coroner Ahearn in the Inquest touching the death of TJB (1989). The received wisdom has been that doctors are in charge of the health care system and the patients. All other staff are subordinate to them and controlled by them. The possibility of challenge by another health care professional, unless similarly qualified, would be unthinkable because they would not be sufficiently meritorious to make the challenge. Yet nowadays many nurses are both highly skilled and qualified, and many are more highly skilled and qualified than the junior doctors who practise in our health services. They are capable of equal participation in health care decision making and are equally as capable of recognising when a patient's treatment is not working.

Yet the criterion for equal participation in clinical decision-making debates has been nothing less than a medical degree. This has been the catchcry of the doctors opposed to the nurse practitioner debate. David Hall (1997) described similar phenomena for blacks as 'the myth of meritocracy'. Murray, on the subject of merit, has this to say:

Merit is defined by white men to reward what white men become. Merit, as we know it, explicitly values particular experiences and abilities—the ones developed by white upper class men—and therefore implicitly devalues others ... [M]eritocracy calls those who conform to these standards 'equal'. Those who are different, it calls 'unqualified'. (1996 p.1078)

Nurses must be recognised as 'equal' and 'qualified' to participate in these discussions. It is totally unacceptable that nurses should shoulder the 'autonomous professional' burden of responsibility without a concomitant exercise of power. They perceive their duty to the patient to be just as real and tangible as the doctors' and, judging by the Morgan polls (Anon 1998a), the public trust nurses to behave morally. But this is not a claim for nurses to practise medicine; rather it is a claim for nurses to practise decision making and to exercise power. It is a claim for nurses to be recognised for what they do. The practice of decision making and the exercise of power have become confused with the practice of medicine, because these activities have been the sole prerogative of doctors.

Neither law nor policy makes provision for nurses to be recognised as 'equal' or 'qualified'. The legislative changes proposed by the implementation of nurse practitioners will go some way to assist nurses working alone in rural and remote areas. Still, the success of the positions will depend on the scope of practice which can be negotiated by the State Steering Committee, which will have representation from the AMA (NSW Branch), the RACGP, and the Rural Doctor's Association. But these changes will not assist the nurses in multidisciplinary clinical situations where they need to challenge the doctors. Nor, incidentally, will they assist the nurses working alone in inner city projects such as the Kirketon Road Sexual Health Centre (a drop-in centre in King's Cross, Sydney which provides health care to prostitutes, street kids, and IV drug users) or the Matthew Talbot Hostel for Homeless Men.

It seems as though the courts and tribunals are only able to focus on nursing issues when nurses come alone beneath the judicial gaze. There is a substantial body of case law in the industrial and disciplinary jurisdictions where judges focus on nursing work and nursing concerns exclusively and coherently. They recognise the qualifications of nurses and their desire as a profession to maintain standards of public safety (Re L and Nurses Registration Board 1989). They acknowledge their concern to see that nurses are adequately qualified to practise in their field (Re Singh and College of Nurses of Ontario 1981), and sometimes express concerns that nurses are over-zealous in their desire to maintain these standards (Pickard v College of Nurses of Ontario 1987, Hefferon v UKCC 1988).

But when nurses are considered alongside doctors, this coherence often breaks down. Nurses are almost disregarded as 'real' players in the health care game. Instead their status tends to be determined not by their own actions or accounts, but by the descriptions of them which are provided either by counsel for the doctors or the hospitals, by medical expert witnesses, or by medical witnesses of fact. It is as though the judges become dazzled by the presence of the doctors, and the nurses slip into some sort of professional shadow land where their contribution to health care is in some way dimmed. Then there is a very real sense that the nurses are little more than extensions of the doctors, and their actions are often only given weight when the doctors say they carry weight, such as in the defence of reliance.

CONCLUSION

This chapter has discussed the consequences of the juxtaposition of the five images which emerged from the case law. These are: the acceptance that doctors can represent and/or substitute for nurses; acceptance of medical control over patient care; fragmentation of the nursing role and the subsequent devaluation of nursing care and privileging of delegated medical work; poor living and working conditions and poor remuneration; reciprocal use of the defence of reliance, lack of support for independent moral agency in nursing; and the invisibility of nurses when the courts and tribunals are dazzled by doctors.

As one solution, it has been suggested that a health care form of 'crew resource management' could be introduced to provide a clear framework and expectation for nurses to be involved in clinical decision making, and to enable them legitimately to intervene if they felt the patient was at risk.

12

Speaking out from the shadows

INTRODUCTION

Before this book concludes, let us return to where it began, at Wilcannia Hospital on the banks of the Darling River in outback New South Wales in the middle of the night. The nurse, you will remember, was Sr Heathcote. She had with her an untrained wardsmaid, one elderly and two child patients, and a new admission, a disorientated young man who kept wandering off. Because she had no facilities to restrain the young man, she arranged for him to be detained in a police cell, after seeking endorsement by telephone with the matron and the doctor. There he hanged himself. It is a story of assumptions and misunderstandings, most of which relate to the role, status and responsibilities of Sr Heathcote.

At the inquest into the young man's death (Inquest touching the death of MAQ) Dr Ryan testified that he relied on Sr Heathcote and expected her to make a provisional diagnosis. She may well have been able to do so in acute medical/surgical emergencies. She would have had a strong grounding in medical/surgical nursing, having trained and worked at the Radcliffe Infirmary, Oxford. But the management of alcohol withdrawal requires special skills which this nurse did not have.

If she did make a diagnosis (and the doctor expected her to do so) there was no law, nor even any policy, to support her in this behaviour. Quite the contrary. In Heathcote v NRB & Walton (1991, p.11) Ward DCJ pointed out that the policy manual explained (somewhat superfluously) that she was 'not the doctor' which meant that she was 'not to perform any treatment on her own initiative'. The authors of the policy manual, who were in all probability nurses, corroborate the doctor's handmaiden story. If one were 'not the doctor', one would naturally be unable to take any initiative, as nurses are (according to that stock story) only extensions of doctors.

However, in reality the nurses (and patients) at Wilcannia would never survive if the nurses really were doctors' handmaidens, given that the doctors are so far away in Broken Hill. When a patient has a cardiac or respiratory arrest on arrival at the hospital, nurses have to initiate resuscitation before they ring the doctor, otherwise the patient would suffer irreversible brain damage due to the delay. Likewise, when a patient is admitted with an excruciating injury, nurses have to apply a temporary dressing and provide analgesia before they ring the doctor to avoid unnecessary suffering. Of course they are 'not the doctor', but they *are* nurses, and they must initiate these procedures for patient safety. To live within the constraints imposed by such a policy would be farcical, and contrary to good practice. Nurses in such situations actually live outside the policy (NSW Health Department, 1992), and (still, at the time of writing) outside the law.

But the Heathcote cases also serve to highlight that nurses know that they are 'not the doctor', and that, as professional nurses, they are aware of the limitations of their competence. On this occasion Sr Heathcote knew that she was out of her depth. She did what experienced nurses well know how to do. She referred the matter to more experienced staff for assistance. She woke up the matron and she contacted the doctor. She said to Dr Ryan, 'I just don't know' (Healthcote v NRB & Walton, 1991, p.6).

But here the policy was silent on the possibility that a nurse *might* know what to do in a given situation, whereas the reality was that both the doctor and the nurse knew that she often *did* know what to do. In such situations there will always be a lack of clarity as to why the nurse contacted the doctor. Was the referral a matter of form or substance?

In this situation, Sr Heathcote did not ring the doctor because the policy said she must. The Coroner accepted the doctor's evidence that she was wont to act on her own initiative on many occasions. She rang the doctor because, as a professional practitioner, she knew when to refer for help. But there is little, if any, room for such a suggestion within the stock story, and the resultant situation can only be described as a farce.

THE END OR THE BEGINNING?

This part of the book has concluded that the five images which have emerged from analysis of the case law demonstrate that the nursing role is, of necessity, highly flexible. However, it can be seen that the more 'basic' aspects of nursing care are often undervalued and delegated to non-nurses, whereas the medically derived aspects are often privileged.

The recognition of professional status for nurses is influenced by the five images that have emerged from the case law analysis, all of which, to some extent still, coexist today. Because of the continuation of the stock story images, professional status is not unequivocal, although there is greater recognition now than there was for most of the last century.

The ability of nurses to exercise power in their professional lives improved significantly over the last century, although financial constraints in health care have curtailed nursing's managerial autonomy of late. However, from a clinical perspective, the issue is much less satisfactory. The clinical responsibilities which nurses shoulder and the authority which they exercise arise in a climate of medical permission or abrogation, rather than one of nursing entitlement. This book has demonstrated that this creates considerable moral dilemmas for nurses when clinical care is unsatisfactory.

The images which have emerged from the case law do not portray a uniformly positive picture of any of the groups, nurses, doctors or lawyers, who come under scrutiny. This is despite the fact that the intent of the book was to use 'outsider' scholarship to address the status of nurses. Lawyers who use outsider scholarship are in the unusual position of being 'insiders' to the law by dint of their legal qualifications, but 'outsiders' to the area of jurisprudence (in the case of this book, health law) which they seek to scrutinise, by dint of some other identifying characteristic (in this case, being also a nurse). A book which is written, inter alia, to enable the voices of outsiders to be heard will inevitably be somewhat controversial, as it begins from the premise that the existing order is deficient in some way. As a result of this, the legal system and the medical dominance of health care and health law have on occasions received strong criticism. But the book has not shied away from criticising nursing as the outsider group if it has seemed necessary to do so.

There is no coherent body of law which addresses the status and responsibilities of the registered nurse in Australia. The same could be said for all the countries whose law and writings have featured in this book. There is no coherent body of law because the role of the nurse in health care is neither recognised nor legitimised. Nurses are outsiders to the health care and the health law system. Even as I write these words, nurses in remote clinics and small hospitals will be making provisional diagnoses, prescribing medications, ordering pathology and radiology and referring patients onto doctors when they know they are out of their depth. The nurses at Matthew Talbot Hostel for Homeless Men will be doing the same in Woolloomooloo. Tonight patients will die in nursing homes and on wards and in many of those cases nurses will not wake the doctors to confirm that the patient is dead, simply because there will be no need to do so. They will contact the relatives, lay out the patients and help the family to grieve. Today or tomorrow or the next day, a nurse may or may not intervene to stop a doctor from making a mistake which might harm the patient. It will not depend on the law. It will depend on the courage of the nurse. Nurses operate inside (or outside) a legal framework which insufficiently recognises their work and their presence. The developing body of jurisprudence which calls itself health law will not be complete until it addresses the problems and difficulties encountered by nurses, the majority group of health workers, and recognises their central role in health care delivery. If this book has achieved anything, this is not the end, but only the beginning.

Appendix
The five images of the nurse

The nurse as a ministering angel

- Nursing is a quasi-religious calling, and nurses are most like women in holy orders, therefore:
  - Nurses are unlike witches, and unlike Sarey Gamp;
  - Nurses are expected to demonstrate high moral standards and to be abstemious and sober; they embody all that is good and proper and their lives must be strictly controlled;
  - Because nursing is a practical skill which comes from the heart, it is better learnt 'at the bedside';
  - Nurses must be asexual beings, because the work they do involves them in extremely intimate physical activities;
  - Because nurses are so good, their acts or omissions could not be malicious.
- It is a privilege to serve as a nurse, and therefore nurses should not complain about poor living and working conditions and huge workloads.

The nurse as a domestic worker

- Nurses are domestic workers to the extent that they do cleaning and cooking, undertake tasks which provide personal comfort, and get their hands (and clothes) dirty. These domestic tasks are to be viewed as separate from, and intrinsically inferior to, 'true' nursing work—rather than as an integral element of holistic nursing care.
- Such tasks could not possibly be performed by professional, upper or middle class people; they could only be undertaken by domestic workers or people of the lower classes.
- People who do such work would be less likely to give reliable evidence in court than professional medical men, so this should be imputed to nurses generally.

- People such as nurses who do such work do not deserve the same pay or living conditions as professional, middle or upper class people.

The nurse as the doctor's handmaiden

- Nursing is an extension or component part of medicine;
  - Nurses are physical extensions of doctors;
  - Nursing work is solely delegated medical work under the close control of a doctor;
  - Nursing is a part of medicine's business, and doctors can speak for nurses.
- Because the nurse is no more than a participant in medical care, the nurse is expected to obey the doctor.
- Nurses are not expected to challenge doctors even if they believe the doctor to be making mistakes which are endangering the patient's life.
- If the nurse carries out the orders of the doctor without question the nurse will not be at fault even if (s)he believes on reasonable grounds that the doctor's orders are incorrect or immoral and may endanger the patient.
  - Even if the nurse performs activities which s(he) knows to be morally wrong the nurse can be exonerated if s(he) were ordered to do so by a doctor.

The nurse as subordinate professional

- Nurses are acknowledged to possess specialised skills, although much of the nursing work which is regarded as specialised is delegated medical work.
- Nurses are expected to be able to perform these specialised skills without direct supervision by a doctor.
- However, nurses are still under the control of doctors; BUT
- Nurses are expected to be able to bring specific problems to the attention of the doctor; AND
- Nurses are expected to challenge doctors when the doctor appears to be wrong.
- Nurses may only substitute for doctors with the doctor's permission.

The nurse as autonomous professional

- The nursing profession must be self-regulating;
  - Entry to the nursing profession must be restricted and governed by their own regulatory authority;
  - Nurses must be able to control standards for the practice of nursing, which should be recognised by the courts and tribunals;
  - Nursing must be able to control continuance in the profession.
- Nurses must manage and control the nursing workforce and nursing work on a day-to-day basis.
- Nursing has a unique body of specialist knowledge;
  - Nursing education is the formal theorising of women's work (early argument);
  - Nursing is a scientific discipline with the same characteristics of knowledge as medicine, just different content areas (later argument);
  - Although nursing and medicine are separate and distinct disciplines, there is an overlap of workload, due to the fact that the two operate so closely together;
  - Nursing is a caring discipline based on research, which has created a distinct body of nursing knowledge (current argument);
  - The practice of nursing requires specialised training and education;
  - Nursing as a profession requires proper professional remuneration.
- Clinical nursing knowledge and expertise should be given equal weight to that of medicine in clinical decision making.

References

[Anonymous]. Shock. UNA J Royal Victorian College of Nursing 1938. May 2nd: 134

[Anonymous]. 'The way we were' (reprint from The Lamp June 1947). The Lamp 1997; 54 (5): 46

[Anonymous]. Nurses once again top the polls. The Lamp 1998a; 55 (5): 35

[Anonymous]. Nurses take back cleaning and disinfection. ANJ 1998b; 6 (1): 6

Abel-Smith B. A history of the nursing profession. London: Heinemann; 1960

Adam-Smith P. Australian women at war. Ringwood: Penguin; 1996

Adrian A, O'Connell J. Nurse practitioners. In Lumby J, Picone D eds. Clinical challenges. Sydney: Allen & Unwin; 2000

Albon A, Lindsay G, eds. Occupational regulation and the state. Sydney: Public Interest Centre for Independent Studies; 1984

Alexander J. The changing role of clinicians: their role in health reform in Australia and New Zealand. In: Bloom A. ed. Health reform in Australia and New Zealand. Melbourne: Oxford University Press; 2000

Anastasopoulos C, Vale S. Nurses threaten to 'take to streets' Aus Doc 1997; 31st October: 5

ANCI. Code of Ethics for nurses in Australia. Canberra: ANCI; 1993. revised 2001

ANCI. Code of Professional Conduct for nurses in Australia. Canberra: ANCI; 1995

ANCI. National competency standards for the registered and enrolled nurse. Canberra: ANCI; 1994, revised 1999

Armstrong D. The first fifty years. Sydney: Australasian Medical Publishing; 1965

Arnold P. Nursing paper not the answer. NSW Doctor 1992; August: 5

Austin A. Deconstructing voice scholarship. Houston Law J 1993; 30: 1671

Australian Confederation of Operating Room Nurses. Revised standard for cleaning in the operating suite. ACORN J 1996a; 9(3): 14

Australian Confederation of Operating Room Nurses. Competency standards for perioperative nurses Sydney: ACORN J; 1996b

Australian Medical Association (NSW) Ltd. Policy statement on the role of nurse practitioners. Sydney: AMA, 1992

Australian Medical Association (NSW) Ltd. Media release 24th April: nurse practitioner project flawed. Sydney: AMA; 1996

Australian Medical Association (NSW) Ltd. Media release 25th August: government's cave-in to nurses: a black day for rural health. Sydney: AMA; 1998

Australian Medical Association, Rural Doctors Association, Australian College of Remote & Rural Medicine, Royal Australian College of General Practitioners. NSW Government prescribes peril for patients and health care. Joint media release May 22nd 2000

Australian Medical Association. Handbook of resolutions. Sydney: AMA; 1997

Australian Nursing Federation. Competency standards for advanced nursing practice. Melbourne: ANF; 1997

Bandman EL, Bandman B. Critical thinking in nursing. Norwalk: Appleton & Lange; 1988

Barber J, Shadbolt A. Some mutiny, some bounty: psychohistory of Lucy Osburn. In Covacevich et al, eds. History, heritage and health. Proceedings of the Fourth Biennial conference of the Australian Society of the History of Medicine; 1996

Barnes RD. Black women law professors and critical self-consciousness: a tribute to Professor Denise S Carty-Benia. Berkeley Womens Law J 1990-1991; 6: 57

Baume P, ed. The tasks of medicine: an ideology of care. Sydney: MacLennan & Petty; 1998

Beazley M. Evidence or Intuition: the anatomy of a medico-legal trial. Paper delivered to the annual conference of the Australasian Association for Quality in Health Care. June 19th 1998. Sydney

Bell D. The Supreme Court, 1984 term—Foreword: The civil rights chronicles. Harv Law Rev 1985; 99: 4

Bell D. Faces at the bottom of the well: the permanence of racism. New York: Basic Books; 1992

Bendall E, Raybould E. A history of the General Nursing Council for England and Wales 1919-1969. London: HK Lewis; 1969

Benner P. From novice to expert. Am J Nurs 1982; March: 402

Benner P. From novice to expert: excellence and power in clinical nursing practice. California: Addison Wesley; 1984

Benner P, Wrubel J. The primacy of caring: stress and coping in health and illness. California: Addison Wesley; 1989

Bloom A, ed. Tooheys medicine for nurses 9th edn. Edinburgh: E&S Livingstone; 1969

Bloom A, ed. Health reform in Australia & New Zealand. Melbourne: Oxford University Press; 2000

Bonawit V. The image of the nurse: the community's perception and its implications for the profession. In: Gray G, Pratt R, eds. Issues in Australian nursing II. Melbourne: Churchill Livingstone; 1989

Bonnet R. The assault. In: Tattam A, ed. From the heart: true stories by Australian nurses. Melbourne: Lothian Books; 1997

Bowd D. Lucy Osburn. Sydney: Hawkesbury Press; 1968

Brennan B. The perioperative nurses role/rights/responsibilities in coroners' inquiries. ACORN J 1994; 7 (1): 19

Brennan TA, Leape, LL, Laird N et al. Incidence of adverse events and negligence in hospitalised patients: results of the Harvard medical practice study. New Eng J Med 1991; 324: 370–376

Brewer AM. Nurses, nursing and new technology: implications of a dynamic technological environment. Sydney: UNSW; 1983

Briggs A. Report of the committee on nursing. London: Department of Health and Social Services; 1978

Brindle D. Nurses snuff out Lady of the Lamp image. Guardian Weekly May 9th 1999

Bromberger B, Fife-Yeomans J. Deep sleep: Harry Bailey and the scandal of Chelmsford. Sydney: Simon & Schuster; 1991

Bryon PD, Johnson A. Impact of the change of education preparation on clinical practice and recruitment patterns. In: What, if anything, ails nurses? Proceedings from Western Sydney Area Health Service nursing colloquium 1990: 58

Buhagiar A. The time has come to pull up our socks. Aus Doc 1992a; August 4th: 6

Buhagiar A. Eyeing off the patients is not on. Aus Doc 1992b; September 11th: 6

Buhagiar A. General practice must repel invaders. Aus Doc 1992c; August 28th: 6

Burnard P, Chapman C. Professional and ethical issues in nursing. Chichester: John Wiley; 1988

Burns L, Goodnow J. The use of dilemma situations to analyse industrial action by nurses. Collegian 1995; 3 (2): 26

Callan Park Report 1961—see McClemens 1961

Calmore J. Close encounters of the racial kind: pedagogical reflections and seminar conversations. Uni of San Francisco Law Rev 1997; 31: 903

Cameron S. Competencies for registration of nurses in Australia. In: Gray G, Pratt R, eds. Issues in Australian nursing IV. Melbourne: Churchill Livingstone; 1995

Chelmsford Report 1990—see Slattery 1990

Chesterman M. Accident compensation: proposals to modify the common law. Research Paper: New South Wales Law Reform Commission Reference on Accident Compensation. November 1983

Chesterman M. Charities, trusts and social welfare. London: Weidenfield and Nicholson; 1979

Chiarella M. Nursing process—tool or rule? NT 1983; 78: 13

Chiarella M. Monitoring the nursing process. Nursing Mirror 1985; 160 (20): 40

Chiarella M. Towards an atomic theory of nursing. Senior Nurse 1988: 8 (4): 25

Chiarella M. Imaging nursing—reflecting and projecting. Aus Health Rev 1990; 13 (4): 299

Chiarella M. Frontiers in nursing. Proceedings of the Royal College of Nursing, Australia National Forum, Darwin 1994

Chiarella M. Regulatory mechanisms and standards: nurses friends or foes? In: Gray G, Pratt R, eds. Issues in Australian Nursing IV. Melbourne: Churchill Livingstone; 1995

Chiarella M. Extending life. In: Lumby J, Picone D, eds. Clinical challenges. Sydney: Allen & Unwin; 2000

Chinn P. Feminist pedagogy in nursing education in curriculum revolution: reconceptualising nursing education. Proceedings of the National League for Nursing's 5th Annual Conference 1998

Chulov M. Set for country practice. Sunday Telegraph 1998; 23rd August

Clark G. To be or not to be—its time to market nursing's image. In: Gray G, Pratt R, eds. Issues in Australian Nursing II. Melbourne: Churchill Livingstone; 1989

Clulow M. A closer look, disposable gloves—an assessment of the value of vinyl, latex and plastic gloves. Professional Nurse 1994; February: 234

Confederation of Australian Critical Care Nurses Inc. Competency standards for specialist critical care nurses. Perth: Ink Press; 1996

Cordery C. Military influences on Nightingale's reforms of modern nursing: the dominance of ritual and tradition. In Covacevich et al, eds. History, heritage and health. Proceedings of the Fourth Biennial conference of the Australian Society of the History of Medicine; 1996

Cott NF. The bonds of womanhood. New Haven: Yale University Press; 1977

Cotterell R. The sociology of law. London: Butterworths; 1984

Cox E. Leading women. Sydney: Random House; 1996

Crenshaw K. Demarginalising the intersection of race and sex: a black feminist critique of anti-discrimination doctrine, feminist theory and antiracist policies. Uni of Chicago Legal Forum 1989; 139: 167

Currie CT. The nursing process: revolutionary philosophy or passing phase? BMJ 1984; 3rd November: 1219

Daniel A. Medicine and the state. Sydney: Allen & Unwin; 1990

Davies M. Asking the law question. Sydney: Law Book; 1993

De La Cuesta C. The nursing process: from development to implementation. JAN 1983; 8: 365

Delacour S. The construction of nursing: ideology, discourse and representation. In: Gray G, Pratt R, eds. Towards a discipline of nursing. Melbourne: Churchill Livingstone; 1991

Delgado R. Storytelling for oppositionists and others: a plea for narrative. Mich Law Rev 1989; 87: 2411

Delgado R. The Rodrigo chronicles: conversations about America and race. New York: NYU Press; 1995

Demou T. Determined nurses worry AMA. Aus Doc 1992; Aug 21: 2

Department of Health. Report of the Select Committee on registration of nurses 1904. London: Department of Health; 1905

Dickenson M. An unsentimental union. Sydney: Hale & Iremonger; 1993

Dingwall R, Rafferty A-M, Webster C. An introduction to the social history of nursing. London: Routledge; 1991

Dock LL, Stewart IM. A short history of nursing . 4th edn. New York: WB Saunders; 1938

Dolan JA, Goodnow S. History of nursing. 11th edn. Philadelphia: WB Saunders; 1963

Dowling R. The morals of the story: narrativity and legal ethics. Indiana Law Rev 1993; 27: 191, 214

Duckett S. Financing of health care. In: Gardner H, ed. Health policy: development, implementation and evaluation in Australia. Melbourne: Churchill Livingstone; 1992

Duffy E. Horizontal violence: a conundrum for nursing. Collegian 1995; 2 (2): 5

Easson M. Opening address, Nurses and medications, examining roles and partnerships. ANF, RCNA, PHARM Committee of the DHSH, Proceedings of the nurses and medications, examining roles and partnerships conference, November 1994. 1995

Ehrenreich B, English D. Witches, midwives and nurses: a history of women healers. New York: Feminist Press; 1973

Emden C. Ways of knowing in nursing. In: Gray G, Pratt R, eds. Towards a discipline of nursing. Melbourne: Churchill Livingstone; 1991

Employment Studies Centre of the University of Newcastle. Productivity and nurses' pay: proposal for a framework agreement Stage 2 of research project for the NSWNA. Newcastle: University of Newcastle; 1992

Espinoza L. Legal narratives, therapeutic narratives: the invisibility and omnipresence of race and gender. Mich Law Rev 1997; 95: 901

Fanon F. The wretched of the earth. New York: Grove Press; 1963

Festinger L. A Theory of cognitive dissonance. Southern California: Stanford University Press; 1957

Field D, Taylor S, eds. Sociological perspectives on health, illness and health care. Carlton, Victoria: Blackwell Science; 1998

Finley L. Breaking women's silence in law: the dilemma of the gendered nature of legal reasoning. Notre Dame Law Rev 1989; 64: 886

Fisher S. Gender, power, resistance: is care the remedy? In: Fisher S, Davis K, eds. Negotiating at the margins. New Jersey: Rutgers University Press; 1993

Fisher W. Human communication as narration: toward a philosophy of reason, value and action. Colombia: University of South Carolina Press; 1987

Flexner A. The Flexner Report on medical education in the United States and Canada 1910. New York: Carnegie Foundation for the Advancement of Teaching; 1910

Flexner A. Is social work a profession? Proceedings of the National Conference of Charities and Correction. 1915

Flight Safety Foundation website. Online. http://www.flightsafety.org/ap_2000.html

Foucault M. The archaeology of knowledge., trans AM Sheridan Smith. London: Tavistock Publications; 1972

Friedson E. Profession of medicine. New York: Dodd Mead; 1970

Gardner H, ed. The politics of health: The Australian experience. Melbourne: Churchill Livingstone; 1989

Gardner H, ed. Health policy: development, implementation and evaluation in Australia. Melbourne: Churchill Livingstone; 1992

Gardner H, ed. The politics of health: The Australian experience. 2nd edn. Melbourne: Churchill Livingstone; 1995

Gardner H, McCoppin B. Emerging militancy? The politicisation of Australian allied health professionals. In: Gardner H, ed. The politics of health; the Australian experience Melbourne: Churchill Livingstone; 1989

Gaze H. Sweeping changes. NT 1992; 86: 24

Gerber P. Employees and independent contractors revisited. ALJ 1999; 73: 29

Gillespie R. Handmaidens & battleaxes. ABC television program. True Stories. 10th June 1990

Gilligan C. In a different voice: psychological theory and women's development. Cambridge: Harvard University Press; 1982

Ginzberg E. The economics of health care and the future of nursing. JONA 1981; 11 (3): 32

Gladwin M. Ethics: talks to nurses. Philadelphia: WB Saunders; 1930

Godden J. Silence and stereotypes. In: Covacevich et al, eds. History, heritage and health. Proceedings of the Fourth Biennial conference of the Australian Society of the History of Medicine; 1996

Goodman-Draper J. Health care's forgotten majority: nurses and their frayed white collars. London: Auburn House; 1995

Gordon M. Nursing diagnosis and the diagnostic process. Am J N 1976; 76 (8): 1298

Gray AM. The economics of nursing: a literature review. Coventry: University of Warwick; 1987

Gray G, Pratt R, eds. Towards a discipline of nursing. Melbourne: Churchill Livingstone; 1991

Gray G, Pratt R, eds. Issues in Australian nursing IV. Melbourne: Churchill Livingstone; 1995

Graycar R. Hoovering as a hobby: the Common Law's approach to work in the home. Refractory Girl 1985; 28: 22

Graycar R. Womens work: who cares? Syd Law Rev 1992; 14: 70

Graycar R, Morgan J. The hidden gender of law. Sydney: Federation Press; 1990

Griffin GJ, Griffin JK. Jensen's history and trends of professional nursing. St Louis: CV Mosby; 1969

Grillo T. Tenure and minority women law professors: separating the strands. USF Law Rev 1997; 31: 47, 749

Grosz E. Space, time and perversion: the politics of bodies. Sydney: Allen & Unwin; 1995

Hall D. Reflections on affirmative action: halcyon winds and minefields. N E Law Rev 1997; 31: 941

Hallam J. Nursing the image: media, culture and professional identity. London: Routledge; 2000

Haralambos M, Heald RM. Sociology: themes and perspectives. 2nd edn. Suffolk: Chaucer Press; 1985

Harris AP. Foreword: the jurisprudence of reconstruction. Cal Law Rev 1994; 82: 741

Hart A. Who cares? package in action: teaching the nursing process. Southampton: Department of Teaching Media, University of Southampton; 1986

Hart G, Montgomery L, Bull R. Peer consultation: a strategy to support collegial practice. In: Gray G, Pratt R, eds. Issues in Australian nursing IV. Melbourne: Churchill Livingstone; 1995

Hayman RL, Levitt N. The tales of white folk: doctrine, narrative and the reconstruction of racial reality. Cal Law Rev 1996; 84: 377

Hayward J. Information: a prescription against pain. London: RCN; 1981

Health Care Complaints Commission. Health Care Complaints Commission Annual Report Sydney: HCCC; 1999

Heenan A. Uneasy partnership. NT 1990; 87 (10): 25

Heerey P. Truth, lies and stereotype: stories of Mary and Louis. Newcastle Law Rev 1996; 1 (3): 1

Henderson V. Basic principles of nursing care. Geneva: ICN; 1969

Hills B. The sacrifice of Sister Sophia. The Lamp 1990; 46 (11): 26

Hindwood B. Nurse in profile. The Lamp 1991; 48 (8): 48

Hines N. Strategies for strength. Closing address to the Eighth World Congress of Operating Room Nurses, Adelaide 6-10 September 1993. ACORN J 1993; 6 (4): 23

Holmes C. Theory: where are we going? In: Gray G, Pratt R, eds. Towards a discipline of nursing. Melbourne: Churchill Livingstone; 1991

Home Care Services of New South Wales, The Australian Council of Community Nursing Services (NSW Branch), and The New South Wales Nurses Association. Joint statement on personal care. The Lamp 1991; 48 (10): 20

Hon. Dr Andrew Refshauge MLA. The Health Minister's speech to delegates. The Lamp 1995; 52 (8): 6

Hughes D. When nurse knows best: some aspects of doctor-nurse interaction in a casualty department. Sociology of Health and Illness 1988; 10 (1): 1

Humphries D. Medical profession divided as nurses diagnose and prescribe. Sydney Morning Herald 1998; 26th August: 3

Information Australia, surgeon ordered to retrain. Health Law Update 1998; 5(50): 3

International Council of Nurses. Nurses and nursing. Proceedings of the 15th Quadrennial Congress of the International Council of Nurses: Mexico City 13–18 May; 1973

International Council of Nurses. Statement on nursing education, nursing practice and service and the social and economic welfare of nurses. Geneva: ICN; 1969, revised 1975

Jamer KS. Nursing the surgical patient. UNA: J of the Royal Victorian College of Nursing 1938; 1st April: 113

Jenkins E. Nurses' control over nursing. In: Gray G, Pratt R. eds. Issues in Australian nursing II. Melbourne: Churchill Livingstone; 1989

Joanna Briggs Institute for Evidence Based Nursing Practice. Pressure sores—Part II: management of pressure related tissues damage. Vol. 1: 2; 1997

Johnstone L. The impact of medical technologies on stress and job satisfaction amongst perioperative nurses. ACORN J 1997; 10 (2): 23

Johnstone M-J. Nursing and the injustices of the law. Sydney: WB Saunders/Baillière Tindall; 1994

Johnstone M-J. Bioethics: a nursing perspective. 2nd edn. Sydney: WB Saunders/Baillière Tindall; 1995

Kalisch B, Kalisch P. Image of the nurse in motion pictures. Am J N 1982; 82 (4): 605

Kalisch B, Kalisch P, Clinton J. The world of nursing on prime time 1950–1980. Nursing Research 1982; 31 (6): 359

Keatinge D. Collegiality or collaboration: attitude or structure? In: Gray G, Pratt R, eds. Issues in Australian nursing IV. Melbourne: Churchill Livingstone; 1995

Kennedy I, Grubb A. Medical law: text with materials. 2nd edn. London: Butterworths; 1994

Knepfer G, Johns C. Nursing for life. Sydney: Pan Books; 1989

Kokowski S. Editorial. The Lamp 1991; 48 (10): 3

Kwong AYM. Four years not enough. Aus Doc 1992; August 14: 9

Lane V, Sivaram A. Innovative referencing: crediting nurses professional activities beyond the bedside. The Lamp 1999; 56 (1): 36

Lather P. Getting smart: feminist research and pedagogy with/in the postmodern. New York: Routledge; 1991

Lawler J. Behind the screens: nursing, somology and the problem of the body. Melbourne: Churchill Livingstone; 1991

Lawrence III CR. Each others' harvest: diversity's deeper meaning. USF Law Rev 1997; 31

Legge A. Born to nurse. NT 1998; 94 (14): 44

Leininger M. Caring: the essence of nursing and health. Wayne State University Press: Detroit; 1984

Little M. Humane medicine. Cambridge: Cambridge University Press; 1995

Lumby J. Threads of an emerging discipline: praxis, reflection, rhetoric and research. In: Gray G, Pratt R, eds. Towards a discipline of nursing. Melbourne: Churchill Livingstone; 1991

Lumby J, Zetler J. The image of the nurse in the Nineties—1890 or 1990? In: Proceedings of the Royal College of Nursing Australia conference, Nursing in the Nineties. Sydney 24th & 25th May 1990

Luntz H, Hambly D. Torts: cases and commentary. 4th edn. Melbourne: Butterworths; 1995

Lupton G, ed. Sociology of health and illness: Australian readings. 2nd edn. Melbourne: MacMillan Education Australia; 1995

Luxford Y. Birth of a nation: convict midwives. In: Mutiny and medicine: proceedings of the Fourth Biennial Conference of the Australasian Society of the History of Medicine; 1996

Luxton RW. New lamps for old. Australasian Nurses J 1947; 45 (2): 29

MacFarlane J, Castledine G. A guide to the practice of nursing using the nursing process. St Louis: CV Mosby; 1982

Mackay D. Politics of reaction. In: Gardner H, ed. The politics of health: the Australian experience. 2nd edn. Melbourne: Oxford University Press; 1995

Mackay L. Conflicts in care: medicine and nursing. London: Chapman & Hall; 1993

MacKinnon C. Feminism, Marxism, method and the state: toward feminist jurisprudence. Signs 1983; 8: 35

MacKinnon C. Feminism unmodified: discourses on life and law. Cambridge, Massachusetts: Harvard University Press; 1987

MacLennan JG. The evolution of nursing apparel. In: Covacevich et al, eds. History, heritage and health. Proceedings of the Fourth Biennial conference of the Australian Society of the History of Medicine; 1996

Madjar I. The body in health, illness and pain. In: Lawler J, ed. The body in nursing. Melbourne: Churchill Livingstone; 1997

Marriner A. The nursing process: a scientific approach to nursing care. St Louis: CV Mosby; 1975

Matasar R. Storytelling and legal scholarship. Chicago-Kent Law Rev 1992; 68: 353

Matsuda M. Looking to the bottom: critical legal studies and reparation Harvard Civil Rights-Civil Liberties Law Rev 1987; 22: 323

Matsuda M. Pragmatism modified and the false consciousness problem. Southern California Law Rev 1990; 63: 1763

Mauksch IG. The development of collegiate nurse education in the United States. NT 1984; 80 (5): 56

McClemens J. Report of the Royal Commission into certain matters affecting Callan Park Mental Hospital; 1961

McCrystal Culp Jr J. Telling a black legal story: privilege, authenticity, "blunders" and transformation in outsider narrative. Virginia Law Rev 1996; 82: 69

McKenzie K. The way we were. The Lamp 1998; 55 (7): 11

McKenzie SC. Storytelling: a different voice for legal education. Uni Kansas Law Rev 1992; 41: 251

Menkel-Meadow C. Excluded voices: new voices in the legal profession making new voices in the law. Uni Miami Law Rev 1987; 29: 42

Meyer P. Convicts, criminals, prisoners and outlaws: a course in popular storytelling. J Legal Ed 1992; 42: 129

Miller D. A surgeon's story. Sydney: John Ferguson; 1985

Miller J. Nurses must be stopped. Aus Doc 1992; 18th September: 8

Millette BE. Using Gilligan's framework to analyze nurses stories of moral choices. Western J of Nursing Research 1994; 16 (6): 661

Minda G, ed. Postmodern legal movements: law and jurisprudence at century's end. New York: New York University Press; 1995

Ministry of Health, Board of Education. Inter-Departmental Committee on nursing services Interim Report (Chairman: The Right Hon. The Earl of Athlone). London: Ministry of Health; 1939

Mitchell JA. Is nursing any business of doctors? A simple guide to the "nursing process". BMJ 1984: 228

Moait S. General Secretary's report. The Lamp 1998; 55 (6): 5

Moait S. The nurse and the electronic media. The Lamp 1998; 55 (2): 5

Montgomery J. Professional regulation: a gendered phenomenon? In: Sheldon S, Thomson M, eds. Feminist perspectives on health care law. Sydney: Cavendish Publishing; 1998

Morgan M. Images of organisation. London: Sage Publications; 1997

Murray YM. Merit teaching. Hastings Constitutional Law Quarterly 1996; 23: 1073

Name and address supplied. Bullying needs to be addressed now. ANJ 1998; 6(1): 3

Napier R. cited In: Rotherham S. Extra training sought. Aus Doc 1998a January 16: 11

Napier R. Nurse practitioners–costly politics? Health Management Bulletin 1998b; 4: 8–10

National Expert Advisory Group on Safety and Quality in Australian Health Care. Final Report. 1999

National Health and Medical Research Council. The role of the nurse in Australia. Canberra: NHMRC; 1991

National Health and Medical Research Council. Guidelines for the development and implementation of clinical practice guidelines. Canberra: NHMRC; 1995

New South Wales Parliamentary Debates. Legislative Assembly 4th November 1924

New South Wales Parliamentary Debates. Legislative Assembly 2nd September 1953

New South Wales Parliamentary Debates. Legislative Assembly 20th March 1991

Neyle D, West S. In support of a scientific basis. In: Gray G, Pratt R, eds. Towards a discipline of nursing. Melbourne: Churchill Livingstone; 1991

Nicholson M. Plan keeps nurse practitioners in check. NSW Doctor 1993; October 9: 5

Nightingale F. Nursing the sick. In: Quain Sir R, ed. A dictionary of medicine. London: Macmillan; 1882

Nightingale F. Notes on nursing: what it is and what it is not. London: Camelot Press; reprinted 1952

NSW Health Department. Circular 97/483 Patient information and consent to treatment

NSW Health Department. Final report of the women's health policy review Committee on women's health services in NSW. Sydney: NSW Health Department, 1985

NSW Health Department. The role and function of nurse practitioners in New South Wales: Discussion Paper. Sydney: NSW Health Department; 1992

NSW Health Department. Interim guidelines for dying with dignity. Sydney: NSW Health Department; 1993

NSW Health Department. Nurse practitioner review Stage 2, Vols I & II. Sydney: NSW Health Department; 1993

NSW Health Department. Issues relating to specialty nursing vacancies. Sydney: NSW Health Department; 1995

NSW Health Department. Final report of the nursing recruitment and retention Taskforce. Sydney: NSW Health Department; 1996a

NSW Health Department. Report of the stage three pilot project on nurse practitioners in New South Wales. Sydney: NSW Health Department; 1996b

NSW Health Department. Nurse practitioner services in New South Wales. Sydney: NSW Health Department; 1998

NSW Health Department. Government Action Plan for Health, Bulletin 1; 2000

NSW Health Department. Nursing workforce research project report. Sydney: NSW Health Department; 2001

NSWNA. Those who can do, those who can't, bully. The Lamp 1999; 56 (9): 12

Nurses Board of South Australia. Position statement: The role of the registered nurse in delegating nursing care to care workers in the community; 1993

Nurses Registration Board of NSW, University of Newcastle and Central Coast Area Health Service. Project to review and examine expectations of beginning registered nurses in the workforce. Newcastle: University of Newcastle; 1997

O'Byrne S. Legal criticism as storytelling. Ottawa Law Re 1991; 23: 487

O'Connor DJ. A critical history of Western philosophy. Houndmills: MacMillan; 1964

Osburn L. Letter to Florence Nightingale November 1868, Held in the British Museum Reference Add. Mss 47,757 ff. 92–94

Papke DR. Discharge as denouement: appreciating the storytelling of appellate opinions. Narrative and the Legal Discourse: a Reader in Storytelling and the Law; 1991

Parker J. Being and nature: an interpretation of person and environment. In: Gray G, Pratt R, eds. Towards a discipline of nursing. Melbourne: Churchill Livingstone; 1991

Parker J. Identified aspects of practice knowledge communicated in the nursing handover. Proceedings of the Royal College of Nursing, Australia Third National Nursing Forum, Frontiers in Nursing; 1994

Partlett D. Professional negligence. Sydney: Law Book; 1985

Percival E. Achieving national standards for the regulation of nursing. In: Gray G, Pratt R, eds. Issues in Australian nursing IV. Melbourne: Churchill Livingstone; 1995

Pereira L, Lee GM, Wade K. The effect of surgical handwashing routines on the microbial counts of operating room nurses. Am J Infection Control 1990; 18 (6): 354

Petersen A, Wadell C, eds. Health matters: a sociology of illness, prevention and care. Sydney: Allen & Unwin; 1998

Picard E. Legal liability of doctors and hospitals in Canada. 2nd edn. Toronto: Carswell Legal Publications; 1984

Picone D. The Presidents report to the 1990 annual conference. The Lamp 1990; 47(8): 15

Powell JA. The colorblind multiracial dilemma: racial categories reconsidered. USF Law Rev 1997; 31: 789

Pratt R. Controlling the profession's destiny. In: Gray G, Pratt R, eds. Issues in Australian nursing IV. Melbourne: Churchill Livingstone; 1995

Price LC. Political ecologies of nurse practitioners in four countries. Unpublished Masters Thesis, School of Nursing and Department of Epidemiology and Public Health, Yale University; 1998

Pringle R. Sex and medicine: gender, power and authority in the medical profession. Cambridge: Cambridge University Press; 1998

Probert B. Working life. Melbourne: McPhee Gribble; 1989

Pyne R. On being accountable. Health Visitor 1988; 61: 173

Queensland Nursing Council (QNC). Scope of nursing practice decision making framework; 1998

Rafferty A-M. The politics of nursing knowledge. London: Routledge; 1996

Reason J. Human error. New York: Cambridge University Press; 1990

Redfern S. Myths and rituals in the operating suite related to infection control: effects on patient care. Proceedings of the 1997 World Conference of Operating Room Nurses Toronto, Canada, Sept 8–12; 1997

Riach P. Equal pay and opportunity. J Ind Rel 1969; 11: 99

Ride T. Do we understand the process? Nursing Mirror 1983; 17th Aug: 12

Riehl CJ, Roy C. Conceptual models for nursing practice. New York: Appleton Century Crofts; 1980

Robinson V. White caps: the story of nursing. Philadelphia: JB Lippincott; 1946

Roper N, Logan WW, Tierney AJ. Using a model for nursing. Edinburgh: Churchill Livingstone; 1983

Royal Australian College of General Practitioners, Position statement on nurse practitioners; 1999

Royal Commission into Aboriginal Deaths in Custody 1991—see Wooten 1991

Royal Commission into Deep Sleep Therapy 1990—see Slattery 1990

Russell RL. From Nightingale to now: nurse education in Australia. Sydney: WB Saunders/
Baillière Tindall; 1990

Russell RL, ed. Off the record: the life and times of Muriel Knox Doherty 1896–1988.
An autobiography. Sydney: New South Wales College of Nursing; 1996

Sachs A, Hoff Wilson J. Sexism and the law. Oxford: Martin Robertson; 1978

Sadler C. Soap opera. NT 1990; 86: 24

Salvage J. The politics of nursing. London: Heinemann; 1985

Sarat A, Felstiner WLF. Law and strategy in the divorce lawyers office. Law and Society Rev
1986; 20 (1): 93

Sarmas L. Storytelling and the law: a case study of Louth v Diprose. Melbourne Uni Law Rev
1994; 19: 701

Sawyer LM. Nursing Code of Ethics: an international comparison. Int Nurs Rev 1989; 36 (5):
145

Sax S. Organisation and delivery of health care. In: Gardner H, ed. The politics of health:
the Australian experience. Melbourne: Churchill Livingstone; 1989

Scheppele K. Foreword: telling stories. Mich Law Rev 1989; 87: 2073

Schultz B. A tapestry of service Vol. 1, 1788-1900. Melbourne: Churchill Livingstone; 1991

Scutt J. The sexual gerrymander. Melbourne: Spinifex Press; 1994

Serghis D. No respite from skill shortages. ANJ 1998; 6 (1): 17

Seymer L. A general history of nursing. London: Faber & Faber; 1949

Sheehy E. Personal autonomy & the criminal law: emerging issues for women. Background
Paper, Canadian Advisory Council on the Status of Women. Ottawa: September 1987

Short S, Sharman E. Dissecting the contemporary nursing struggle in Australia. In: Lupton G,
ed. Sociology of health and illness: Australian readings. 2nd edn. Melbourne: MacMillan
Education; 1995

Smith FB. Florence Nightingale: reputation and power. London: Croom Helm; 1982

Speedy S. The contribution of feminist research. In: Gray G, Pratt R, eds. Towards a discipline
of nursing. Melbourne: Churchill Livingstone, 1991

Spence D. Tender loving academics. The Independent Monthly 1989; September: 41

Staunton P. Editorial. The Lamp 1989; 46 (6): 2

Staunton P. There, but for the grace of God. The Lamp 1990; 46 (11): 24

Staunton P. The vindication of Sister Sophia. The Lamp 1991; 48 (4): 17

Staunton P. Editorial. The Lamp 1991a; 48 (5): 3

Staunton P. Nurses: fighting for a decent health system in New South Wales. The Lamp
1991b; 48 (8): 20

Staunton P. Editorial. The Lamp 1993; 50 (4): 3

Staunton P. Editorial. The Lamp 1994; 51 (9): 3

Staunton P. Industrial reports. The Lamp 1995a; 52 (5): 13

Staunton P. Industrial reports. The Lamp 1995b; 52 (6): 9

Staunton P, Whyburn R. Nursing and the law. 4th edn. Sydney: WB Saunders/Baillière
Tindall; 1997

Stein L, Watts DT, Howell T. The doctor-nurse game revisited. NEJM 1990; 322 (8): 546

Stein-Parbury J. Patient and person. 2nd edn. Melbourne: Churchill Livingstone; 2000

Stewart IM, The science and art of nursing (1929) 2(1) Editorial Nursing Education Bulletin, 1

Street A. Inside nursing: a critical ethnography of nursing. New York: State University of
New York Press; 1992

Strzlecki LR, Nelson JH. Evaluation of closed container flash sterilisation system.
Orthopaedic Nursing 1989; 8 (1): 1

Sweet S, Norman I. The doctor-nurse relationship: a selective literature review. JAN 1995; 22
(1): 165

Taylor B. Being human: ordinariness in nursing. Melbourne: Churchill Livingstone; 1994

The Honourable JH Wooten AC QC. Regional Report on Inquiry in New South Wales,
Victoria and Tasmania of Royal Commission into Aboriginal deaths in Custody. Canberra:
AGPS; 1991

The Honourable Mr Acting Justice JP Slattery AO. Report of The Royal Commission into
Deep Sleep therapy. Sydney: HMSO; 1990 (cited as The Chelmsford Report)

Thornton M. Dissonance and distrust: women in the legal profession. Melbourne: Oxford
University Press; 1996

Toomer P. Crying with shame. ANJ 1998; 6 (2): 14

van Manen M. Doing phenomenological research and writing monographs. Alberta: Faculty of Education and Public Service, University of Alberta; 1984

Venamore J. On the front line: nursing and complementary therapies. The Lamp 1997; 54 (6): 3

Vicinus M, Nergaard B, eds. Ever yours, Florence Nightingale: selected letters. London: Virago; 1989

Walker K. On what it might be to be a nurse: a discursive ethnography. Unpublished PhD thesis, La Trobe University; 1993

Walker K. Dangerous liaisons: thinking, doing nursing. Collegian 1997; 4 (2): 4

Walker K. Nursing, narrativity and research: towards a poetics and politics of orality. In: Rolfe G, ed. Research, truth & authority. Hampshire: Macmillan Press; 2000

Weekes P. Nurses face sex harassment. Australian, 18th May 1995

Whitty N. 'In a Perfect World:' feminism and health care resource allocation. In: Sheldon S, Thomson M, eds. Feminist perspectives on health care law. Sydney: Cavendish Publishing; 1998

Whitworth J. The direction of medical research in Australia. Collegian 1994; 1 (1): 26

Wicks D. Nurses and doctors at work: rethinking professional boundaries. Sydney: Allen & Unwin; 1999

Williams G, Hepple BA. Foundations of the law of torts. 2nd edn. London: Butterworths; 1984

Williams PJ. The alchemy of race and rights: diary of a law professor. Cambridge, Massachusetts: Harvard University Press; 1991

Willis E. Illness and social relations. Sydney: Allen & Unwin; 1994

Wilmore H. Who cares for you? The Lamp 1997; 54 (3): 17

Wilson R, Runciman W, Gibberd R et al. The quality in Australian health care study. MJA 1995; 163: 458

Winter S. The cognitive dimension of the agon (sic) between legal power and narrative meaning. Mich Law Rev 1989; 87: 2225

Yeo J. Act now or suffer later. Open letter from Dr John Yeo to the Minister for Health. Letters Page, Sydney Morning Herald, March 26 1990

Zwickler B. Sheep. In: Tattam A, ed. From the heart: true stories by Australian nurses. Melbourne: Thomas C. Lothian; 1997

Index